Evidence-Based Electrotherapy

Pieter van Kerkhof

Evidence-Based Electrotherapy

Theory and Practice

Springer

Pieter van Kerkhof
Medicine and Public Health
Physiotherapy, Occupational Therapy
Pleudaniel, Bretagne, France

ISBN 978-3-662-73018-8 ISBN 978-3-662-73019-5 (eBook)
https://doi.org/10.1007/978-3-662-73019-5

This book is a translation of the original German edition "Evidenzbasierte Elektrotherapie," 2nd edition, by Pieter van Kerkhof, published by Springer-Verlag GmbH, DE in 2025. The translation was done with the help of an artificial intelligence machine translation tool. A subsequent human revision was done primarily in terms of content, so that the book will read stylistically differently from a conventional translation. Springer Nature works continuously to further the development of tools for the production of books and on the related technologies to support the authors.

This Springer imprint is published by the registered company Springer-Verlag GmbH, DE, part of Springer Nature.
The registered company address is: Heidelberger Platz 3, 14197 Berlin, Germany

Preface

Yet another new book on electrotherapy. One might wonder whether we really need it. Is this book any different? Well, I believe it is, particularly in that I will not be citing pioneers like Kowarschik and Edel as references for treatments. With all due respect for what these individuals have contributed to the development of electrotherapy: Our knowledge and understanding of the explanations for how and why certain applications work—or do not work—have expanded enormously over the past 15–20 years. Names like Bjordal, Draper, Lundborg, Rosén, Sluka, Louw, and Butler are known only to a handful of "enthusiasts," but that is sure to change.

The aim of this book is to provide the reader with a solid theoretical foundation for the most common electrotherapy procedures, based on current scientific knowledge. In other words: applied science, "evidence-based." From theory to practice, from the laboratory to the patient. These fundamentals, complemented by a thorough physiotherapeutic assessment, are intended to enable readers not only to select the appropriate electrotherapeutic intervention for a particular patient, but also to determine the correct dosage. In addition, the detailed references are intended to enable readers to justify the choice of a specific electrotherapy application to relevant third parties.

Please do not expect a cookbook! The author asks for your understanding that, on occasion—and clearly indicated—a personal opinion may appear. Please take this opinion for what it is, namely, almost the lowest level of evidence. Nevertheless, there will be no ready-made recipes.

Level IV: Opinions and beliefs of respected authorities (based on clinical experience).

On SpringerLink you will find several forms available for download: an information sheet on TENS application for patients, assessment forms, a very brief summary of the applications, and a checklist for the treatment procedure.

Another distinctive feature of this book is that it addresses aspects of quality management, particularly risk management as it relates to electrotherapy. Some of this will seem familiar to you, and I will undoubtedly be preaching to the choir. You are certainly already doing many things intuitively right. However, you will see that a systematic approach to risk management offers significant advantages! Not least because electrotherapy is clearly associated with certain risks.

Apart from preaching to the choir a few sacred cows will also meet their end—but after all, that's what new books are for.

At this point, I would like to extend a heartfelt thank you to Eva-Maria Kania and Hiltrud Wilberts from Springer Verlag, who supported me throughout this project with great patience and expertise. Thanks also to my colleague Michael Seubert from Hamburg, who got me involved in this work in the first place. And of course, a special thank you to my patient wife, who was actually quite pleased that I had something meaningful to do during the Covid-19 period.

I wish you much enjoyment and success with this book! For better readability, the generic masculine form is used in the following text.

Pleudaniel/Brittany, France Pieter van Kerkhof
March 2021

Contents

About the Author

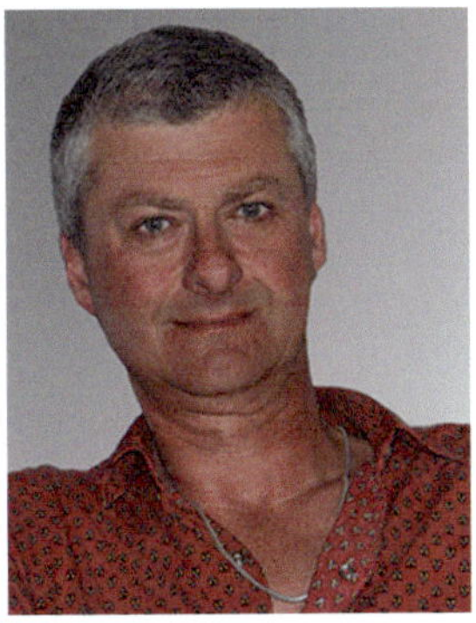

- Born 1957 in Arnhem, Netherlands
- Physiotherapy diploma in 1979, Academie voor Fysiotherapie in Arnhem, Netherlands, Bachelor's degree
- Subsequently in the service of Her Majesty until the end of 1980
- 1981–1987 Physiotherapy at Regional Hospital Langenthal, Switzerland, last 2 years as head physiotherapist
- 1987–1994 Chief Head Physiotherapist at Cantonal Hospital Winterthur, Switzerland
- 1994–2003 Self-employed in private practice
- 2001–2006 Lecturer in electrotherapy at the Physiotherapy School, Stadtspital Triemli, Zurich, Switzerland
- 2007 Lecturer in electrotherapy at the Physiotherapy School of the Zurich University of Applied Sciences in Winterthur, Switzerland
- 2008–2010 Master of Science (Physiotherapy) program, Philipps University, Marburg, Germany. Master's thesis on risk management in electrotherapy
- 2005–2013 Electrotherapy courses for physiotherapists and occupational therapists in Germany and Switzerland
  Resident in Brittany since 2014

1 Pain and Pain Inhibition

1.1 A Bit of History

Electrotherapy is by no means new!

We know that as early as 400 years before our era, electric rays were caught and used to treat conditions such as gout or "bleeding." The Torpedo torpedo (spotted electric ray), for example, can deliver 60 V/50 A. Divers describe the shock as "a very powerful punch," and the shock is said to knock an adult man off his feet. For treatment, the animals were held near the painful part of the body (with body contact). The rays then produced—defensively, of course, and normally also to stun or kill their prey—series of electric shocks, which reduced the pain. Galen explained that it did not help to eat the ray; one had to hold the living animal to the painful spot, which would then use its bioelectrical weapon… Not for the faint of heart.

Among the ancient Egyptians, electric catfish (also "electric catfish," Malapterus electricus, capable of 350 to 500 V) were already known 6000 years ago. Whether they were used therapeutically or simply eaten is unknown. In some African regions, the electric organs are still used for healing purposes today.

In 46 BCE, a Roman physician, Scribonius Largus, advocated a treatment method for gout. A quote from Scribonius (Schonack 1913):

> "For both types of podagra (gout attack in the metatarsophalangeal joint of the big toe, 'the gout,' very painful, author's note), one must place a living black electric ray under the feet when the pain approaches, standing not on a dry shore, but on one washed by the sea, until one notices that the entire foot and the shin up to the knees are numb. This remedy relieves the pain immediately and also cures for the future. In this way, Anteros, the freedman of Tiberius, the procurator of inheritances, was cured."

Well then, that sounds like a pretty intense TENS application.

Even anal prolapse or even hemorrhoids were apparently treated with these little creatures. This probably represents the first electrical muscle stimulation. How this treatment was carried out, I am happy to leave to the reader's imagination.

Here is a quote from Scribonius regarding the treatment of headaches (Schonack 1913):

> "Even the oldest and most unbearable headaches are immediately relieved and permanently cured by the black electric ray [author's note: Torpedo nigra], if it is placed alive on the painful spot until the pain stops and that part becomes numb. As soon as this is felt, the remedy should be removed so that the sensation in that area is not destroyed. However, one must obtain several rays of this kind, because the cure sometimes occurs only with two or three, that is, the numbness, the sign of healing."

Since no significant progress was made in the field of electricity over the following 2000 years, the electric ray was able to easily maintain its position in therapy during this time. There are even descriptions from the Middle Ages of tables on which the patient was tied down before being given the Ichtho-therapy.

P. van Kerkhof, *Evidence-Based Electrotherapy*, https://doi.org/10.1007/978-3-662-73019-5_1

In 1745, E. von Kleist, and then in 1746 in Holland, Pieter van Musschenbroek invented the "Leyden jar" (the precursor of the capacitor), and this jar revolutionized the use of electric current: people were no longer dependent on the capricious fish.

In 1756, the Briton Richard Lovett treated sciatica, headaches, kidney stones, gout, and "hysteria" with electricity.

In 1825, the French physician Sarlandière was the first to use Leyden jars connected to needles for electroacupuncture.

In 1799, Volta developed the first battery, and later, around 1850, the induction coil was invented, and with it, induction current.

Now things really got exciting. People became mobile.

1.2 General Remarks on Pain

The International Association for the Study of Pain defines pain as follows: "Pain is an unpleasant sensory and emotional experience associated with actual or potential tissue damage, or described in terms of such damage." Pain, therefore, is what the patient perceives as pain, not what the therapist makes of it. If the patient says it feels like 1000 knives, then it is not a "severe stabbing pain." It is like 1000 knives, period. And if, after therapy, it is 50% better, then it is only 500 knives. It greatly benefits patient interaction to use the same vocabulary as the patient. It builds trust.

The following will discuss some important pain theories in more detail. As this is about conveying basic knowledge, the subject cannot be explored in great depth. Those who wish to delve deeper into the material should consult the bibliography at the end of the chapter.

1.3 Pain Inhibition Through Information

The effectiveness of so-called Pain Neuroscience Education (PNE) in patients with chronic pain has been proven, especially when the method is combined with conventional physiotherapeutic interventions (Moseley 2002, 2003; Louw et al. 2011, 2016; Rufa et al. 2019). The method has been shown to reduce pain, disability, and pain catastrophizing, and even improve overall mobility. In the following, I will discuss individual elements of PNE. I would like to encourage the reader to search the internet for names such as Moseley, Butler, Louw, and Gifford in connection with PNE. Many of their publications are freely available online and will provide more information about this exciting method than I can offer here due to space constraints. Some aspects will remind the reader of the implementation of a so-called back school. The major difference lies in the explanatory model underlying the didactic concept.

PNE aims to change patients' preconceived notions about chronic pain. Unlike the biomechanical-anatomical explanatory model, PNE describes the pain experience as a function of the nervous system and not in relation to tissue pathology. The knowledge imparted about the biology and physiology of the nervous system is intended to enable the patient to understand why pain can exist without or with very little structural pathology.

Topics addressed include pain as an alarm signal, the influence of pain on emotions, stimulus transmission, the influence of brain activity, the impact of experiences and beliefs, decoupling of pain and pathology, plasticity of the nervous system, and much more.

The patient is encouraged to engage with his problem. Questions such as "What do you think is going on with your back?", "What do you think should happen to your back?", and "Where do you see yourself in 5 years?" are intended to provide both the therapist and the patient with a basis for treatment planning. A very good introduction to PNE is, for example, "Has anyone ever explained to you why you (still) have pain?" Answers such as "Of course, I have a disc protrusion" should, if possible, not be answered confrontationally with "Yes, but you know, 40% of people without back pain have that too and lead completely normal lives."

It may seem trivial, but the statement "Your nervous system is reacting like a misadjusted alarm system. If you have pain, it does not mean you are doing something wrong" has different consequences for the patient than "You have a disc injury, please do not bend over anymore." Here, chronification is already preprogrammed.

The comparison of the nervous system to an alarm system is generally well understood. Especially when you explain how the alarm can be set too sensitively and therefore is triggered by even minor deviations. The treatment goal would accordingly be to "turn down" the sensitivity of the alarm system. I am happy to leave it to the readers to come up with further analogies, and at this point, I would like to refer to the book *Explain Pain* by Butler and Moseley.

Therapists who use PNE combine it with interventions such as general exercise, aerobic activity, manual therapy such as mobilisation and soft tissue techniques, mobilisation of neural structures, electrotherapy, relaxation techniques, and breathing exercises. Instruction in an appropriate home program is, of course, essential.

The patient's level of knowledge is continuously checked by the therapist through targeted questioning. Uncertainties are discussed, questions are answered, and further relevant knowledge is provided in a measured way using images (of the nervous system, please NOT of disc herniations), examples, metaphors, and brochures or books (Butler and Moseley 2016).

This all sounds like a lot of "talk time" during a therapy session. Experience shows that the first session usually lasts up to an hour, follow-up sessions last about 30 to 40 min (Louw et al. 2016). Of course, much can be discussed while the patient demonstrates their home exercises or warms up on the ergometer. Sometimes, the knowledge is not imparted during the therapy session but in separate information sessions.

Incidentally, the method works better in a 1:1 setting than in a group (Moseley 2003).

1.4 The Specificity Theory

This theory, also known as the "labeled line" theory, states that each somatosensory modality has its own dedicated pathway. According to this theory, pain is an independent sensation with its own sensors, pathways, and central nervous system centers. This theory dates back to ideas that are thousands of years old and was formally proposed and tested in the 19th century (Mendell 2014; Moayedi and Davis 2013).

Most of us are familiar with the illustration from Descartes' (1596–1650) posthumously published work *Traité de l'Homme (1662).* This illustration more or less depicts the contemporary understanding of the nociceptive system: particles from the fire move the skin and pull on a hollow "thread," this pull opens a "gate" in the brain. Through the open gate, an "animal spirit" can now flow into the hollow thread and thus activate the muscles so that the foot can be withdrawn from the fire (Fig. 1.1).

Descartes' idea was not new; it goes back to Claudius Galenus (129–199 CE). Galenus, or Galen, postulated that an organ must be able to receive a stimulus and that there must be a connection between the organ and the brain. Furthermore, there must be a processing system that converts the stimulus into conscious perception (Ochs 2004). Galen based his theories on

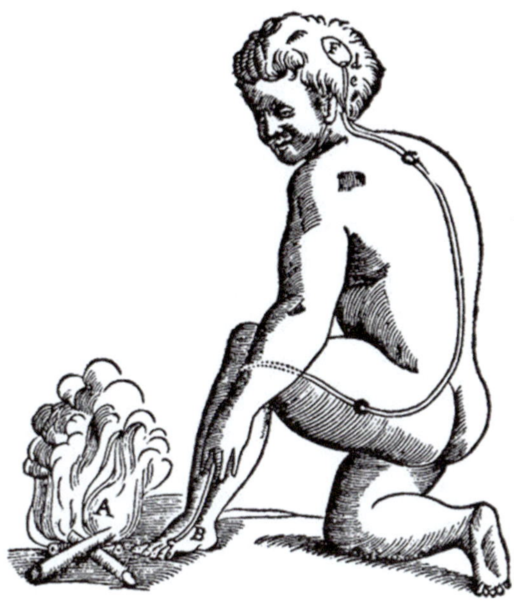

Fig. 1.1 Descartes' concept of pain conduction. Wikipedia.commons. https://upload.wikimedia.org/wikipedia/commons/8/8a/Descartes-reflex.JPG

ideas from the Greek Herophilos of Chalcedon (ca. 335–280 BCE), who demonstrated the existence of sensory and motor nerves. Galen based his work on the investigations of a certain Erasistratus (ca. 305–250 BCE), who was able to show that the brain influences motor activities. The latter conducted experiments on living humans, so one might wonder where he got this knowledge.

However, Descartes also believed that the brain received information about the intensity and quality of a stimulus depending on how the aforementioned thread was pulled. In more modern terms: stimulus patterns and stimulus frequency determine the brain's response.

The specificity theory gained real momentum in the 19th century after Pacini, Meissner, Merkel, and Ruffini discovered various specific tactile organs in the skin. Unfortunately, no pain-specific receptors had been discovered by then, so the debate about what pain actually was continued. Pain was considered an emotion—a theory that goes back to Plato and Aristotle—and therefore pain was thought to be a property of the soul and not a physical perception.

The evidence for the specificity theory accumulated, but only discoveries such as the identification of specific pathways in the spinal cord by Schiff and Woroschiloff (Rey 2005) and the four basic somatosensory modalities by Max von Frey (of the aesthesiometer): cold, heat, pain, and touch (Rey 2005) will be mentioned here. It is also worth noting that Sherrington, in addition to terms such as synapse and proprioception, coined the term nociceptor many years *avant la lettre* in 1906. In 1967, Burgess and Perl were the first to identify myelinated afferent nerve fibers that respond only to noxious stimuli; in 1969, Bessou and Perl discovered nociceptive unmyelinated fibers: polymodal nociceptors and high-threshold mechanoreceptors.

The specificity theory remained the most important pain theory for many years until it lost popularity after 1965 with the formulation of the Gate Control Theory of Pain (Melzack and Wall).

1.5 The Intensity Theory

The second pain theory discussed here is the intensity theory (Moayedi and Davis 2013). It was Plato, in the 4th century BCE, who suggested that pain is an emotion that occurs when a stimulus is stronger than normal. Many centuries later, it was Erasmus Darwin (Charles's grandfather) who supported this concept, and 100 years later Wilhelm Erb proposed that pain could occur in any sensory system if the stimulus was sufficiently intense. A certain Arthur Goldscheider, in 1898, based on studies by Bernhard Naunyn, proposed a kind of summation effect, whereby repeated stimulation could trigger pain and the stimuli would converge and sum in the spinal cord. In 1859, Naunyn had conducted experiments with syphilis patients: in these patients, the spinal cord was damaged, and repeated subsensory stimulation of the skin led to unbearable pain. Naunyn therefore already suspected a kind of summation effect, an idea that Goldscheider later developed further. The theory never became truly popular, partly because the then very popular Sherrington strongly supported the specificity theory with his assumption that nociceptors existed.

1.6 The Pattern Theory

The third theory reviewed here is the so-called pattern theory (Moayedi and Davis 2013). This theory was proposed in 1929 by the American psychologist John Paul Nafe as the "quantitative theory of feeling" (Nafe 1929). The theory ignores findings about specialized nerve endings and many other observations that support the specificity and intensity theories. It states that every somesthetic sensation arises from certain temporal and spatial patterns of nerve conduction, which encode the sensation in terms of type and intensity.

The pattern theory formed the basis for the Gate Control Theory of Melzack and Wall.

1.7 The Gate Control Theory

The Gate Control Theory (GCT), which continues to shape pain research to this day, was formulated in 1965 by Ronald Melzack and Patrick Wall (Fig. 1.2). The theory accepts the findings of the specificity theory and the pattern theory and proposes a model that explains the apparent contradictions between these theories. The GCT states that the transmission of pain from the peripheral nerve to the spinal cord is subject to modulation by both neurons in the spinal cord and the brain. No more and no less. And that is what makes this theory so elegant (Melzack and Wall 1965; Dickenson 2002; McMahon et al. 2013; Mendell 2014; Moayedi and Davis 2013).

More specifically, the two investigators initially claimed that there is a modulating control at the first synaptic connection between primary afferents and transmission cells (T-cells) in lamina II of the substantia gelatinosa (SG) of the spinal dorsal horn.

The theory essentially comprises three aspects:

1. When the neural activity of myelinated, fast-conducting non-nociceptive afferent fibers predominates, this inhibits the activity of the thin, slow-conducting nociceptive afferent fibers via activation of inhibitory interneurons in the substantia gelatinosa. This leads to hypoalgesia or analgesia.
2. When the activity mediated by slow-conducting, nociceptive afferent fibers predominates, it exacerbates pain by deactivating the inhibitory SG interneurons.
3. This process—or: the "gating"—is dynamically modulated by segmental or descending central control.

In 1968, Melzack and Casey refined the GCT by formulating a multidimensional, complex description of pain with three components that influence each other. The adapted theory assumes that the physical and psychological processes involved

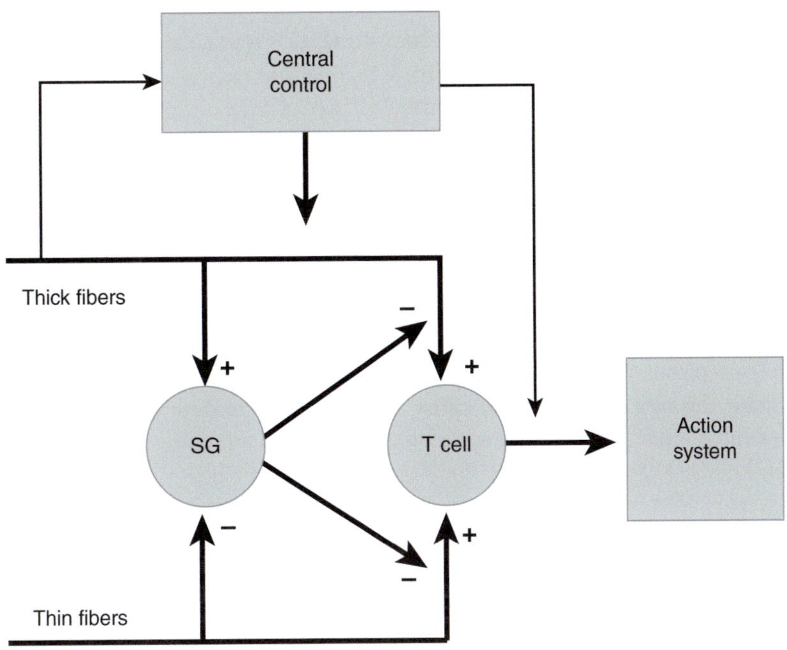

Fig. 1.2 The first version of the Gate Control Theory

in pain perception must be understood as a unit. This unity determines the pain experience.

- **Sensory-discriminative component:** We can describe pain in terms of location, intensity, quality, and duration. This processing takes place in the thalamocortical structures.
- **Affective-motivational component:** A cold bath on a hot summer day elicits a very different sensation than the same bath in the middle of winter when the heating has broken down. At least in Northern and Central Europe. Thus, a sensory experience can evoke pleasurable or unpleasant feelings depending on the situation. This is true for sensations with the ear, eyes, or nose as well. What is special, however, is that pain (almost) always disturbs our well-being, whereas other sensations can remain neutral. Processing takes place in the limbic system.
- **Cognitive-evaluative component:** Depending on the context, we can perceive pain as mild, unpleasant, worrying, or unbearable, among other things. In evaluating pain, we compare current pain with pain from the past and the experiences associated with it. There is ample evidence that pain is influenced by these central nervous cognitive processes. These include, for example, anxiety, attention, anticipation, suggestion, placebos, nocebos, cultural background, previous experiences, upbringing, and conditioning. These processes can modulate both sensory and affective responses. A person under hypnosis may feel a potential pain, but the pain bothers them less. This means that by changing the cognitive state through hypnosis, the affective component is altered, but not the sensory component.

These three components interact and influence the motor system, which then leads to an appropriate motor response to the stimulus. For example, if someone almost burns themselves on a lit match, the reaction is very different from when that person picks up an unexpectedly hot but very valuable Ming Dynasty teacup.

1.7.1 Peripheral Pain Perception and Segmental Transfer

In addition to the three components mentioned above, there are two other functional systems involved in nociception: the peripheral pain apparatus and the segmental pain apparatus in the spinal cord. In the periphery, nociceptive stimuli are detected by specialized receptors in the skin, muscles, bones, joints, and internal organs.

In the skin, three groups can be distinguished:

- High-threshold mechanoreceptors, which transmit their impulses to the spinal cord via Aδ fibers
- High-threshold thermoreceptors, which transmit their impulses via C fibers
- Polymodal receptors, which also transmit their impulses to the spinal cord via C fibers

At the level of the spinal cord, at the dorsal horn neurons, there is convergence of two fiber systems (Handwerker et al. 1975; Todd 2010):

- Thick (5–12 mm), myelinated, rapidly (30–70 m/s) conducting nerve fibers of type Aβ, which originate from mechanoreceptors (e.g., Vater-Pacini corpuscles) and transmit pressure, touch, and vibration sensations to the dorsal horn neurons (transmitter or T-cells = interneurons) in lamina II and III.

Some authors prefer a numerical classification. Here, fiber type Aβ (according to Erlanger and Gasser) corresponds to numerical type II, Aδ corresponds to type III, and C fibers correspond to type IV (according to Lloyd-Hunt).

- Somewhat slower (12–30 m/s) conducting nerve fibers of type Aδ. These are thinner (2–5 mm) fibers with a thin myelin sheath. These fibers transmit impulses from nociceptors in the skin to the T-cells in lamina I and V (pain, cold, and touch): the first pain (see below); and thin (0.4–1.2 mm), slowly conducting (0.5–2 m/s) unmyelinated C fibers, which transmit information from polymodal nociceptors to interneurons in lamina II (the substantia gelatinosa): the second pain.

In the SG, a transfer occurs in three directions (Price 2002; Todd 2010):

- to the spinothalamic tract, which transmits impulses to the thalamus
- to a motor anterior horn cell in the same segment, from which impulses for flexor reflexes (protective reflexes) and visceromotor reflexes originate
- to autonomic nerve fibers in the same segment, which trigger autonomic responses to pain

Activity from both thick and thin fibers stimulates interneurons (T-cells) in the dorsal horn of the spinal cord. Impulses conducted by thin fibers inhibit inhibitory enkephalinergic interneurons in the dorsal horn. This is followed by a reduction in the presynaptic inhibition of the interneurons, allowing the information to be transmitted centrally. This ultimately leads to the actual perception of pain.

The inhibitory system for the dorsal horn neurons located in lamina V of the dorsal horn consists of the GABAergic interneurons of the substantia gelatinosa located in lamina II and III (GABA: gamma aminobutyric acid). The inhibitory effect of these interneurons is, for example, enhanced by benzodiazepines such as Valium®.

The inhibitory interneurons are activated by impulses conducted via the fast-conducting fibers. This activation of the interneurons leads to a presynaptic inhibition of impulse transmission, which ultimately results in a "closing" of the spinal "gate." Incidentally, the term "gate" probably does not come from the English "gate" but rather from the circuit diagram of an old-fashioned amplifier tube, in which the grid (i.e., "gate") serves to modulate the electron flow.

Thus, if the Aβ fibers are stimulated, the input from the slow-conducting pain fibers is modulated by the action of the inhibitory interneurons of the SG. The information conducted via the Aβ fibers activates GABAergic inhibitory interneurons.

1.7.2 Adaptation of the GCT

Criticism of the Gate Control Theory focused on the fact that the role of central, higher centers was not taken into account and that the theory did not explain why pain sometimes occurs despite the destruction of thin nerve fibers. Therefore, in 1968, Melzack and Casey proposed an adaptation of the GCT (Melzack and Casey 1968). They additionally incorporated the systems mentioned above: the sensory-discriminative, the motivational-affective, and the central control system (Fig. 1.3).

This central nervous modulation influences, on the one hand, the psychomotor component of pain expression, such as moaning, facial expressions, or the desire for medication, and on the other hand, it also modulates the affective and autonomic components. When a painful stimulus occurs, autonomic reactions arise: blood flow may change (vasodilation or vasoconstriction), heart rate changes, as do blood pressure and respiratory rate. The pupils may dilate or constrict, and there may be increased sweating. These reactions often occur with visceral pain (e.g., biliary colic) and may be accompanied by nausea and vomiting.

Pain assessment depends on social situation, family background, upbringing, and ethnic origin. It is also important under what circumstances pain occurs. If we know that we are going to be pricked during a blood draw, the pain perception is very different from when someone unexpectedly pricks us with a needle. Here, the anticipation of pain already has a pain-suppressing effect.

The Gate Control Theory remains a widely accepted theory of pain, and a multitude of receptors have been discovered on interneurons that are involved in pre- or postsynaptic signal modulation. Several such receptors or channels have proven to be effective targets for pain

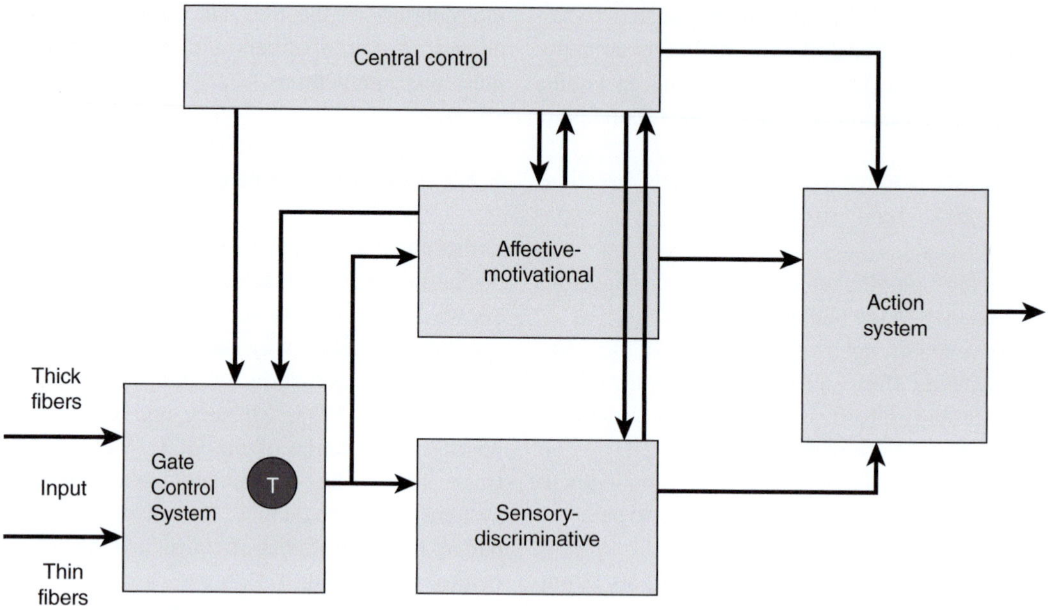

Fig. 1.3 The extended GCT

medications, such as gabapentin, a drug used for neuropathic pain. Gabapentin binds to a specific subgroup of Ca channels, which become more active after persistent ectopic activity from damaged peripheral nerves has increased neural activity in the spinal cord.

These Ca channels produce, among other things, glutamate, an important neurotransmitter in A and C fibers. This local increase in glutamate leads to enhanced stimulation of glutamate receptors such as the NMDA (N-methyl-D-aspartate) receptor, which plays an important role in central sensitization. The latter causes increased excitability of spinal neurons, thereby enlarging their receptive field and likely playing an important role in the development of secondary hyperalgesia or allodynia. Since the NMDA receptor, among other things, has binding sites for ketamine, this explains the effectiveness of this drug in certain pain conditions (Dickenson 2002; McMahon et al. 2013).

Thus, there are many subgroups of receptors on various interneurons that, depending on the coding of neural activity, trigger complex processes (Todd 2010).

It is clear that the simple scheme proposed by Melzack, Wall, and Casey could never correspond to reality, since at the time there were not yet the means and possibilities available as there are today in modern laboratories. This fact only makes the theory more elegant and concise.

1.8 Opioid Receptors

In 1973, various investigators independently discovered opioid receptors (mu = μ, delta = δ, and kappa = κ opioid receptors) in certain brain areas. At first, this discovery seemed rather peculiar: Why does the human body have receptors specifically for a substance whose possession can lead to long prison sentences?

In 1975, John Hughes and Hans Walter Kosterlitz discovered in pig brains a substance with properties similar to morphine: they called it enkephalin (meaning “in the head”). It was thought that this substance would form the basis for a new generation of analgesics. Unfortunately, its analgesic effect was not overwhelming, but it was highly addictive (Kosterlitz and Hughes 1975; Hughes and Kosterlitz 1983; Hughes et al. 1997).

Shortly thereafter, chemist Choh Hao Li from the University of California in San Francisco recalled that he had already isolated β-endorphin from camel pituitary glands in the 1960s, and that this contained enkephalin. At the time, he did not know what to make of this discovery, but now the question arose as to whether this β-endorphin was also involved in pain inhibition. He injected β-endorphin into the brain and found that it was 48 times more potent than morphine. Administered intravenously, it was three times more potent than morphine. And it also had a high addiction potential (Li et al. 1977).

This was the first time an endogenous, central pain inhibition system had been discovered. The next step led to the extraordinarily effective electroanalgesia by local stimulation of these brain areas (stimulation-produced analgesia, SPA) (McMahon et al. 2013).

Stimulation is particularly effective in the periaqueductal gray matter (PAG) and in the periventricular gray matter as well as in certain thalamic regions. The highest concentrations of endorphins and their receptors have also been detected here. It is now known that painful electrical stimulation from the periphery (hyperstimulation analgesia, APL-TENS = acupuncture-like TENS = low frequency high intensity electrical stimulation) and direct, focal stimulation of brain areas lead to increased endorphin release detectable in the cerebrospinal fluid. Endorphins act by blocking the transmission of pain signals at both the spinal and supraspinal levels, just like morphine and its derivatives.

Opiates are those substances that contain opium or opium alkaloids (morphine). Opioids are all substances with morphine-like effects, including those produced by the body itself.

The pathways that conduct nociceptive input centrally synapse along the way with nuclei of the reticular formation. These nuclei send impulses to the periaqueductal gray matter. Stimulation of these nuclei leads to feedback of impulses to the nucleus raphe magnus. From here, monoaminergic (serotonin, noradrenaline) pathways descend through the spinal cord and activate, at the segmental level, enkephalinergic inhibitory interneurons.

Evidence for the existence of these mechanisms includes, among other things, the fact that the analgesic effect is abolished by administration of low doses of naloxone (an antagonist for μ-opioid receptors) and naltrindole (an antagonist for δ-opioid receptors). Similarly, blockade of serotonin (by administration of methysergide, a 5-HT receptor blocker) and transection of the aforementioned pathways lead to a reduction in pain inhibition.

Interestingly, both opiates and SPA long-term treatment can lead to physical dependence and withdrawal syndromes. A comparable effect also occurs with acupuncture, acupressure, hypnosis, and physical exertion. In acupuncture, the Aδ (pin-prick) fibers are stimulated, which make contact at the outer edge of the dorsal horn with enkephalinergic interneurons. These interneurons can inhibit the transmission of nociceptive information via the SG. Thus, stimulation of Aδ fibers at a frequency of about 2–4 Hz can cause analgesia in the treated segment (electroacupuncture, low frequency TENS).

It has been shown that a second mechanism runs in parallel with this inhibition. Activation of descending serotonergic pathways from the brainstem can also activate enkephalinergic interneurons. On this basis, attempts are made to explain the heterosegmental effect of acupuncture and other treatment methods (TENS). Evidence for this hypothesis is that administration of L-tryptophan (5-HT = L-5-hydroxytryptophan), a serotonin precursor, enhances acupuncture analgesia and the analgesic effect of TENS (McMahon et al. 2013).

1.9 Types of Pain

All higher developed animal organisms possess specialized receptors with such high excitation thresholds that they are normally only activated by tissue-damaging or tissue-threatening stimuli (so-called noxae, from Latin "nocere," to harm). These sensors and their afferent nerve fibers are therefore called nociceptors. The neural structures activated by nociceptors are referred to as the nociceptive system. Nociception, on the other hand, refers to the entire process of detection, transmission, and central nervous processing of noxious signals (Handwerker 1998; McMahon et al. 2013; Schaible 2015).

- Inflammatory pain **or** nociceptor pain: Inflammation leads to a characteristic pain symptomatology, referred to as allodynia and hyperalgesia. *Allodynia* refers to pain caused by non-noxious stimuli, i.e., stimuli that would never cause pain in healthy individuals, even with prolonged application. For example, if someone has sunburn, even a light touch of the skin causes pain. *Hyperalgesia*, on the other hand, refers to increased sensitivity to truly noxious stimuli, i.e., potentially harmful stimuli that trigger pain more quickly or at lower intensity than in healthy individuals. The pain can occur as a result of traumatic, inflammatory, or tumorous tissue damage.
  - Primary hyperalgesia is an increased response to a normally painful stimulus at the site of injury or inflammation. This also includes pain due to muscle injury. Primary hyperalgesia usually occurs with both thermal and mechanical stimuli and is (at least partially) caused by primary afferent nociceptor sensitization. Thus, primary hyperalgesia is caused by the direct effects of injury to skin and nerve tissue, while secondary hyperalgesia refers to increased pain sensitivity of the surrounding tissue.
  - Secondary hyperalgesia is defined as an increase in pain sensitivity outside the area of injury or inflammation. Secondary hyperalgesia is due to sensitization of central neural structures and requires continuous nociceptive input from the area of primary hyperalgesia to be maintained. Secondary hyperalgesia affects only mechanical hyperalgesia, i.e., "allodynia" and "pinprick," and not thermal hyperalgesia.
- Projected pain: If a nerve root is compressed and inflamed, for example due to a herniated disc, the resulting impulses in the pain-conducting fibers are projected into the area supplied by the affected nerve. In this type of pain, the site of the pain trigger is therefore not identical to the site where the pain is perceived. The same phenomenon occurs when you hit your elbow and strike the ulnar nerve: the resulting tingling is not felt at the elbow, but in the corresponding area on the ulnar side of the hand. Because impulses generated in this way do not normally occur, it is difficult for the cortex to interpret them. The resulting activity is therefore projected by our consciousness into the innervation area of the affected nerve, because these impulses normally also originate from there. Some authors classify *neuropathic pain* as a subgroup of this type of pain. This arises from spontaneous activity due to damage to the nociceptive system itself and not from stimulation of nerve endings (Gierthmühlen and Baron 2016; Watson and Sandroni 2016; Colloca et al. 2017). Neuropathic pain also frequently leads to allodynia and hyperalgesia. A typical example is phantom pain, which is projected into a body part that no longer exists.
- Referred pain: The occurrence of this type of pain is based on the fact that nociceptive afferents from the skin, muscles, joints, and organs synapse onto the same interneurons. As a result, precise information about the origin of the pain is lost. This explains, for example, why pain from a heart attack is not perceived in the heart, but in the left (or even right) arm. Axon collaterals of primary nociceptive afferents can also branch off at the level of the spinal nerve, innervating structures at different depths. Most often, referred pain is perceived in the same dermatome. Many organs always use the same skin areas for pain projection. These skin areas are called Head zones or Head's zones. They are of diagnostic and therapeutic interest.

- Central pain: This occurs due to functional disturbances or defects of spinal or supraspinal nociceptive systems, which can then lead to spontaneous activity of these structures. Examples include anaesthesia dolorosa after avulsion of the dorsal roots or thalamic pain following damage to the ventral sensory thalamic nuclei. However, such central lesions are not always painful, as can be seen in the case of strokes and brain tumors (Watson and Sandroni 2016).
- Reflex pain: This term refers to pain that occurs due to reflex mechanisms. Muscle tension can trigger pain, and the tension can in turn be exacerbated by the pain, and so on. Pain can also occur due to inappropriate autonomic reflex activity, although this type of pain is more likely to be classified as neuropathic pain.
- Psychosomatic pain: Psychological stress can manifest as physical complaints. Such pain can be influenced by changes in lifestyle or psychotherapeutic interventions.

Some authors distinguish between physiological nociceptor pain (pNS) and neuropathic pain in nociceptor pain (nS). pNS arises from disease or damage to an organ, while nS results from damage to the nerve fibers themselves.

Congenital insensitivity to pain should also be included among the various types of pain. In some of these cases, no defect in the nervous system can be detected, but sometimes either the peripheral nociceptors or the primary nociceptive afferents are missing. Patients do not feel pain, and the many injuries that occur as a result lead to mutilations and infections and almost always to early death.

Pain from the skin is mediated by nociceptors that respond particularly to painful mechanical and heat stimuli. Visceral nociceptors are activated, among other things, by contraction and distension of organs. Pain in the musculoskeletal system is transmitted by nociceptors in muscles, tendons, joints, bones, and periosteum. In addition to the nervous system, nociceptors are found in the human body in the skin and skeletal muscles, tendons, and joints, which respond to both mechanical (pinprick, crushing) and chemical (e.g., bradykinin, prostaglandin) and thermal (heat, cold) stimuli and are therefore referred to as "polymodal," although the term is somewhat misleading: in principle, they only respond to tissue damage. Incidentally, it has been found that polymodal nociceptors can also transmit non-painful sensations. Instead of polymodal nociceptors, the term CMH receptors is now more commonly used: C for chemical, M for mechanical, and H for "heat" (Handwerker 1998).

In addition to the direct stimulation of nociceptors, many endogenous substances influence pain perception. These substances are released by vascular endothelial cells, immune cells (including mast cells), leukocytes, and platelets, as well as by cells of the peripheral nervous system (neuropeptides).

In healthy tissue, the thresholds for nociceptor activation vary. As soon as a pathophysiological change occurs in the tissue, such as inflammation, all nociceptors become sensitized, i.e., their thresholds are lowered. This leads to normally non-painful stimuli now being perceived as painful, a phenomenon known as hyperalgesia. This sensitization is caused by the action of these substances. Important inflammatory mediators are bradykinin, serotonin (which enhances the nociceptor response to bradykinin), and arachidonic acid metabolites (prostaglandins, thromboxane, leukotrienes). Inhibition of prostaglandin production by administration of cyclooxygenase inhibitors (COX inhibitors, for example, Aspirin®) leads to a reduction in inflammation-related pain and is the basis for therapy with nonsteroidal anti-inflammatory drugs (NSAIDs).

The release of neuropeptides from the endings of polymodal nociceptors leads to so-called neurogenic inflammation. This process is of great importance for the development of pain. The topic is discussed in detail in Chap. 2.

1.10 Pain Transmission

The Aδ and C fibers enter the spinal cord via the dorsal root. The spinal cord is composed of several laminae, with the most superficial layer referred to as Lamina I (Alles and Smith 2018). Most Aδ fibers (= type II) synapse with interneurons in Lamina I and V, while most C fibers (= type III) synapse with interneurons in Lamina II. It is here that connections to motor and autonomic efferents also occur, thereby influencing withdrawal reflexes and sympathetic responses. Aβ fibers terminate mainly in Laminae III–VI. Various cells are involved in these connections. There are pain-specific cells that synapse only with C and Aδ fibers, and others that synapse only with Aβ fibers. The most common interneuron, connected to all three types, is the so-called wide dynamic range neuron (WDR). These cells respond to all stimuli, from light touch to severe pain caused by pressure, heat, or chemical changes. WDR neurons discharge in a graded manner depending on stimulus intensity and exhibit so-called wind-up, a form of short-term neuroplasticity. During wind-up, the discharge frequency of the WDR neuron increases with each subsequent stimulation. WDR neurons are very likely involved in the development of neuropathic pain.

In addition to the neurons mentioned, the spinal cord contains excitatory (glutamatergic) and inhibitory (GABAergic) interneurons, which can influence the responses of the neurons described above. These interneurons are under the influence of descending pain modulation mechanisms.

Most, but not all, slowly conducting cutaneous afferents are nociceptive. Among the Aδ afferents, there is a clearly defined group of cold-sensitive sensors, and among the C fibers, warm-sensitive sensors. Other Aδ and C fibers are sensitive mechanoreceptors.

The conduction velocity of C fibers is so slow that one can subjectively distinguish impulse conduction in Aδ and C fibers, at least when the hand or foot is stimulated, since the impulses must then travel a longer distance before reaching the CNS. A needle prick produces the so-called double pain phenomenon: the prick (Aδ) is perceived almost immediately, followed by a brief pain-free interval, and then the second pain, often more burning or drilling in character (C). These are referred to as first and second pain.

Aδ fibers have an inhibitory connection via enkephalinergic interneurons in Lamina II and III with interneurons of the substantia gelatinosa. C fibers probably synapse directly onto the SG in Lamina II and have an excitatory effect there. This circuitry explains the segmental pain-inhibiting effect of acupuncture: the Aδ receptors are stimulated by the acupuncture needle and, via this interneuron, inhibit the afferent C fiber information. The afferents from the fast-conducting Aβ fibers (touch and temperature sensors) enter Lamina IV and are connected to the SG via (probably GABAergic) inhibitory interneurons. This circuitry corresponds to the gate control mechanism.

In Lamina I and V, pain fibers (Aδ) from various structures (skin, muscles, organs, etc.) enter. These afferents sometimes synapse with the same neurons. As a result, information about the origin of the pain signal is partially lost.

This is presumably the reason for sometimes unexpected pain localization. It also explains the occurrence of symptoms in structures that are connected via the same segment in which another structure is symptomatic.

The second-order neurons cross to the contralateral side and ascend centrally via the spinothalamic tract (STT). On the way to the thalamus, the STT has connections with the reticular formation in the brainstem. This allows pain to influence the respiratory and cardiovascular centers. In addition, additional connections to the ascending reticular activating system (ARAS) affect arousal and attention (for more information on the stress response and its consequences for therapy, see Sect. 1.15).

Important thalamic connections include, among others,

- to the primary somatosensory cortex. Here, especially in the somatosensory cortex in the postcentral gyrus, pain localization takes place.
- to the limbic system (e.g., the PAG and the amygdala). Here, the affective-emotional component of pain is perceived. The projection of pain fibers into the limbic system can be considered the basis for the immediate

effect of pain on general well-being. Conversely, the limbic system also influences pain perception and can attenuate or amplify subjective perception. The amygdala is the key relay in the brain for stabilizing mood, aggression, and social behavior.

- to the hippocampus. This plays a central role in the formation and processing of memories.
- to the hypothalamus. This is the fundamental control center for basic biological functions, such as attack and defense behavior ("fight or flight"). The hypothalamus controls the pituitary gland and thus especially the hormonal stress response (the autonomic orientation, see also "alarm phase") (Sect. 1.16).

1.11 Central and Descending Pain Modulation

Impulses from Aδ and C afferents trigger activation of the hypothalamic-pituitary functional complex via the thalamus (Price 2002; Sapolsky 2004; Leung 2012; McMahon et al. 2013). In the hypothalamus, proopiomelanocortin (POMC) is broken down, producing, among other things, β-endorphin. This β-endorphin acts directly on the periaqueductal gray (PAG). The pituitary gland also produces POMC, which is split in two phases into adrenocorticotropic hormone (ACTH = adrenocorticotropin), β-endorphin, methionine-enkephalin, and various other products.

A small portion of this β-endorphin enters the circulation. The larger portion binds to μ-opioid receptors in the PAG, causing pronounced central pain inhibition. ACTH triggers the release of cortisol from the adrenal cortex. The combined action of cortisol and β-endorphin is the reason for the primary suppression of pain in an acute stress reaction.

The PAG also projects to the raphe nucleus (nucleus raphe magnus, NRM) in the medulla oblongata, and the NRM is in turn excited by the PAG through disinhibition of an inhibitory interneuron. The raphe nucleus projects via the monoaminergic (the neurotransmitter here is 5-hydroxytryptamine = serotonin) dorsolateral tract to enkephalinergic interneurons, so-called stalked cells, in Lamina II of the substantia gelatinosa. This circuitry causes presynaptic inhibition of Aδ and C afferents and probably postsynaptic inhibition of the second (spinothalamic tract) neuron.

These inhibitory mechanisms are activated after a few minutes by low frequency TENS, electroacupuncture, and acupuncture, in which the needle is manually, i.e., mechanically, stimulated at a low frequency (Chiang 1974; Li et al. 1977; Han et al. 1991; Le Bars and Willer 2002; Leung 2012). These stimulations cause the release of met-enkephalin, endomorphin-2, and β-endorphin.

Evidence for the involvement of endomorphin-2 and β-endorphin is that analgesia is reversed by administration of naloxone. Naloxone is an antagonist for the endomorphin-2 and β-endorphin binding sites: the μ-opioid receptors. Analgesia from high frequency TENS (100 Hz) is not reversed by naloxone, but by naltrindole (an antagonist for δ-opioid receptors, where enkephalins bind) and by serotonin antagonists. This means that in this application, endomorphin-2 and β-endorphin are not involved, but rather dynorphin (which binds to κ-opioid receptors), enkephalins, and the monoamines serotonin and noradrenaline (Han et al. 1991; Han 2004). Likewise, blockade of serotonin (by administration of methysergide, a 5-HT receptor blocker) and transection of the aforementioned pathways lead to a reduction in pain inhibition.

1.12 Diffuse Noxious Inhibitory Control (DNIC)

Hippocrates already knew it when he said, "If a patient is exposed to two simultaneous pains at different locations in his body, the stronger one dulls the other." Or something to that effect.

Diffuse Noxious Inhibitory Control(s), also called "counterirritation" and "bulbospinal pain control," refers to an inhibitory mechanism that is non-segmentally controlled by painful stimuli at an arbitrary body site. Therefore, the stimulation is referred to as "heterotopic," also "dystopic" or "ectopic," i.e., located at an atypical site. It is probably the evolutionarily oldest pain inhibition system and ensures that the organism focuses on the strongest, i.e., most important, pain.

The theory describes inhibition of multireceptive neurons (wide dynamic range = WDR neurons) in the spinal cord by painful stimuli in an area outside the affected receptive fields (Villanueva and Le Bars 1995; Le Bars et al. 1992; Le Bars 2002). The inhibition works only with intact brainstem function, and involvement of the endogenous opioid system has been demonstrated: the effect is reduced by administration of naloxone (Bing et al. 1990, 1991).

Paradoxically, a small dose of morphine appears to reduce the effect. This is explained by the fact that morphine blocks the afferent part of the DNIC. As a result, the input into the system is too low and it is not activated. The stimulus must be painful for the mechanism to work.

The centers involved are quite well known. The involvement of the subnucleus reticularis dorsalis (SRD) in the caudal medulla is considered certain, as lesions of this structure strongly suppress DNIC. The SRD projects via the dorsolateral funiculus to the substantia gelatinosa in the dorsal horn of all spinal cord segments, i.e., where the afferent Aδ and C fibers also synapse. Administration of serotonin antagonists leads to a reduction in inhibition; the descending pathways in the dorsolateral funiculus are serotonergic and are therefore probably responsible for transmission. The involvement of the locus coeruleus (LC) is also very likely, either directly via the spinothalamic tract or indirectly via the nucleus paragigantocellularis. The LC projects noradrenergically and inhibits the substantia gelatinosa.

DNIC works only if the applied stimulus is actually painful—in contrast to pain inhibition via the GCT, where Aβ fibers are not painfully stimulated. The DNIC mechanism is almost certainly involved in the effect of low frequency TENS, also acupuncture-like TENS (APL), in which Aδ and C fibers are stimulated and an intense but well-tolerated sensation is produced. In addition, involvement in acupuncture-induced analgesia is considered certain (Bing et al. 1990, 1991; Le Bars and Willer 2002). Likewise, the pain-relieving effects of strong heat and cold applications can be explained by this mechanism (Le Bars and Willer 2002).

The theory states that dorsal horn neurons in the spinal cord are inhibited by a painful stimulus applied at an arbitrary location on the body. Therefore, any painful stimulus (such as an acupuncture needle) in extrasegmental areas can relieve pain. This mechanism works in both peripheral and central inhibition systems. The peripheral system works via Aδ and C fibers, and indeed, the spread of the so-called De-Qi sensation is a sign of activation of the Aδ fibers (Leung 2012). The De-Qi sensation (also Deqi, Teh Chi) is a relatively unpleasant dull feeling of heaviness triggered during acupuncture. If this sensation is suppressed by a local intramuscular injection of procaine, acupuncture is ineffective (Chiang 1974). More about the De-Qi sensation under TENS (Sect. 1.12 and 3.4.2.).

Caution: Pitfall

The DNIC mechanism could pose a problem for us physiotherapists. The following example may illustrate this.

Let us assume a patient has lateral elbow pain during a specific movement. The therapist examines the elbow, the shoulder, and very likely also the cervical spine. Suppose the findings at the elbow are not particularly clear, but our therapist, during a targeted localized movement at the front of C5/6, elicits a rather unpleasant local pain and some radiation into the affected arm: Eureka, something found! And it would almost fit.

After our therapist has performed this painful movement at C5/6 for some time, he now asks the patient to repeat the pain-inducing movement (for the elbow), and lo and behold: the pain has decreased.

Is the colleague now justified in postulating a causal relationship?

By no means! It is possible that the local pain at C5/6 was strong enough to trigger the DNIC mechanism. Only the further course of treatment will show to what extent other structures may be involved in the elbow problem.

It would be unreasonable to focus solely on the cervical spine based on such a reaction. Of course, any reputable (manual) therapist will base their hypothesis on more than what has been somewhat exaggerated here, but still: pain inhibition mechanisms have their pitfalls. ◄

1.13 Long Term Depression

It is not entirely clear whether LTD is an independent pain inhibition phenomenon or whether it is part of DNIC (Sandkühler et al. 1997). Studies in primates, cats, and rats (Wagman and Price 1969; Handwerker et al. 1975; Sandkühler et al. 1997; Liu et al. 1998; Nilsson and Schouenborg 1999; Nilsson et al. 2003) have shown that low-frequency electrical stimulation of Aδ fibers (0.1–0.5 ms, 15 min) leads to inhibition of C fibers in the substantia gelatinosa lasting up to 2 h, which is not mediated by GABAergic interneurons. Blockade of NMDA neurons abolished the effect. The authors refer to this as *Long Term Depression* (LTD). As a cause, Sandkühler postulates a long-lasting desensitization of postsynaptic receptors (probably NMDA, see DNIC) due to increased postsynaptic Ca concentration in the substantia gelatinosa. LTD can explain the pain-relieving effect of acupuncture (since needling stimulates Aδ fibers), of APL-TENS, as well as the effect of thermotherapies (ice, heat), in which thermosensitive Aδ fibers are stimulated. LTD would fit nicely into the mechanism of DNIC.

1.14 Special Case: Neuropathic Pain

In nociceptor-mediated pain, the peripheral and central nociceptive systems are intact. This type of pain usually occurs as a result of an inflammatory reaction, for example after an injury or overuse. In the case of chronification, functionally plastic changes can occur at various neural levels. Normally, this type of pain responds well to NSAIDs or glucocorticoids. When treating patients with primarily nociceptive pain, we can assume that the various pain inhibition systems are functioning at all levels (exception: see “Stress Reaction,” Sect. 1.16).

The treatment of neuropathic pain presents a particularly difficult problem. This type of pain occurs when structures of the peripheral or central nervous system themselves are damaged. Nerve injury can lead to structural and anatomical changes in the nervous system, which are often irreversible. The resulting pain is quite characteristic: it is usually burning, persistent pain, often combined with hyperalgesia or allodynia, paresthesias or dysesthesias, or neurological deficits such as hypoesthesia or hypalgesia (Gilron et al. 2015; Gierthmühlen and Baron 2016; Baron et al. 2016; Watson and Sandroni 2016; Colloca et al. 2017; Alles and Smith 2018; St John Smith 2018).

Neuropathic pain responds poorly or not at all to NSAIDs, glucocorticoids, and opioids. Therefore, other medications are used for this type of pain, such as tricyclic antidepressants, SSRIs (Selective Serotonin Reuptake Inhibitors), or anticonvulsants, sometimes opioids like tramadol (Tramal®) or GABA receptor antagonists, among others (Sawynok 2001; Alles and Smith 2018; Otto et al. 2019).

A major problem with the use of these agents is the occurrence of side effects and the fact that the pain can have very different causes. It is now assumed that in a single patient, several mechanisms responsible for pain generation, which mutually influence each other, are at play. Therefore, it is not possible to establish binding treatment protocols.

The following briefly addresses these causes and discusses the possible consequences for electrotherapy.

- Damage to a peripheral nerve and the subsequent Wallerian degeneration triggers an inflammatory reaction. Cytokines are released (interleukins, TNF-α), and inflammatory mediators such as bradykinin and prostaglandins are produced (Handwerker 1998). This leads to sensitization of the still intact nociceptors, which subsequently release increased amounts of neuropeptides (substance P and CGRP). A neurogenic inflammation develops, which further enhances sensitization (Weber et al. 2001; Sommer et al. 2018). This sensitization usually leads to heat hyperalgesia and mechanical hyperalgesia (pressure hyperalgesia). Neurogenic inflammation partially responds to the administration of NSAIDs, as these inhibit cyclooxygenase and thus the formation of prostaglandin. The pain also responds to treatment with capsaicin ointment and patches. Capsaicin desensitizes the C-fibers responsible for burning pain via the same mechanism by which the corresponding receptors in the mouths of regular chili consumers are desensitized (Winter et al. 1995; Simone et al. 1998; Anand and Bley 2011). Low-frequency electrotherapy with hyperemic currents such as direct current or diadynamic current is indicated here, as it can reduce sensitization by depleting neuropeptides (Schnizer et al. 2003) (capsaicin-like effect of the direct current component). It should be noted that in the initial treatments, forced neuropeptide release can lead to an intensification of pain, and that treatment must be carried out in short, initially daily intervals to prevent replenishment of the neuropeptide stores. After each subsequent treatment, there may be a brief increase in pain, as the existing neuropeptides are released again each time. Due to the reflex neurogenic reflex, temporary symptoms may occur on the opposite side. The patient must therefore be particularly well informed about the treatment.

- Due to continuous nociceptive input from the periphery, secondary nociceptive dorsal horn neurons become sensitized. As a result of this increased excitability, these neurons respond to afferent stimuli with an increased firing rate. Therefore, normally non-painful stimuli are perceived as painful (= allodynia). Segmental release of, among others, glutamate and substance P further increases the excitability of dorsal horn neurons, leading to an enlargement of the receptive fields in the periphery—in other words, the pain area increases. For electrotherapy, this means that therapies that are normally perceived as non-painful may be painful or even intolerable for these patients. This must, of course, be taken into account when selecting parameters. When using TENS, (very) short pulses combined with high frequencies and low dosages must be chosen. The frequently occurring allodynia or hyperalgesia may make local treatment impossible, as even light touch can be very painful. In such cases, segmental or non-segmental applications, applications over special points (acupuncture points, nerve points, etc.), or applications on the contralateral side are options.
- Due to a peripheral nerve lesion, both segmental and central pain inhibition can be reduced. There is a reduction in μ- and δ-opioid receptors. In addition, GABA production decreases and the number of associated receptors is reduced. GABAergic interneurons are involved in the gate control mechanism. After a peripheral nerve lesion, there is increased release of cholecystokinin (CCK) (Wiesenfeld-Hallin et al. 1999, 2002). This leads (at least in rats) to a central and peripheral decrease in μ-opioid receptors (the binding sites for β-endorphins), and the δ-opioid receptors (for enkephalins) are also antagonistically influenced by CCK (Heinricher and Neubert 2004; Hebb et al. 2005; Reynolds et al. 2011). As a result, the effect of opioids is reduced—the reason why this group of medications is often ineffective for this type of pain. For physiotherapy, these facts mean that in some patients, neither segmental nor central pain inhibition can be optimally activated. Nevertheless, it is possible to activate the monoaminergic descending inhibition (NRM and NRG) and (perhaps) the DNIC.
- Injury to C-fibers can lead to degeneration of these fibers in the spinal cord in

lamina II (Devor and Wall 1978; Woolf et al. 1992). This triggers so-called sprouting of Aβ-fibers from lamina III and IV into lamina II. Normally non-painful afferent Aβ-fiber information is now interpreted as painful. If one now attempts to specifically stimulate Aβ-fibers in electrotherapy, for example with a high-TENS application, in order to induce segmental inhibition, this therapy may be perceived as (extremely) painful and may produce no effect or even the opposite effect. In this case, it is probably better to stimulate the still intact C-fibers and Aδ-fibers so that the central and descending inhibitory mechanisms are activated.

- A comparable phenomenon occurs with sympathetic nerve fibers. Several investigators have observed that after a peripheral nerve lesion, sympathetic fibers grow into the spinal ganglion (Ramer et al. 1999; García-Poblete et al. 2003). These fibers form so-called baskets around thick myelinated fibers and also form synapse-like structures on the cell bodies. This may result in sympathetic activity stimulating these A-fibers (sympathetically maintained pain, CRPS1). After sympathectomy, the sprouting was prevented, confirming that these were postganglionic sympathetic fibers. The underlying mechanism is unclear. The involvement of cytokines and nerve growth factor is suspected. For therapy, this means that sympathetically active interventions can influence pain behavior. The work of B. Kaada confirms this assumption, as does the effectiveness of a blockade of the stellate ganglion (see the section on Kaada stimulation in Chap. 3).
- Normally, a nerve fiber is only excited by adequate stimulation. No action potentials are generated if the stimulus threshold is not exceeded. However, it has been observed that after a nerve lesion, spontaneous discharges often occur (Han et al. 2000; Devor 2009; North et al. 2018). These discharges are referred to as "ectopic" impulse generation (ectopic = not at the typical site). The discharges sometimes originate in the neuroma (if one has formed), but have also been observed in the spinal ganglion and along the course of the nerve. Ectopic discharges can also stimulate neighboring, intact nerve fibers, resulting in so-called "cross-talk" or "signal jumping" or ephapsis (Greek "ephapse" = contact). This refers to the jumping of signals from one nerve fiber to another, running parallel in the same bundle. This amplifies the effect of individual ectopic discharges. Cross-talk has also been demonstrated in the spinal ganglion between A- and C-fibers. Both damaged and intact nerve fibers can develop ectopic activity. Ectopic activity arises from increased expression of various types of Na and Ca channels on the membrane and in any neuroma. The cause of the increased expression is unclear, but NGF is thought to play a role. The increase in the number of these channels results in increased excitability of the nerve fiber. For electrotherapy, this means that particular caution and low dosages are required. However, as long as, for example, a mild high TENS is running, the nerve fiber is not able to simultaneously conduct ectopic discharges—the phone line is, so to speak, occupied.

1.14.1 Medications for the Treatment of Neuropathic Pain

See also Alles and Smith (2018), Otto et al. (2019).

- Tricyclic antidepressants (TCA) belong to the older generation of antidepressants. Due to side effects, the newer so-called selective serotonin reuptake inhibitors (SSRIs) are now preferred. Incidentally, these medications of course also have their side effects, which simply manifest differently. TCAs block the reuptake of monoaminergic neurotransmitters in the spinal cord and CNS, and do so more effectively than SSRIs. The descending pathways from the NRM use precisely these monoamines as neurotransmitters, and due to the mechanism of action of these agents, the availability of these transmitters is improved. In addition, antidepressants interact with the endogenous opioid system: pain relief is reversed by administration of naloxone. An inhibitory effect on Na, Ca, histamine, and acetylcholine receptors has also been demonstrated. The dose usually administered for neuropathic pain is below the antidepressant dose. This means that pain reduction does not occur due to an antidepressant effect.

- High-dose capsaicin patches (8%) cause a reversible degeneration of nociceptive nerve fibers in the skin and can thus provide pain relief for about 3 to 5 months. The patch is applied to the painful area(s) for 1 h, sometimes after pretreatment with a lidocaine patch to suppress the capsaicin-induced burning pain (Backonja et al. 2008; Clifford et al. 2012; Irving et al. 2012). A 2017 meta-analysis showed that the effect of the patch is comparable to that of medications such as gabapentin and pregabalin, but without the unpleasant side effects such as drowsiness, dizziness, and fatigue (van Nooten et al. 2017). The results of the studies mentioned should be interpreted with caution, as some of the investigators were employed by the manufacturer of the patches.
- Anticonvulsants such as gabapentin, which binds to calcium channels of interneurons in the substantia gelatinosa, pregabalin, which binds to calcium channels on peripheral nerves, and carbamazepine, which binds to sodium channels. Anticonvulsants reduce membrane excitability and thus suppress ectopic impulse generation. Their main area of application is the treatment of epilepsy, with carbamazepine also used for alcohol withdrawal, acute mania, and as maintenance therapy for bipolar affective disorders. It is therefore not surprising that some patients are unsettled after reading the package insert.
- According to German guidelines, opioids are recommended only as second- or third-line medications (Otto et al. 2019). Tramadol is a weak agonist at the μ-opioid receptor and also has a noradrenaline and serotonin reuptake inhibiting effect. Tapentadol is used successfully in diabetic neuropathy and chronic back pain with a neuropathic component. Patients treated with such opioids do not respond or respond only very weakly to low frequency TENS (Chandran and Sluka 2003). Léonard et al. (2010) attribute this to the fact that endomorphin-2, β-endorphin, and opioids bind to the same receptor, the μ-opioid receptor. For these patients, high TENS is therefore recommended.

It is important that physiotherapists have at least a basic understanding of how these medications work. Unfortunately, there are misconceptions about the use and mechanism of action of this group of medications. Statements regarding antidepressants such as "You may still have pain with these medications, but you just don't care as much" or "You gain a bit more distance from the pain" are not helpful and should be avoided. Patients are, of course, always informed that these are psychotropic drugs and that their use does not mean that the patient "just has a psychological problem." However, we all know that some things, even when explained, are not always understood. Here, an informed therapist can contribute to patient education and thus improve compliance and therapy outcomes.

1.14.2 General Principles of Treatment

In general, it must be stated that neuropathic pain is difficult to treat. The same pain can arise in different patients through different mechanisms, and the same mechanism can cause different types of pain. Likewise, a particular pain in a patient may have several different causes, which may even influence each other.

We have a wide range of treatment options at our disposal, which should not go untried. It is important for the therapist to be willing to apply these methods systematically, without giving the patient the impression that one does not know what one is doing and that the patient is a "guinea pig." If the therapist understands which mechanisms may be involved in pain generation, it will be easier to explain this to the patient and motivate them to participate.

Each application should, depending on the patient's response, be used at least 4 to 6 times in order to assess its effect. Even the slightest improvements are important and must be taken into account. If a 30 to 50% improvement is considered a realistic goal in drug treatment, we should certainly not expect more (Otto et al. 2019). If, thanks to our interventions, the patient can get by with a little less medication, that is already a success.

An initially successful therapy application may lose its effect over the course of treatment (see Chap. 3). Here, too, only systematic review can help to increase the effectiveness of treatment, for example by changing electrode placement or varying the stimulation frequency.

Finally, it should be noted that neuropathic pain can also occur in combination with nociceptive pain. It is now assumed that, for example, post-nucleotomy syndrome (failed back syndrome), spinal stenosis, and complex regional pain syndrome (CRPS1) arise from such combinations (Baron et al. 2016). The term "mixed pain syndrome" or "mixed pain concept" is used for these combinations.

1.15 Inhibitory Mechanisms and Consequences for Electrotherapy

The most effective pain therapy is undoubtedly the one in which all three inhibitory systems are activated (Fig. 1.4):

- Segmental inhibition (long term depression) by stimulation of Aδ-fibers with relatively long pulses and low frequencies (2–4 Hz). The Aδ-fibers are stimulated with pulses between 15 and 100 μs, the C-fibers with phase durations of about 150 μs and longer. Stimulation of the C-fibers should be avoided here.

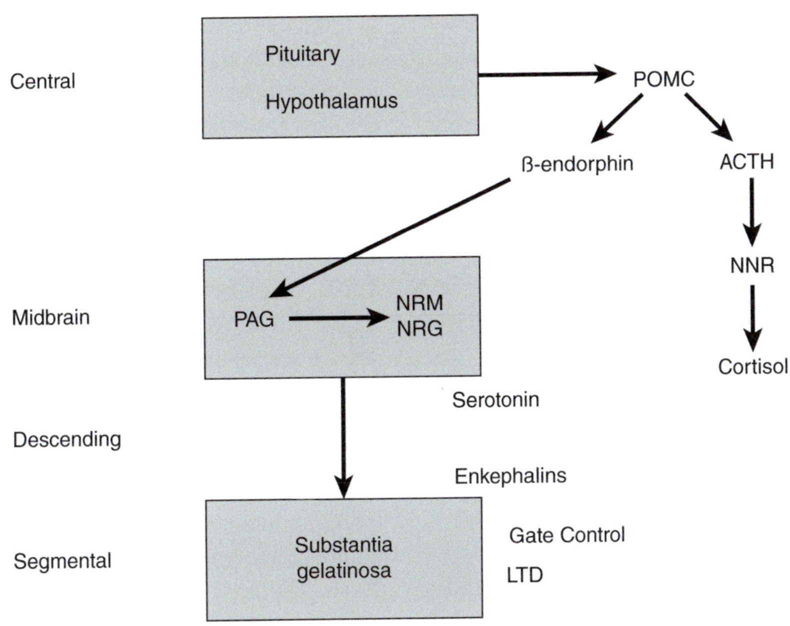

Fig. 1.4 Schematic representation of pain inhibition mechanisms. POMC: pro-opiomelanocortin; ACTH: adrenocorticotropic hormone; NNR: adrenal cortex; PAG: periaqueductal gray; NRM: nucleus raphe magnus; NRG: nucleus raphe gigantocellularis; LTD: long term depression

- Descending segmental inhibition via the PAG with the same stimulation parameters.
- Central (asegmental) inhibition via stimulation of the Aδ-fibers with the same parameters requires at least 20 min of stimulation in healthy subjects before β-endorphin production begins (Salar et al. 1981). In patients, pain relief may occur after just a few minutes.
- The induction of muscle contractions during treatment is a prerequisite for the effect of low frequency TENS. This additionally stimulates the intramuscular Aδ-fibers. Stimulation of these fibers appears to be responsible for the rather unpleasant heavy sensation that is also known from acupuncture and EAP, the De-Qi sensation (Chiang 1974).

The TENS method of choice would therefore be low frequency TENS (= APL-TENS).

If, for reasons such as those described under "Alarm Phase" (Sect. 1.16), these inhibitory systems cannot be activated, it is possible to influence pain via the gate control mechanism. Here, higher frequencies are required (around 100 Hz) and shorter pulses, up to 75 μs, so that only the Aβ-fibers are stimulated. Muscle contractions should be avoided. In this case, so-called conventional TENS = high TENS = high frequency low intensity TENS is used.

A better effect through electronic tricks, in which low and high frequencies alternate in imaginative ways or are delivered via two separate channels, has not been proven to date, with one exception. More on this in Chap. 3.

1.16 Ergotropic and Trophotropic Tuning: The Stress Reaction and Its Influence on Therapy Choice

The choice of which pain inhibition system to activate depends on how the activity of the nervous system is oriented. If the autonomic nervous system, and thus the patient, is in the so-called alarm or orientation phase, the sympathetic nervous system is activated, and *ergotropic* functions predominate. These functions are geared toward fight and flight ("fight or flight"). Due to the activity of the ascending reticular activating system (ARAS), consciousness is heightened so that all information can be absorbed. There is no inhibition of afferents, because every bit of information could be important for the individual's survival.

The ARAS consists of a system of nerve fibers originating in the reticular formation and, via connections to the thalamus and cortex, exerts a relatively nonspecific activating influence on large parts of the neocortex and mediates effects on the autonomic nervous system and the musculoskeletal system. The ARAS is therefore also referred to as a nonspecific sensory subsystem.

Excitation of the ARAS causes a general activation of the organism, a so-called arousal. It thus appears to be responsible for the transition from a state of relaxed wakefulness to one of general alertness. Morphologically, the ARAS, like the entire reticular formation, is difficult to define. Although biochemically and morphologically defined areas can be differentiated, no specific functions of the nuclei can be established, only an association with certain systems (e.g., motor function).

1.17 Course of the Stress Reaction

The course of the stress reaction is as follows: If the amygdala has classified a situation as threatening, the entire organism is put on alert. In the autonomic nervous system, activation of the sympathetic system (ergotropic orientation) predominates (for a very detailed and highly recommended account, see Sapolsky 2004). Epinephrine (adrenaline), norepinephrine (noradrenaline), and dopamine (all three together are so-called catecholamines) are released immediately, and very shortly thereafter, corticotropin-releasing hormone (CRH; formerly CR factor = CRF) from the hypothalamus, which prompts the pituitary gland to release adrenocorticotropic hormone (ACTH, also called corticotropin). ACTH is produced, along with several other hormones (LPH: lipotropic hormone, MSH: melanocyte-stimulating hormone), as well as β-endorphin and methionine-enkephalin, by proteolysis from a common precursor protein, proopiomelanocortin (fully: pro-opio-melano-cortico-tropin = POMC). ACTH stimulates the adrenal cortex to produce glucocorticoids, such as cortisol; see also Fig. 1.4.

Glucocorticoids influence metabolism and the immune system. Cortisol increases the blood levels of metabolizable molecules, i.e., glucose, amino acids, fatty acids, and glycerol, to provide energy sources. The organism needs energy to flee (or to fight, depending on personal disposition).

The effects of adrenaline and glucagon are enhanced and prolonged, leading to increased gluconeogenesis and glycogen breakdown in the liver, proteolysis and lipolysis in the periphery. Cortisol and synthetic glucocorticoids (e.g., prednisone, dexamethasone, triamcinolone) suppress the immune response and inflammatory processes. This occurs by reducing the production of pro-inflammatory and maintenance cytokines, decreasing cell migration, and especially by inhibiting the synthesis of eicosanoids (inflammatory mediators such as prostaglandins and leukotrienes). Cortisol also acts on connective tissue, inhibiting collagen synthesis and wound healing and reducing calcium absorption.

All this primarily leads to activation of central pain inhibition and, among other things, to the following reactions:

- increased alertness, increased processing speed of the brain with simultaneous fixation on the pain-inducing situation
- heightened perception (pupils dilate—mydriasis due to contraction of the dilator pupillae muscle—vision and hearing are enhanced)
- increased muscle tension, increased reaction speed
- increased heart rate, increased contractile force, elevated blood pressure
- shallower and faster breathing, relaxation of the tracheal and bronchial musculature
- vasoconstriction of skin and mucosal vessels (one becomes pale)
- reduced saliva production (dry mouth)
- reduced activity in the gastrointestinal tract, sphincter contraction
- energy supply in muscles and nerve cells: increased glycogenolysis and gluconeogenesis in the liver, along with decreased insulin production
- increased lipolysis in fat cells

The increased activity in the cortex has, among other things, the following effects:

- It forms the basis for an increase in arousal.
- It enhances the uptake and transmission of sensory and motor signals to the cortex; for this purpose, various inhibitory mechanisms are suppressed.

These sensible reactions normally subside relatively quickly after the end of the threatening situation. In the case of prolonged stress, as is often the case in so-called modern humans, increased cortisol production leads, via negative feedback, to a decrease in ACTH production and thus to a decrease in β-endorphin production: the central pain inhibition mechanisms do not function or function inadequately. Metabolism remains catabolic, cardiovascular activity remains elevated, digestive activity decreases. No tissue building (wound healing!) takes place. At maximum depletion of all reserves, a wide variety of physical and psychological changes can occur (Sapolsky 2004) (Fig. 1.5).

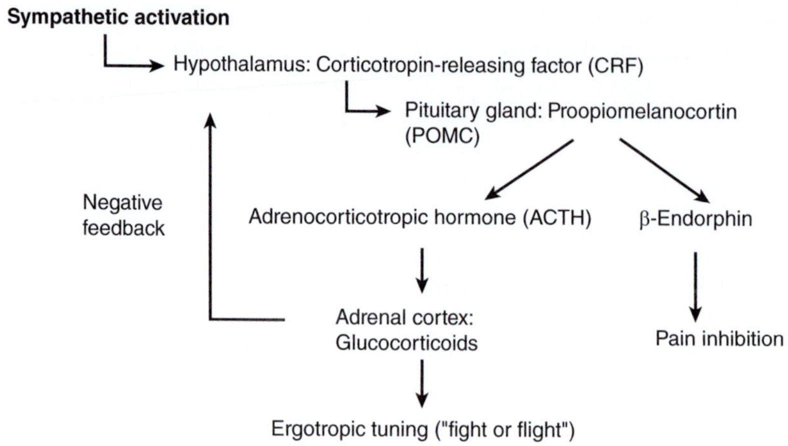

Fig. 1.5 Course of a normal stress reaction

1.18 Consequences for Therapy

In such a fixed ergotropic situation, the almost painful stimulation of Aδ and C fibers with centrally acting TENS modalities is pointless and probably even counterproductive. It should be noted that these TENS modalities exhibit a certain aggressiveness because it is precisely these Aδ and C fibers that are being stimulated. The patient (their CNS) cannot distinguish whether these stimuli are being applied for good or ill. In the ARAS, stimulus specificity is not maintained, so it is not possible to differentiate between individual sensory modalities. Any type of stimulus conducted centrally via Aδ and C fibers can be interpreted as threatening to the organism and thus maintain or even intensify the ergotropic state. However, in these patients, High TENS can certainly be used, and it appears sensible to gradually increase the dosage until the desired intensity—"clearly perceptible, but just not painful"—is reached.

Only when the CNS, in the so-called adaptation or defense phase, functions selectively again and operates trophotropically (parasympathetic activity, oriented toward anabolic functions, i.e., recovery, rest, regeneration = *wound healing*, "rest and digest"), is non-relevant information once again inhibited. The supraspinal pain modulation system can be activated via Aδ and C fibers, leading to the production of endomorphins and β-endorphins, and the transmission of nociceptive afferents is suppressed.

A thorough medical history, which should also include aspects such as family situation, workplace environment, leisure activities, etc., provides initial indications of possible psychosocial overload. This concerns issues such as unemployment, divorce, death in the family, building a house, and much more, as well as how the patient copes with these situations.

These insights should definitely be taken into account when choosing therapy. In addition, this could be a possible reason why certain forms of therapy sometimes work and sometimes do not.

For very detailed information on the impact of chronic stress on the human organism, the book *Why Zebras Don't Get Ulcers* by Robert Sapolsky (Professor of Biology and Neurology at Harvard University, USA) is recommended. Please do not be misled by the unusual title! The man is a solid scientist and a good storyteller.

References

Alles SRA, Smith PA (2018) Etiology and pharmacology of neuropathic pain. Pharmacol Rev 70:315–347

Anand P, Bley K (2011) Topical capsaicin for pain management: therapeutic potential and mechanisms of action of the new high-concentration capsaicin 8% patch. Br J Anaesth 107(4):490–502

Backonja M, Wallace MS, Blonsky ER, Cutler BJ, Malan P Jr, Rauck R, Tobias J (2008) NGX-4010 C116 Study Group. NGX-4010, a high-concentration capsaicin patch, for the treatment of postherpetic neuralgia: a randomised, double-blind study. Lancet Neurol 7(12):1106–1112

Baron R, Binder A, Attal N, Casale R, Dickenson AH, Treede RD (2016) Neuropathic low back pain in clinical practice. Eur J Pain 20(6):861–873

Bing Z, Villanueva L, Le Bars D (1990) Acupuncture and diffuse noxious inhibitory controls: naloxone-reversible depression of activities of trigeminal convergent neurons. Neuroscience 37(3):809–818

Bing Z, Cesselin F, Bourgoin S, Clot AM, Hamon M, Le Bars D (1991) Acupuncture-like stimulation induces a heterosegmental release of Met-enkephalin-like material in the rat spinal cord. Pain 47(1):71–77

Butler DS, Moseley GL (2016) Schmerzen Verstehen, 3. Aufl. Springer, Berlin/Heidelberg, ISBN-13: 978-3662486573

Chandran P, Sluka KA (2003) Development of opioid tolerance with repeated transcutaneous electrical nerve stimulation administration. Pain 102(1–2):195–201

Chiang C (1974) A physical theory of acupuncture anesthesia. Physiol Chem Phys 6(1):85e86

Clifford DB, Simpson DM, Brown S, Moyle G, Brew BJ, Conway B, Tobias JK, Vanhove GFA (2012) Randomized, double-blind, controlled study of NGX-4010, a capsaicin 8% dermal patch, for the treatment of painful HIV-associated distal sensory polyneuropathy. J Acquir Immune Defic Syndr 59(2):126–133

Colloca L, Ludman T, Bouhassira D, Baron R, Dickenson AH, Yarnitsky D, Freeman R, Truini A, Attal N, Finnerup NB, Eccleston C, Kalso E, Bennett DL, Dworkin RH, Raja SN (2017) Neuropathic pain. Nat Rev Dis Primers 3:17002

Devor M (2009) Ectopic discharge in Aβ afferents as a source of neuropathic pain. Exp Brain Res 196(1):115–128

Devor M, Wall PD (1978) Reorganisation of spinal cord sensory map after peripheral nerve injury. Nature 276(5683):75–76

Dickenson AH (2002) Gate control theory of pain stands the test of time. Br J Anaesth 88(6):755–757

García-Poblete E, Fernández-García H, Moro-Rodríguez E, Catalá-Rodríguez M, Rico-Morales ML, García-Gómez-de-las-Heras S, Palomar-Gallego MA (2003) Sympathetic sprouting in Dorsal Root Ganglia (DRG): a recent histological finding? Histol Histopathol 18:575–586

Gierthmühlen J, Baron R (2016) Neuropathic pain. Semin Neurol 36(5):462–468

Gilron I, Baron R, Jensen T (2015) Neuropathic pain: principles of diagnosis and treatment. Mayo Clin Proc 90(4):532–545

Han HC, Lee DH, Chung JM (2000) Characteristics of ectopic discharges in a rat neuropathic pain model. Pain 84(2–3):253–261

Han JS (2004) Acupuncture and endorphins. Neurosci Lett 361:258–261

Han JS, Chen XH, Sun SL, Xu XJ, Yuan Y, Yan SC, Hao JX, Terenius L (1991) Effect of low- and high-frequency TENS on met-enkephalin-arg-phe and dynorphin a immunoreactivity in human lumbar CSF. Pain 47(3):295–298

Handwerker HO (1998) Einführung in die Pathophysiologie des Schmerzes. Springer Verlag, Berlin/Heidelberg, ISBN-13: 978-3540627982

Handwerker HO, Iggo A, Ogawa H (1975) Dorsal horn neurones responding to cutaneous afferent input. J Physiol 244(1):1P–2P

Hebb ALO, Poulin JF, Roach SP, Zacharko RM, Drolet G (2005) Cholecystokinin and endogenous opioid peptides: interactive influence on pain, cognition, and emotion. Prog Neuro-Psychopharmacol Biol Psychiatry 29:1225–1238

Heinricher MM, Neubert MJ (2004) Neural basis for the hyperalgesic action of cholecystokinin in the rostral ventromedial medulla. J Neurophysiol 92:1982–1989

Hughes J, Kosterlitz HW (1983) Opioid peptides: introduction. Br Med Bull 39(1):1–3

Hughes J, Kosterlitz HW, Smith TW (1997) The distribution of methionone-enkephalin and leucine-enkephaline in the brain and peripheral tissues. Br J Pharmacol 120(4 Suppl):428–436; discussion 426-7

Irving G, Backonja M, Rauck R, Webster LR, Tobias JK, Vanhove GF (2012) NGX-4010, a capsaicin 8% dermal patch, administered alone or in combination with systemic neuropathic pain medications, reduces pain in patients with postherpetic neuralgia. Clin J Pain 28(2):101–107

Kosterlitz HW, Hughes J (1975) Some thoughts on the significance of enkephalin, the endogenous ligand. Life Sci 17(1):91–96

Le Bars D (2002) The whole body receptive field of dorsal horn multireceptive neurones. Brain Res Rev 40(1–3):29–44

Le Bars D, Willer JC (2002) Pain modulation triggered by high-intensity stimulation: implication for acupuncture analgesia. In: Sato A, Li P, Campbell J (Hrsg) Acupuncture – is there a physiological basis? International congress series, Bd 1238. Elsevier, Amsterdam, S 11–29

Le Bars D, Villanueva L, Bouhassira D (1992) Willer. Diffuse Noxious Inhibitory Controls (DNIC) in animals and in man. JC Patol Fiziol Eksp Ter 4:55–65

Léonard G, Goffaux P, Marchand S (2010) Deciphering the role of endogenous opioids in high-frequency TENS using low and high doses of naloxone. Pain 151(1):215–219

Leung L (2012) Neurophysiological basis of acupuncture-induced analgesia – an updated review. J Acupunct Meridian Stud 5(6):261–270

Li CH, Yamashiro D, Tseng LF, Loh HH (1977) Synthesis and analgesic activity of human beta-endorphin. J Med Chem 20(3):325–328

Liu XG, Morton CR, Azkue JJ, Zimmermann M, Sandkühler J (1998) Long-term depression of

C-fibre-evoked spinal field potentials by stimulation of primary afferent Aδ-fibres in the adult rat. EJN 10(10):3069–3075

Louw A, Diener I, Butler DS, Puentedura EJ (2011) The effect of neuroscience education on pain, disability, anxiety, and stress in chronic musculoskeletal pain. Arch Phys Med Rehabil 92:2041–2056

Louw A, Zimney K, O'Hotto C, Hilton S (2016) The clinical application of teaching people about pain. Physiother Theory Pract 5:385–395

McMahon S, Koltzenburg M, Tracey I, Turk DC (2013) Wall & Melzack's textbook of pain. W B Saunders Co Ltd, 6th Revised Edition, ISBN: 9780702040597

Melzack R, Casey KL (1968) Sensory, motivational, and central control determinants of pain. In: Kenshalo DR (Hrsg) The skin senses. Thomas, Springfield, S 423–443

Melzack R, Wall P (1965) Pain mechanisms: a new theory. Science 150:3699

Mendell LM (2014) Constructing and deconstructing the gate control theory of pain. Pain 155(2):210–216

Moayedi M, Davis KD (2013) Theories of pain: from specificity to gate control. J Neurophysiol 109:5–12

Moseley L (2002) Combined physiotherapy and education is efficacious for chronic low back pain. Aust J Physiother 48:297–302

Mosely L (2003) Unraveling the barriers to reconceptualization of the problem in chronic pain: the actual and perceived ability of patients and health professionals to understand the neurophysiology. J Pain 4:184–189

Nafe JP (1929) A quantitative theory of feeling. J Gen Psychol 2(2–3):199–211

Nilsson HJ, Schouenborg J (1999) Differential inhibitory effect on human nociceptive skin senses induced by local stimulation of thin cutaneous fibers. Pain 80:103–112

Nilsson HJ, Psouni E, Schouenborg J (2003) Long term depression of human nociceptive skin senses induced by thin fibre stimulation. Eur J Pain 7(3):225–233

van Nooten F, Treur M, Pantiri K, Stoker M, Charokopou M (2017) Capsaicin 8% patch versus oral neuropathic pain medications for the treatment of painful diabetic peripheral neuropathy: a systematic literature review and network meta-analysis. Clin Ther 39(4):787–803

North RY, Lazaro TT, Dougherty PM (2018) Ectopic spontaneous afferent activity and neuropathic pain. Neurosurgery 65(1):49–54

Ochs S (2004) A history of nerve functions: from animal spirits to molecular mechanisms. Cambridge University Press, Cambridge, ISBN 052124742X

Otto J, Forstenpointner J, Binder A, Baron R (2019) Pharmakologische Therapie chronischer neuropathischer Schmerzen. Internist 60:711–723

Price DD (2002) Central neural mechanisms that interrelate sensory and affective dimensions of pain. Mol Interv 6:392–403

Ramer MS, Thompson SW, McMahon SB (1999) Causes and consequences of sympathetic basket formation in dorsal root ganglia. Pain Suppl 6:S111–S120

Rey R (2005) A history of pain. Harvard University Press, Cambridge, MA, ISBN 0674399676

Reynolds J, Bilsky EJ, Meng ID (2011) Selective ablation of mu-opioid receptor expressing neurons in the rostral ventromedial medulla attenuates stress-induced mechanical hypersensitivity. Life Sci 89(9–10):313–319

Rufa A, Beissner K, Dolphin M (2019) The use of pain neuroscience education in older adults with chronic back and/or lower extremity pain. Physiother Theory Pract 35(7):603–613

Salar G, Job I, Mingrino S, Bosio A, Trabucchi M (1981) Effect of transcutaneous electrotherapy on CSF β-endorphin content in patients without pain problems. Pain 10:169–172

Sandkühler J, Chen JG, Cheng G, Randić M (1997) Low-frequency stimulation of afferent Adelta-fibers induces long-term depression at primary afferent synapses with substantia gelatinosa neurons in the rat. J Neurosci 17(16):6483–6491

Sapolsky R (2004) Why zebras don't get ulcers, 3. Aufl. Holt paperbacks, Ney York, ISBN-10: 0805073698

Sawynok J (2001) Antidepressants as analgetics: an overview of central and peripheral mechanisms of action. J Psychiatry Neurosci 26:21–29

Schaible HG (2015) Pain control. Springer, Heidelberg, ISBN 978-3-662-46449-6

Schnizer W, Kröling P, Claussen A, Magyarosy I (2003) Die Abschwächung (Desensibilisierung) des Galvanischen Erythems durch wiederholte Gleichstromreizung. Phys Rehab Kurort Med 13(3):145–148

Schonack W (1913) (Übersetzer) Die Rezepte des Scribonius Largus (Scribonii Largi Compositiones). Gustav Fischer, Jena

Simone DA, Nolano M, Johnson T, Wendelschafer-Crabb G, Kennedy WR (1998) Intradermal injection of capsaicin in humans produces degeneration and subsequent reinnervation of epidermal nerve fibers: correlation with sensory function. J Neurosci 18(21):8947–8959

Sommer C, Leinders M, Üçeyler N (2018) Inflammation in the pathophysiology of neuropathic pain. Pain 159(3):595–602

St John Smith E (2018) Advances in understanding nociception and neuropathic pain. J Neurol 265(2):231–238

Todd AJ (2010) Neuronal circuitry for pain processing in the dorsal horn. Nat Rev Neurosci 1(12):823–836

Villanueva L, Le Bars D (1995) The activation of bulbo-spinal controls by peripheral nociceptive inputs: diffuse noxious inhibitory controls. Biol Res 28(1):113–125

Wagman IH, Price DD (1969) Responses of dorsal horn cells of M. mulatta to cutaneous and sural nerve A and C fiber stimuli. J Neurophysiol 32(6):803–817

Watson JC, Sandroni P (2016) Central neuropathic pain syndromes. Mayo Clin Proc 91(3):372–385

Weber M, Birklein F, Neundörfer B, Schmelz M (2001) Facilitated neurogenic inflammation in complex regional pain syndrome. Pain 91(3):251–257

Wiesenfeld-Hallin Z, de Araúja LG, Alster P, Xu XJ, Hökfelt T (1999) Cholecystokinin/opioid interactions. Brain Res 848(1–2):78–89

Wiesenfeld-Hallin Z, Xu XJ, Hökfelt T (2002) The role of spinal cholecystokinin in chronic pain states. Pharmacol Toxicol 91:398–403

Winter J, Bevan S, Campbell EA (1995) Capsaicin and pain mechanisms. Br J Anaesth 75(2):157–168

Woolf CJ, Shortland P, Coggeshall RE (1992) Peripheral nerve injury triggers central sprouting of myelinated afferents. Nature 355:75–78

2 Low-Frequency Electrotherapy

Nerves conduct action potentials and thereby transmit information. The following explains how an action potential is generated and how it is propagated. For those who want to know all the details, please consult one of the following physiology textbooks: Pape et al. (2019), Schmidt et al. (2011), or Urry et al. (2016).

2.1 Resting Membrane Potential

There is a difference in the type of electrically charged particles (ions) and their concentrations between the intracellular and extracellular fluids. The K^+ ion concentration is about 40 times higher inside the cell than outside. For Na^+, the situation is different: the intracellular concentration of Na^+ ions is about 10 times lower than extracellularly. Thus, there is a concentration gradient for both ions: for K^+ from inside to outside, and for Na^+ from outside to inside.

The anions are also unevenly distributed: the extracellular Cl concentration is about 50 times higher than intracellularly, and so-called protein anions are found only inside the cell because they cannot cross the membrane.

Due to these concentration differences, K^+ ions continuously diffuse out of the cell and Na^+ ions into the cell. This movement of particles occurs via so-called sodium and potassium channels. To maintain the concentration gradients, active pump mechanisms, known as Na-K pumps or Na^+/K^+ ATPase, constantly transport the incoming Na^+ ions out of the cell and K^+ ions into the cell.

These pump mechanisms consume adenosine triphosphate (ATP) during their operation. With each cycle, three Na ions are pumped out and two K ions are pumped in—a process that repeats about 30 times per second. For example, a small nerve cell typically has 1 million Na-K pumps, which pump 200 million ions in and out per second—a process that consumes about 70% of the cell's energy expenditure.

Due to selective membrane permeability and the pump mechanisms, the distribution of charged particles across the membrane is not uniform. The intracellular fluid contains high concentrations of K^+ ions and anions and low concentrations of Na^+ and Cl^-. The extracellular environment, on the other hand, contains low concentrations of K^+ and high concentrations of Na^+ and Cl^-. The permeability of the cell membrane and the concentration gradient for K^+ ions is particularly pronounced. Therefore, many of these K^+ ions leave the cell. However, each positively charged K^+ ion is paired with a negatively charged protein anion, which cannot leave the cell. Thus, positive and negative ions are separated at the membrane, resulting in an excess of negative charge on the inside of the membrane compared to an excess of positive charge on the outside.

P. van Kerkhof, *Evidence-Based Electrotherapy*, https://doi.org/10.1007/978-3-662-73019-5_2

Such a charge difference (charge gradient) is referred to as an electrical voltage difference or potential difference. Since this voltage difference appears at the cell membrane, it is called the membrane potential or resting potential.

- K^+ ions: intracellular 100,000, extracellular 2000
- Na^+ ions: intracellular 10,000, extracellular 108,000
- Cl^- ions: intracellular 2200, extracellular 110,000
- Proteins (−): intracellular 107,800, extracellular 0

The cause of the resting potential is therefore the unequal distribution of ion types inside and outside the cell. The resting potential is about −90 mV for muscle tissue and about −75 mV for nerve tissue.

2.2 Action Potential

The Na and K channels in the membrane allow diffusion of these ions into and out of the cell. Normally, these channels are closed, and diffusion is not very pronounced. However, the channels can be opened under certain conditions. There are *voltage-gated* channels (e.g., in nerve cells), which open at a specific membrane voltage (threshold or threshold potential). There are also *chemically or ligand-gated* channels, which open after the action of a specific chemical substance (= ligand), such as a neurotransmitter binding to its receptor (e.g., channels at a synapse) (Figs. 2.1 and 2.2).

A stimulus, such as an externally applied negative electric shock, leads to a (relative) increase in positive charge inside the cell (the outside becomes less positive). This causes a

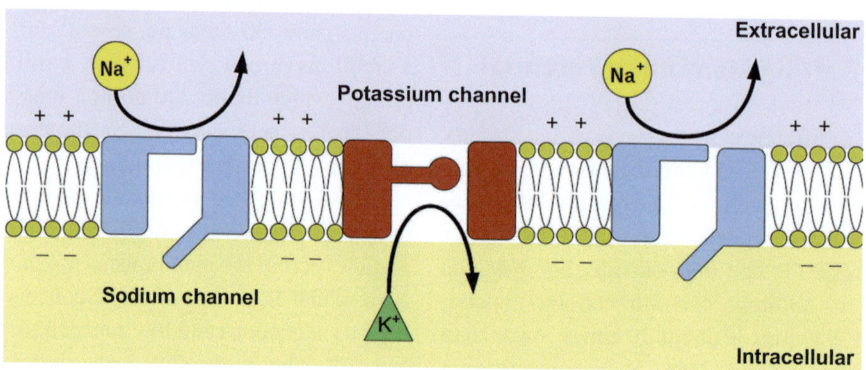

Fig. 2.1 Action potential, resting phase. The Na channels are activated but closed

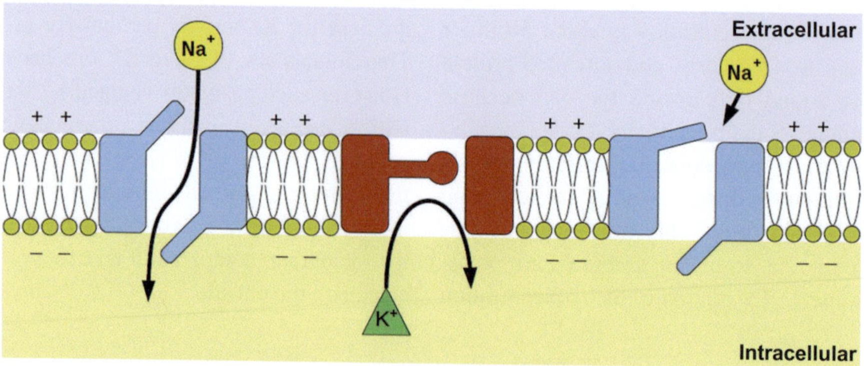

Fig. 2.2 Action potential, before the threshold is reached. Some Na channels open

reduction in the resting potential; the electrical voltage across the membrane decreases. This is referred to as depolarization of the membrane. When a certain threshold is reached, this depolarization acts as a signal on the voltage-gated Na channels.

These now open abruptly, and Na ions can now enter the cell following their concentration gradient. Near the membrane, these Na ions bind to the protein anions located there. This further depolarizes the membrane, and the membrane potential continues to decrease. At a certain point, the membrane potential reaches 0 mV, as the anions on the inner side of the membrane are neutralized by the incoming positively charged Na ions.

However, Na ions continue to flow into the cell, so that the inside of the cell becomes up to 30 mV positive relative to the outside. The membrane's outer surface becomes negative. Thus, a reversal of charge has occurred: the membrane at this site has become *reversed in polarity* (Fig. 2.3).

Now the Na channels close again and the K channels open. As a result, K ions (also following their concentration gradient) flow out of the cell. This causes the positive charge on the inner side of the membrane to decrease again until it eventually becomes negative. The outside becomes correspondingly positive, and the normal state is restored. The membrane has been *repolarized* (Fig. 2.4).

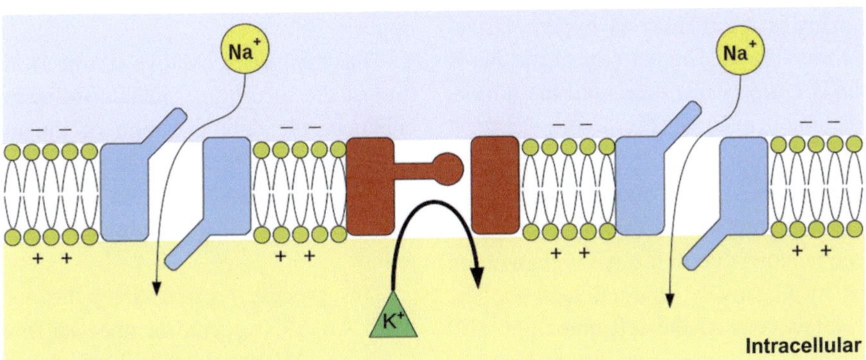

Fig. 2.3 Action potential, depolarization phase. The threshold has been exceeded, all Na channels (locally) open

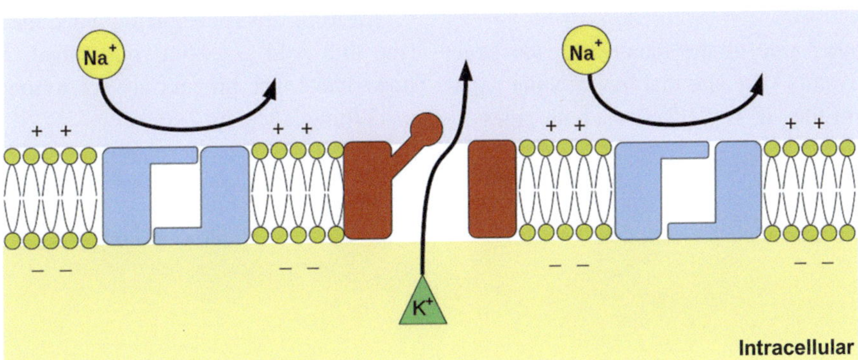

Fig. 2.4 Action potential, repolarization phase. The Na channels are closed and deactivated. The membrane is absolute refractory

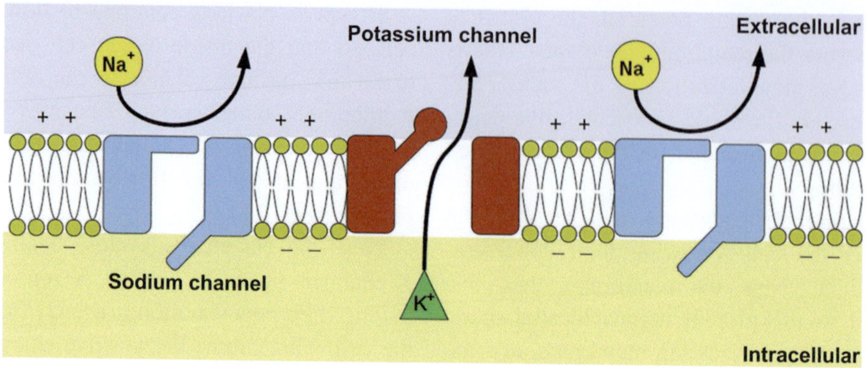

Fig. 2.5 Action potential, end of the repolarization phase. The Na channels are closed but active. The membrane is relative refractory

Since the K outflow initially overshoots, the voltage difference becomes for a short time (0.5–1 ms) somewhat greater than the resting potential. This is referred to as hyperpolarization of the membrane. The activity of the Na-K pump quickly corrects this state until the normal resting potential is restored (Fig. 2.5).

Propagation of an Action Potential (AP)
The site on the inner side of the membrane that has become positive due to the AP is flanked on both sides by negatively charged regions. The negative protein ions of the left and right, still negatively charged regions now attract Na ions, which migrate to these negatively charged sites. *Thus, an electric current flows*. As a result, these sites become more positive (neutralized), causing the membrane to depolarize anew.

On the outer side of the membrane, the exact opposite occurs. The site that has become negative due to the AP is flanked on both sides by positive K ions. Positive charges flow to the negatively charged membrane site, so an electric current also flows on the outside, but in the opposite direction.

The removal of positive charge from the section of the membrane outside following the AP enhances the depolarization of the membrane. As soon as the threshold is reached, an action potential is generated at this site: the Na channels open, and the membrane is reversed in polarity.

This process repeats along the entire nerve fiber. An AP triggered at one site thus triggers a second AP in its immediate vicinity, which in turn triggers a third, and so on. In this way, action potentials (propagated impulses) travel from the nerve cell body along the nerve fiber (neurite) to the terminal boutons.

An AP is always triggered when the threshold (the threshold potential) is reached, no matter how. The entire process always follows the all-or-nothing law (Fig. 2.6).

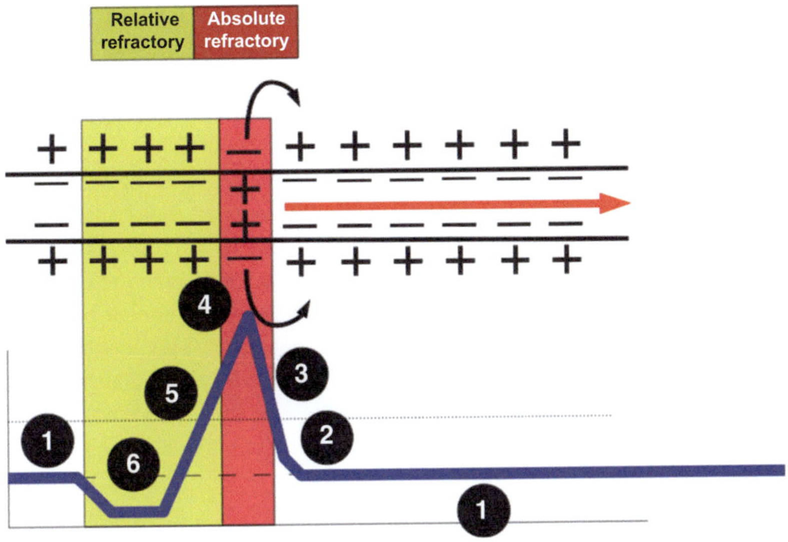

Fig. 2.6 Propagation of an action potential. 1 = resting potential, 2 = threshold potential, 3 = depolarization phase, 4 = overshoot, 5 = repolarization phase, 6 = undershoot. The AP travels to the right. Dotted line = 0 mV

2.3 Effect of the Action Potential at the Fiber End

Where neurites connect with their target cells, at the so-called presynaptic terminal or terminal bouton, the nerve cells are specially structured. This is referred to as an end bulb. In this end bulb are small synaptic vesicles that contain a transmitter substance (neurotransmitter). The vesicles can release the neurotransmitter to the outside by moving toward the membrane and fusing with it. The impulse necessary for this is triggered by an AP.

As soon as the AP reaches the membrane at the synaptic end bulb, it causes the opening of voltage-gated calcium channels. Ca^{+} ions, which have a much higher extracellular concentration than intracellularly, flow into the cell and trigger the release of the vesicles.

Between the end bulb and the target cell (= synapse) is a gap of about 10–50 nm (n = nano = 1 billionth), the so-called synaptic cleft. On the nerve fiber side, it is formed by the presynaptic membrane, and on the target cell side by the postsynaptic (more precisely: subsynaptic) membrane.

2.4 Stimulation of the Target Cell

The AP in the neurite triggers the release of vesicles at the presynaptic membrane. The neurotransmitter (e.g., acetylcholine) is released into the synaptic cleft and reaches the post- or subsynaptic membrane of the target cell. This membrane carries specific receptors that fit the neurotransmitter like a lock and key. As soon as the transmitter molecules have bound to their receptor, this contact triggers a reaction in the target cell. In the case of the muscle fiber, Na channels open, causing the muscle fiber membrane to depolarize. This depolarization ultimately leads to muscle contraction.

The movement of the transmitter across the cleft to its receptor takes only fractions of a millisecond. The contact of the transmitter with its receptor can also last only a short time, otherwise the target cell would be continuously excited, and repolarization between two APs would no longer be possible. In the case of acetylcholine, the enzyme cholinesterase (= acetylcholinesterase), which is present in the synaptic cleft, ensures immediate dissociation of acetylcholine at the receptor into acetic acid (acidum aceticum) and choline. This renders it inactive and it is reabsorbed by the presynaptic membrane. In the end bulb, it is then reassembled into active acetylcholine.

A synaptic vesicle contains about 4000 molecules of acetylcholine. This amount is called a quantum. A single quantum can, via a corresponding number of receptors on the subsynaptic membrane over a membrane area of 1 μm^2, open over 2000 Na channels. After the influx of Ca ions, triggered by an incoming AP, many hundreds of vesicles are released simultaneously.

Transmission at the synapses can be influenced by chemical substances (poisons and drugs), e.g., botulinum toxin, curare, atropine.

Low-frequency electrotherapy covers the range from 0–1000 Hz. This is the range of so-called period-synchronous stimulation, so called because each impulse—or each period—triggers an action potential. Well, almost every impulse. Actually, no one knows for sure. When asked, several specialists had no answer to the question of what the maximum depolarization frequency of a human peripheral nerve might be. Assuming an absolute refractory phase of 1 ms and a relative refractory phase of 2 ms, one arrives at a maximum depolarization frequency of about 330 Hz by calculation. The old master Edel added the mid-frequency range to the two-part division of the grand old master Kowarschik, thus creating a three-part classification, with 1000 as the boundary probably chosen because it is a nice round number. This classification has been retained to this day in the German-speaking world.

A wide variety of applications are included under low-frequency therapy, not all of which will be discussed in detail in this book. The reasons for this are explained in the relevant chapters. Before we get to the applications, the reader will have to digest a bit of theory. There is really no way around it. Let's get started.

2.5 What is Electrotherapy?

Simply put, electrotherapy is the therapeutic application of electricity.

This includes the use of direct current and pulsed currents in various forms. Electrotherapy procedures in the low-frequency range (= LF range) are also referred to as stimulation current therapy procedures.

The application of electrical and electromagnetic forces triggers physical-chemical processes and/or initiates neurophysiological mechanisms in the body for therapeutic purposes.

All cells in the human body possess a membrane potential. This membrane potential can be influenced by the application of electric currents. Since this is an electrical stimulus, it can be considered an adequate stimulus in this case. This is especially true for structures specialized in the generation and conduction of excitations (action potentials), such as nerve cells, various receptors, and muscle cells.

The effects of low-frequency electrotherapy are demonstrably based on the following physiological phenomena:

- Stimulation of 80% of C fibers and 30% of Aδ fibers leads to erythema formation, desensitization and reversible destruction of these fibers, and consequently to pain inhibition.
- Stimulation of Aβ fibers leads to segmental and descending pain inhibition.
- Stimulation of Aδ fibers leads to segmental, descending, and central pain inhibition.
- Stimulation of C fibers leads to descending and central pain inhibition.

2.6 Direct Current

A direct current is a flow of charge carriers that does not change its **direction** or its **strength** during the period of flow. In a technical conductor such as a metal, this is a flow of electrons, whereas in humans, as in a solution in a vessel, it is a flow of ions. A metal is referred to as a "first-order conductor" or "type 1," "class 1," and humans, like a liquid, as a "type 2 conductor." The transport of charged particles (of any kind) is called an electric current.

Instead of direct current, the term galvanic current is often used, in honor of Luigi Galvani.

He lived from 1737 to 1798 and was an Italian anatomist and obstetrician. He is, not entirely justifiably, considered the founder of electrophysiology because of his frog leg experiment. While dissecting a dead frog lying on a metal surface, he observed that when he (or his assistant—there are several versions) touched the frog's leg with his scalpel, the leg twitched. Muscle activity was thus somehow related to electricity. He believed that animals generated electricity in their bodies and that a fluid in their nerves transported electricity to the muscles, causing movement. He also believed that electric eels could build up additional amounts of this fluid and use it to deliver electric shocks. Quite an idea. Mary Shelley then used these findings in 1817 as the basis for her story about a certain Victor Frankenstein. The true founder of electrophysiology should actually be considered Alessandro Count Volta, as he invented the voltaic pile, the precursor of the battery, in 1799–1800. Volta's battery made it possible for the first time ever to apply a constant electric current. Volta's battery was an absolutely crucial invention in the development of our technology-based civilization. Volta's pile consisted of zinc-copper plates connected in series, with felt discs soaked in saline or lye (the electrolyte) in between (Fig. 2.7).

The elegant construction was mounted on glass rods set into wood. Over the following years, Volta improved his battery by initially using tin, brass, or silver as electrode materials. The best results were obtained with the metal pairs silver-zinc and copper-zinc. Volta also discovered that the flow of energy could be reversed—in other words, that the pile could be recharged by supplying current. Thus, with his pile, he had invented not only the electric cell, but also the battery (several electric cells combined) and the accumulator (rechargeable battery). The great advantage of his invention was that anyone with a pair of silver or copper coins and some zinc could build their own battery. To honor Volta's contribution to science, it was decided in 1881 to name the unit of electric potential the "volt."

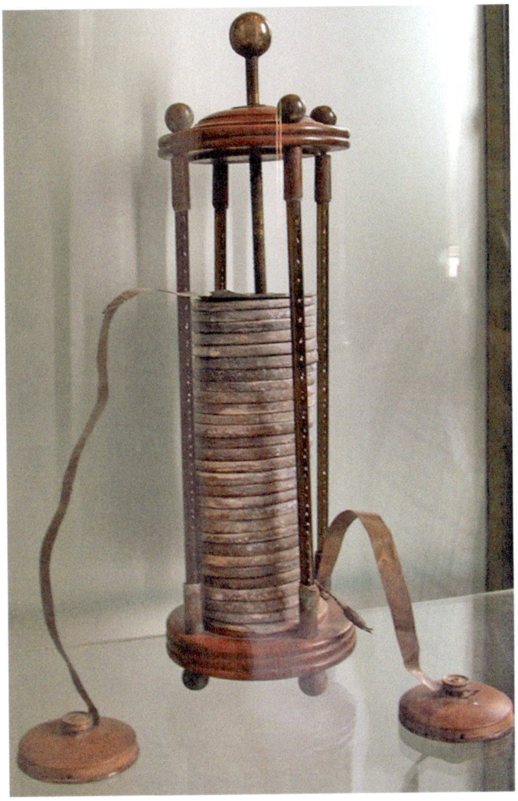

Fig. 2.7 Volta's pile

What actually happens?

During a course, the author was told by a participant that a hip endoprosthesis is a contraindication for a two-cell bath application on both legs. Let's take a closer look. In humans, electrons do not flow from the cathode to the anode or vice versa: any free electron would immediately be captured by an ion. Directly under and near the respective electrodes, ion displacement occurs due to electrical forces. The anions migrate a few centimeters toward the anode and give up their electron(s) there. The cations migrate toward the cathode and receive an electron (or more, depending on the charge). The anode also repels positive ions, and the cathode does the same with negative ions (Fig. 2.8). Thus, there is always an ion current flowing in two directions. The concept of a descending or ascending current is therefore physically nonsensical.

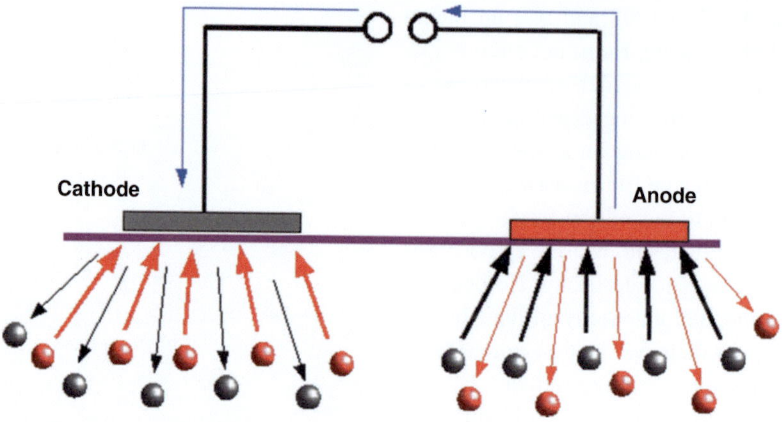

Fig. 2.8 This is how ions flow in the human body. Black: anions, red: cations

Why is it not recommended to apply direct current directly over or very close to metal? Well, the electric field affects all charge carriers within its range. The electrons in the implanted metal are attracted by the anode and repelled by the cathode. This causes a displacement of charge in the metal near the electrodes by induction, which is the spatial displacement of electric charge due to the influence of an electric field. This charge displacement concentrated at the implant can lead to undesirable electrochemical processes in the surrounding tissue. In electrotherapy, it is not the current itself that causes problems, but the chemical reactions induced by the current. (Incidentally: thermal damage due to non-therapeutic applications is not discussed here.) The chemical reactions lead to a change in pH, which is potentially damaging to tissue. More on this later. The electric field is actually extremely weak. Nevertheless, all authors of electrotherapy textbooks agree that metal located in the direct treatment field or in the *vicinity* of two electrodes is a contraindication for direct current applications. However, how "vicinity" should be defined has unfortunately never been precisely determined. 5 cm? 10 cm? From iontophoresis, we know that ions are transported only about 2 cm through tissue after 40 min of application (Panus et al. 1999). This suggests that the influence of such a weak electric field is limited to a few centimeters from the electrodes. The situation mentioned above (cell bath–hip endoprosthesis contraindication) is therefore completely harmless. Unfortunately, there are no measurements regarding where and when actual damage occurs.

Here, common sense is required.

If metal is present in the treatment area during a local application of direct current or a pulsed current with a direct current component (= imbalanced pulsed current), this is definitely a contraindication for such an application. "Local" refers to an application, for example, on a knee, with the electrodes placed medially and laterally to the knee. If, for example, there is a screw in the tibial tuberosity after a tuberosity transfer, direct current application (or treatment with a current form with a direct current component) is absolutely contraindicated.

If the patient has no metal in the knee but a hip endoprosthesis, this is *not* a contraindication for treatment at the knee. If a patient is treated locally on the forefoot for forefoot problems and has a screw in the lateral malleolus (on the same leg, of course), this is *not* a contraindication for foot treatment. If, in this patient, one electrode is on the forefoot and the other on the calf, things get interesting: who can say with certainty what happens 15–20 cm from the electrodes? Fortunately, there are enough other therapeutic options, so let's err on the side of caution and choose something else.

2.7 Physical Principles

To better understand the processes involved, the following section provides a detailed discussion of various physical principles.

2.7.1 Electrolysis

Substances can be broken down under the influence of electricity. This process is called electrolysis, and it is of particular interest to us because of its potentially harmful effects. In aqueous solutions of salts, acids, and bases, electrolytic dissociation into ions occurs. This means that a salt, such as NaCl, does not exist as NaCl in solution, but rather as Na^+ ion and Cl^- ion. This applies to solutions in a vessel as well as to solutions in the human body. When a direct current of sufficient strength is applied to such a solution (and in the body), ion migration occurs (which is actually a tautology, since "ion" in ancient Greek means "going, wandering"). The positively charged Na ions will migrate toward the cathode (negative pole) under the influence of this direct current, which is why they are called cations. The negatively charged Cl ions migrate toward the anode (positive pole) and are therefore called anions.

By the way: This also comes from Greek: kata = down, hodos = way, so the way down; ana = up, so the way up.

Electrically speaking, humans are second-order conductors. This means that current in the human body is not carried by electrons, but by ions. In other words: electrical currents in the human body are always ionic currents. In technical systems, charges are, by definition, transported from the positive pole (anode) to the negative pole (cathode) when using direct current, from plus to minus. However, the cathode has an excess of electrons, the anode a deficit, so in a first-order conductor, electrons actually flow from the cathode to the anode. This contradiction exists because the actual direction of electron movement was not known in the past—for us, this is unimportant, but it can be a bit confusing.

Now to electrolysis: Electrolysis is thus the breaking down of a substance under the influence of electric current. When current is passed through pure water using electrodes, oxygen and hydrogen are produced, and pH changes occur. Exactly the same reactions take place when current is applied to humans, and the pH changes are potentially dangerous because they can cause local tissue damage.

These reactions occur in the sponge used and partly in the tissue under the electrodes. Therefore, the following section discusses these reactions in considerable detail. The reactions that take place in tissue during direct current application are extremely complex, especially in situations where the tissue pH is already lower due to inflammation-like processes. It is therefore likely that, in addition to the reactions described, many other reactions also occur.

2.7.2 Electrolysis of Water

Pure water does not consist solely of H_2O. One out of every 10,000,000 water molecules is dissociated (broken down) according to the equation $2\ H_2O = H_3O^+ + OH^-$

For this reason, water is a second-order conductor (electrolytic conductor). When an electric current is applied to a vessel of water via two electrodes, the H_3O^+ ions migrate to the cathode and the OH^- ions to the anode. The reactions described below occur at the electrodes. Electrolysis is described as it occurs in separate chambers, because this corresponds to the situation in electrotherapy, where two separate electrodes are used.

2.7.2.1 Cathode

The cathode is (of course, only when a voltage is applied) negatively charged due to its excess of electrons. Water molecules at the cathode take up electrons, producing hydrogen and hydroxide ions (OH^-). The H_3O^+ ions (= hydronium ions; "naked" protons practically do not occur) that have migrated to the cathode take up an electron at the cathode and are reduced to H atoms.

These H atoms immediately combine to form H_2 molecules (hydrogen), which rise as gas bubbles at the cathode. The hydroxide ions remain, so the solution becomes increasingly alkaline (basic), and the pH value rises.

Equations:

$$4H_3O^+ + 4e- \rightarrow 2H_2 + 4H_2O$$

and

$$4H_2O + 4e- \rightarrow 2H_2 + 4OH^-$$

2.7.2.2 Anode

There is an electron deficit at the anode. Water molecules give up electrons, producing oxygen and hydronium ions. The OH^- ions (hydroxide ions) that have migrated to the anode give up their electron and are oxidized to OH. Four such OH compounds immediately form water molecules and oxygen atoms. These oxygen atoms combine to form O_2 molecules, which rise as gas bubbles at the anode. The H_3O^+ remains, so the solution becomes increasingly acidic, and the pH value decreases.

Equations:

$$6H_2O \rightarrow O_2 + 4H_3O^+ + 4e^-$$

and

$$4OH^- \rightarrow O_2 + 2H_2O + 4e^-$$

If these reactions occur in a vessel with separate chambers, the OH^- ions remain in solution at the cathode and the H_3O^+ ions at the anode. Over time, they accumulate and cause a change in pH. At the cathode, the pH increases, especially as the H_3O^+ ions disappear from the solution: the solution thus becomes increasingly alkaline. At the anode, the pH decreases, analogous to the reaction at the cathode: for this reason, the solution here becomes increasingly acidic. The equations show that twice as many bubbles are produced at the cathode as at the anode. This fact can be used if you do not know which electrode is the cathode. Hang both electrodes in a glass of water, set direct current, turn up the current. Where there are the most bubbles, that's the cathode.

In a saline solution, you find H_2O, H_3O^+ and OH^-, Na^+ and Cl^-. If you apply current to this mixture, the cathode reaction mentioned above proceeds exactly the same way. Since hydrogen is more noble than sodium, it "readily" accepts an electron. In other words: H_3O^+ is more easily reduced than Na^+. So no sodium is produced, fortunately.

At the anode, however, in addition to oxygen, some chlorine gas can be produced. If a solution contains several types of anions that can be oxidized, those that are closest to the zero point of the redox series, i.e., have a weaker positive standard potential, are oxidized first. The standard potential of O is +1.23, that of Cl is +1.36. Since these potentials are very close together, some chlorine gas can be produced at the anode in addition to oxygen. This chlorine gas reacts with water, producing additional H_3O^+.

2.7.2.3 Device switched off, patient still feels current

Shortly after switching off the current during electrolysis, an ammeter can detect a current spike in the opposite direction. In this brief phase, the reverse process of electrolysis occurs, namely the formation of a galvanic cell. Here, current is not consumed, but is briefly generated. Patients perceive this phenomenon as tingling after the current has been switched off, for example after iontophoresis. And more than one colleague has feared that the device was defective …

2.7.3 Chemical Burns

Let us now assume that electrolysis does not take place in a container, but in a sponge on, and in the skin of a patient during electrotherapy.

The OH^- and H_3O^+ ions can, if present in sufficient concentration, cause what is known as a *chemical burn*: an unsightly, painful injury to the skin. The chemical burn caused by the alkali under the cathode is called liquefaction necrosis (the burned tissue is relatively moist). The burn that occurs under the anode (due to the acid) is called coagulation necrosis. Here, the tissue remains firmer and the skin dries out somewhat.

A chemical burn is always malpractice. Period.

It only occurs if the sponges used are not wet enough, if the intensity is set too high, or if the electrodes are in direct contact with the skin. It occurs very frequently in patients with sensory disturbances, trophic skin disorders in diabetics, or if the patient thinks that a little pain can be tolerated. Immediate measures in the event of a chemical burn are rinsing, wound care, and, if necessary, consultation with a physician. The site should be photographed for documentation. An apology to the patient is also appropriate (Fig. 2.9).

This phenomenon does not occur only with direct current applications, but can also occur with pulsed current methods such as diadynamic current. The longer the pulse duration, the more pronounced the chemical reaction and the greater the risk of chemical burns. With the very short compensated pulses in medium-frequency procedures or with compensated TENS pulses, the situation is different. Since the polarity of the electrodes is constantly changing, the chemical changes that have occurred during one phase are compensated in the next phase; thus, the risk of chemical burns here is almost, but not quite, zero. Tissue damage can still occur (see Fig. 2.9). More on this in Chap. 3.

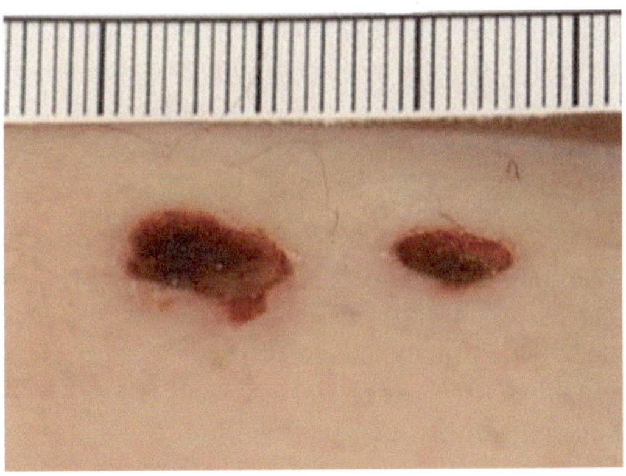

Fig. 2.9 Chemical burn

2.7.4 Direct Current Component or Galvanic Component

Technically, a non-compensated pulsed current is equivalent to a compensated pulsed current (alternating current) superimposed with a direct current, since any pulsed current can be broken down into an alternating current component and a direct current component. The term "direct current component" or "direct current proportion" (also "galvanic component") thus refers to the difference between a non-compensated pulsed current and a compensated pulsed current of the same form, in modern English "AC current with DC offset." Since every non-compensated pulsed current has a direct current component, a corresponding effect occurs in tissue as with normal direct current. The longer the phase duration of a pulsed current, the more pronounced this direct current-like effect. A pulsed current with a frequency of 100 Hz, such as diadynamic current with a phase duration of 10 ms, will produce a greater direct current-like effect than with a phase duration of 2 ms, as in 2–5 (Träbert or, in German, Ultrareiz) stimulation. However, since much higher intensities are used in the latter, the risk of chemical burns is not lower.

2.7.5 Definitions

The current *I* is the amount of charge carriers Q transported within a certain time t. Formula: I = Q/t. Unit C/s = ampere A. "C" stands for coulomb = 6.24 × 10^{18} electrons.

Electric power in watts is the product of voltage (in volts) and current (in amperes), i.e.: 1 W = 1 V × 1 A (1 VA)

Resistance is expressed in ohms (Ω). Skin resistance is not constant and is influenced, among other things, by the thickness of the epidermis, subcutaneous fat, skin moisture and blood flow, and trophic status. In addition, pulse duration, pulse shape, and frequency affect resistance. The literature cites values of about 500 Ω to 1.3 kΩ.

The unit of measurement for *current* is the ampere, abbreviated "A," while *voltage* is given in volts, i.e., "V." In electrotherapy, milliamperes (mA) are used.

Voltage in volts is the force required to make a current flow.

There is a relationship between resistance, voltage, and current. This relationship is described by Ohm's law: the strength of the electric current flowing through an object is proportional to the electric voltage.

In formula: R (resistance) = U (volts): I (amperes) = constant

2.7.6 Constant Current and Constant Voltage

A particular setting of many clinical devices can be explained using Ohm's law: constant current and constant voltage setting, in modern English Constant Current (CC) and Constant Voltage (CV). An example: You perform iontophoresis and set an intensity of 3 mA. At the beginning, the skin has a certain high resistance. After a few minutes of treatment, resistance decreases due to changes in skin blood flow. Ohm's law states that the relationship between R, U, and I must remain constant. If resistance decreases, either the voltage (in volts) or the current (in mA) in the device must be adjusted. If you had chosen a constant voltage setting (which is not possible for iontophoresis on European devices, but this is just for illustration), then as resistance decreases, the current, i.e., the intensity in mA, would increase. This is highly undesirable, as it could cause damage. The device therefore automatically switches to constant current operation (CC). As a result, the 3 mA setting remains unchanged. It is different if you want to use an application where you want to move an electrode, or even gently lift and reapply it, for example in trigger point treatment or muscle stimulation with a small stimulating electrode. Here, you select the constant voltage setting on the device (CV). If you now gently lift the electrode while current is flowing, reducing the contact area, the device measures an increasing resistance. R goes up, something must go down. If the voltage in volts remains constant on the device (CV), the intensity (in mA) must go down. Consequently, the patient (almost) does not get a shock. The ability to set CC or CV operation allows you to search for areas where skin resistance is lower. This is called galvanopalpation.

2.7.6.1 Galvanopalpation or Electropalpation for Pain Point Detection

A large, indifferent anode is attached somewhere on the body. The current for the search electrode is set to be just perceptible. The current form does not matter; TENS currents are the most comfortable. The device is set to Constant Voltage so that the intensity (current) increases where skin resistance is lower.

At suspected pain points, you move a smaller cathode (since the cathode, depending on the pulse form, is somewhat more stimulating) evenly and slowly over the skin. The best way to do this is with a conductive rubber electrode, either with some ultrasound contact gel or in a wet sponge pocket. If you encounter a pain point (trigger point, acupuncture point), the patient will feel a more intense current sensation locally, provided the skin resistance is lower, due to the constant voltage. Goal achieved: point found. The method is a bit cumbersome, but the points found in this way can be treated immediately afterwards.

With *constant current* (CC) devices or CC settings, this method does not work, since the intensity (current in mA) is kept constant despite resistance fluctuations. However, these devices ensure a constant charge to the tissue being stimulated, which is especially important in iontophoresis. If the intensity increases during iontophoresis (due to decreasing resistance as a result of improved blood flow), the risk of a chemical burn and electrolysis of the medication would be greater. In general, one can say: for static treatment: Constant Current; for dynamic treatment: Constant Voltage.

There is a second method for finding areas of lower skin resistance. This method is not without its fun factor for students, but is nevertheless very instructive. Or perhaps because of that. The following example refers to an examination of the back.

- Choose a rather comfortable current form such as High TENS and place a large, indifferent electrode in a convenient location, say, on one shoulder.
- Set the device to Constant Voltage (CV) so that the intensity (the current) increases in areas of lower skin resistance.
- The differential electrode (the cathode for asymmetrically compensated pulses) is placed on your own forearm, on the side you use to palpate. So on the therapist, NOT the patient.
- Now moisten the fingers of the palpating hand and touch the patient somewhere you will not be searching later.
- While maintaining contact with the patient with your palpating fingers, slowly increase the intensity until you feel the current in your (own!) fingertips. Don't worry! Nothing will happen.
- Now slowly move up or down the back. In areas where skin resistance is lower, the intensity increases slightly, and the therapist now feels this in their own fingertips. Voilà!

2.7.6.2 General Information

The easiest way to imagine the key parameters is to compare them to a water pipe. The current describes the amount of electrons flowing per unit of time—in this analogy, the amount of water flowing per unit of time.

Voltage in this analogy describes the pressure under which the water is held. As with water, there can be high voltage (= high water pressure) without any current flowing (= tap closed). Conversely, a very large amount of water can flow per unit of time at very low pressure, as is the case with a wide river.

It is the same with electric current: a 9-V battery can produce a current strong enough to easily trigger strong muscle contractions. But the thing will be empty very quickly.

If electrons flow in only one direction, this is called direct current (galvanic current). The best-known sources of direct current are batteries and accumulators, but also so-called power supply units.

With **alternating current**, the direction of current changes in a certain rhythm (= frequency). A frequency of, for example, 50 Hz (mains electricity) means that the current changes direction 100 times per second (50 times back and forth).

An alternating current always has a mean value = 0, so no net current flows. The often-heard term "compensated alternating current" is incorrect. If the alternating current were asymmetric, i.e., not compensated, it would be an "AC current with DC offset."

The best-known example of an alternating current source is the power outlet, which is part of a 230-V installation. At first glance, it may seem pointless to send current first in one direction and then shortly after in the other. However, this is technically necessary because only with alternating current can voltages be easily transformed. High-voltage transmission lines, for example, operate at 380,000 V (= 380 kV), while main distribution lines in cities operate at 10,000 or 20,000 V (= 10 kV or 20 kV), and the "lighting network" at 230 V. These voltages must be converted into one another, which can be done easily and almost without loss with a transformer in the case of alternating current, but not at all directly with direct current.

2.8 Special Physiological Principles of Direct Current

2.8.1 Relevant Studies

Direct current has traditionally been (and continues to be) used for a variety of indications. Not without reason, as experience and studies show that its use can indeed be successful in certain cases. The mechanism of action is usually explained in relatively simple terms: due to "complex processes," improved blood flow and pain relief are achieved. The cathode locally increases excitability by lowering the membrane potential, a phenomenon known as catelectrotonus. The anode has the opposite effect. A so-called longitudinal current application, with the cathode placed proximally, is traditionally referred to as ascending galvanization, which is thought to have an excitatory effect. If the anode is placed proximally, it is called descending galvanization, which is believed to have a calming effect. The problem with this claim is that the underlying studies were conducted on fish, frogs, and worms. Holzer and Scheminsky conducted studies on humans in 1942/1943. The investigators found that the patellar tendon reflex was enhanced after an ascending Stanger bath application (cathode at the head) and diminished after a descending application (anode at the head) (Falkenbach and Wendt 1993).

A study on healthy subjects by Falkenbach and Wendt (1993) found no difference between ascending and descending Stanger bath applications regarding their influence on the sympathetic nervous system (blood pressure and heart rate), concentration ability, reaction times, or subjective well-being. The authors note as a positive result that driving after a descending treatment is safe. Trnavsky investigated the effect of a descending direct current application on the Hoffmann reflex in the triceps surae muscle and found no change (Trnavsky 1984). More on this in the section on the Stanger bath.

However, the improvement in blood flow is evident, especially under the cathode, where a very pronounced reddening occurs after just a few minutes. According to Edel (1977), pain relief occurs during treatment under the anode, because hyperpolarization temporarily causes a conduction block, the so-called anelectrotonus. Interestingly, pain relief also occurs under the cathode, and this has traditionally been explained by the improved blood flow, which is thought to flush out more inflammatory mediators. Wagner (1995) disagrees, considering the cathode to be the more effective electrode for pain relief and relating this to hyperemia. Unfortunately, a major disadvantage of direct current is the risk of burns. Compensated TENS currents would be much more convenient to use and can even be applied at home. Moreover, there are now numerous publications demonstrating the efficacy of TENS, which is essential in the era of EBM. Should we therefore abandon direct current? By no means!

The following is a rehabilitation of direct current based on scientific literature. In the 1990s, several authors pointed out the capsaicin-like effect of direct current, but the author has the impression that this idea never really caught on. Let us first look at the literature.

- Schnizer et al. (1993) demonstrated that pretreatment with capsaicin suppresses the direct current erythema. Parameters: electrodes 30 cm^2, 0.1 mA/cm^2, 10 min. The erythema after heat treatment and CO_2 bath remained unchanged. The authors suspect a neurogenic component in the mechanism of erythema formation, presumably capsaicin-like.
- Using Doppler flowmetry, Berliner demonstrated that in healthy subjects, skin blood flow under the cathode was 700% of baseline, and under the anode 120%. The direct current was applied using a two-cell bath, 14 min, 7–18 mA (Berliner 1997).
- Schöps et al. (1998a, b) conducted a study to objectify the improvement in blood flow during a direct current application to the back in healthy subjects, measuring the development of erythema in the skin under the electrodes using laser Doppler flowmetry. Parameters: self-adhesive, conductive rubber electrodes (56 × 56 mm), 0.1 mA/cm^2, 30 min. The cathode erythema was already maximal after 15 min and amounted to 1200% of baseline. The anode erythema increased to 871% after 30 min, with a rising trend. The authors attribute the different erythema development to the varying stimulus conditions in the tissue due to the polarity-dependent changes in the ionic environment.
- In another study, Schöps et al. anesthetized areas on the back of healthy subjects with Emla® cream and then applied direct current (15 min, 0.05 mA/cm^2). At the same

time, current was applied to untreated control sites. At the anesthetized sites, erythema was barely visible and reached a maximum of 27% of the control erythema. The authors assume that direct current treatment involves neural structures of the axon reflex, as with capsaicin application (Schöps et al. 1998a, b).

- Fietz-Rubusch studied two methods of pain suppression using the two-cell bath in 26 healthy subjects (Fietz-Rubusch 2000). She compared a 10-min application, clearly perceptible but not painful, with double the duration, i.e., 20 min, but at half the previously used intensity, subsensory. Based on increased ischemia tolerance times, she demonstrated that the longer application with half the intensity and double the duration was significantly more effective, despite the same total current dose. She assumes a primarily neurogenic mechanism in connection with the more pronounced cathode erythema and questions the pain-relieving effect of the anode (Rusch et al. 1988; Wagner 1995). Supporting this is the fact that capsaicin-induced erythema is inhibited by prior direct current application (Rusch et al. 1988; Schnizer et al. 1993). Fietz-Rubusch explains the better effect with longer treatment times by the more effective depletion of neuropeptides stored in the C fibers. It simply takes time for the vesicles to release their contents.
- Wallengren and Sundler (2001) used a special application that specifically stimulates C fibers (cutaneous field stimulation, more on this later) and demonstrated in humans that after 5 weeks of application, the density of nerve terminals in the skin had significantly decreased (0.8 mA, 20 min, once daily, 5 weeks). The result is comparable to that of Nolano et al. (1999). These authors applied capsaicin (0.075%) to the skin of healthy subjects for 3 weeks and also took biopsies. After 3 days, a 74% reduction in nerve fibers in the epidermis was already detectable; after 3 weeks, it was 82%. This was accompanied by reduced sensitivity to heat stimuli and pressure pain. After 6 weeks, sensitivity was almost back to normal.
- Schnizer and Kröling showed that erythema under the anode is pH-dependent, but cathode erythema is not (0.15 mA/cm^2, 20 min) (Schnizer and Kröling 2001). If the pH is kept constant, anode erythema does not occur. Since cathode erythema remains unchanged, it must have a different mechanism of origin.
- Schnizer et al. (2003) found using Doppler flowmetry that daily repeated direct current application led to about a 50% reduction in cathode and anode erythema after 7 treatments (0.15 mA/cm^2, 15 min). A treatment series of 9 times in one day, every 2 h, led to the same result. After a 10-day break, normal erythema could be induced again. The authors in their own words: "The phenomenon of attenuation can be interpreted as desensitization based on depletion and impoverishment of vasoactive mediators."

Conclusions:

- With direct current, the cathode produces the stronger erythema.
- The cathode has the stronger pain-suppressing effect.
- Direct current erythema is neurogenic and is based on the release of vasoactive neuropeptides, comparable to the effect of capsaicin.
- Repeated direct current application leads to a local decrease in the mentioned neuropeptides due to depletion of neuropeptide stores in the involved nerve fiber terminals.
- Repeated direct current application leads to desensitization (also called defunctionalization) of the involved nerve fibers and ultimately to their reversible destruction.

We will now discuss in detail the background and clinical consequences of these findings.

2.8.2 Hyperemic Effect

This is the most therapeutically significant effect of direct current (Fig. 2.10). This effect is not tied to either pole, although erythema is more

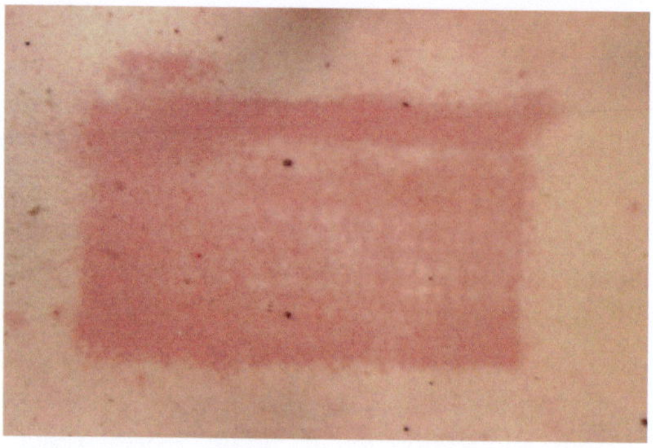

Fig. 2.10 Cathode erythema

pronounced and appears more quickly under the cathode (Schöps et al. 1998a, b). Such erythema occurs not only with classical direct current, but also with so-called uncompensated pulsed currents that have a direct current component, such as diadynamic current, high-voltage stimulation, and uncompensated TENS currents.

In response to electrical stimulation of the TRPV1 receptor (Transient Receptor Potential Vanilloid), which is found on many C fibers and some Aδ fibers, and to the potentially harmful stimulus (the pH change caused by the current), substances are released that influence local blood flow and cell growth. This reaction is known as "neurogenic inflammation." The mechanism is quite well understood and will be discussed in detail below.

Schnizer et al. (2003) showed that direct current erythema under both the cathode and the anode decreases significantly over the course of a treatment series (0.15 mA/cm^2, 15 min, after 7 applications less than 50% of baseline). The phenomenon is reversible: after a treatment break of less than 10 days, normal erythema can be induced again. This phenomenon occurs not only with continuous direct current, but also with pulsed current containing a direct current component (Pierau and Szolcsányi 1989: 2 Hz, 200 µs; Wallengren and Sundler 2001: 4 Hz, 1 ms). It is believed that this is due to depletion of neuropeptides stored in the nerve terminals. In addition, desensitization of the involved receptors and reversible destruction of the C fiber terminals (and some of the Aδ terminals) have been demonstrated in this context. This is an effect known from the use of capsaicin (Ainsworth et al. 1981; Wall and Fitzgerald 1981; Serra et al. 1998; Simone et al. 1998; Nolano et al. 1999; Ringkamp et al. 2001; Sasamura and Kuraishi 1999; Fattori et al. 2016).

If the skin is pretreated with capsaicin and then direct current is applied, the direct current erythema is attenuated. Conversely, pretreatment with direct current inhibits the erythema caused by capsaicin (Rusch et al. 1988). If the skin is anesthetized and then direct current is applied, only a weak erythema is induced (Schöps et al. 1998a, b). These facts are considered evidence that direct current erythema is neurogenic and triggered by capsaicin-sensitive afferents.

If a current with a direct current component, after repeated application, actually inhibits neurogenic inflammation like capsaicin, this provides an explanation for the effectiveness of certain electrotherapy applications, especially those that are no longer so popular today. It also shows that it is not always sensible to work with compensated pulsed currents, as is common in standard TENS applications today. These current forms do not induce erythema due to the lack of a direct current component and therefore may have less effect on processes involving neurogenic inflammation.

Interestingly, erythema under the anode arises in part by a different mechanism than under the cathode. Schnizer and Kröling (2001) showed that erythema under the anode is pH-dependent, but cathode erythema is not: If the pH under the electrodes is kept constant (by using a NaCl solution in the sponges under the electrodes), erythema appears only under the cathode, while anode erythema is almost completely absent. When demineralized or normal tap water is used, H_3O^+ ions are produced under the anode by electrolysis. If, on the other hand, a NaCl solution is used, Na^+ ions carry the current at the anode. The reaction $2\ Cl^- \rightarrow Cl + 2e-$ supplies the anode with electrons. Hardly any H_3O^+ is produced, so the pH remains relatively constant.

Erythema under the anode can be attenuated or completely suppressed by taking acetylsalicylic acid (Aspirin®) (Berliner 1997). Cathode erythema is somewhat reduced, but still occurs (Durand et al. 2002a, b). Aspirin inhibits cyclooxygenase (COX), so inhibition of erythema formation under the anode implies involvement of prostaglandins. A single 1000 mg dose (1 tablet of Aspirin usually contains 500 mg) can inhibit erythema formation under the anode for up to 7 days (Durand et al. 2002a, b). Pretreatment with capsaicin and local anesthesia prevent the development of both cathode and anode erythema (Durand et al. 2002a, b). Thus, erythema depends on intact innervation and an aspirin-sensitive mechanism.

Direct current erythema is located under the electrodes, but is usually not sharply demarcated. Due to the axon reflex (see below, Sect. 2.9.1.), neuropeptide release occurs throughout the innervation area of the stimulated nerves, and these innervation areas are not always directly under the electrode. The erythema can remain visible for hours after treatment. It is sometimes accompanied by flares near the electrodes. An attenuated or disappeared erythema can, as a sign of sensitization, be intensified again after treatment by exposure to cold or heat (showering, sun exposure, or even excitement → mast cells can react to stress).

The improved blood flow in the skin is easily demonstrable and, depending on treatment duration, amounts to over 700 to 1200% under the cathode and still 120 to 871% under the anode (Berliner 1997; Schöps et al. 1998a, b). A consensual improvement in blood flow also occurs on the untreated side (Lissner 1963). The persistent claim that improved blood flow also occurs in deeper tissues (muscle) has not been confirmed to date (Schnizer and Manert 1980).

2.9 Neurogenic Inflammation

It has been over a century since it was discovered that activation of dorsal horn ganglia can cause vasodilation. This observation suggests that the nerve fibers involved not only conduct afferent information but also efferent signals (Bayliss 1901). Since then, evidence has accumulated that stimulation of certain peripheral nerve endings leads to the release of bioactive substances at the nerve terminals (Chal 1988; Koltzenburg and Handwerker 1994; Herbert and Holzer 2002a, b; Richardson and Vasko 2002; Yaksh and Di Nardo 2018). These substances act on cells such as mast cells, immune cells, and muscle cells in the vessel wall, causing an inflammatory reaction. This reaction is characterized by redness and warmth (secondary to vasodilation), swelling (secondary to plasma extravasation), and increased sensitivity (secondary to changes in the excitability of certain nerve fibers): rubor, calor, tumor, and dolor, the classic signs of inflammation (Kowalski and Kaliner 1988; Herbert and Holzer 2002a, b).

This neuropeptide-mediated reaction is referred to as "neurogenic inflammation." The term "neurogenic" is used because the reaction originates from neurogenic structures and occurs only in tissues with intact innervation. Inflammation here is meant as a collective term for the complex, nonspecific defense mechanisms of the organism against injury (Handwerker 1999; Scott et al. 2004).

The erythema is found at the site of stimulation and is often accompanied by a so-called flare response. This is an erythema that extends more or less into the surrounding area and, for example, is often visible as redness around the electrodes during electrotherapy and appears as irregular redness around the needle during acupuncture and dry needling (Serra et al. 1998).

The neuropeptides calcitonin gene-related peptide (CGRP) and substance P (SP) are definitely involved. The involvement of other neuropeptides is still unclear; the release of glutamate and ATP (adenosine triphosphate) is also suspected. To date, CGRP, VIP (vasoactive intestinal peptide), substance P, somatostatin, bombesin, galanin, PACAP (pituitary adenylate cyclase-activating peptide), and neurokinin A have been detected in the terminals of the involved nerve fibers (Levine et al. 1993; Richardson and Vasko 2002; Herbert and Holzer 2002a, b). These neuropeptides are synthesized in the cell bodies of nociceptive C fibers and

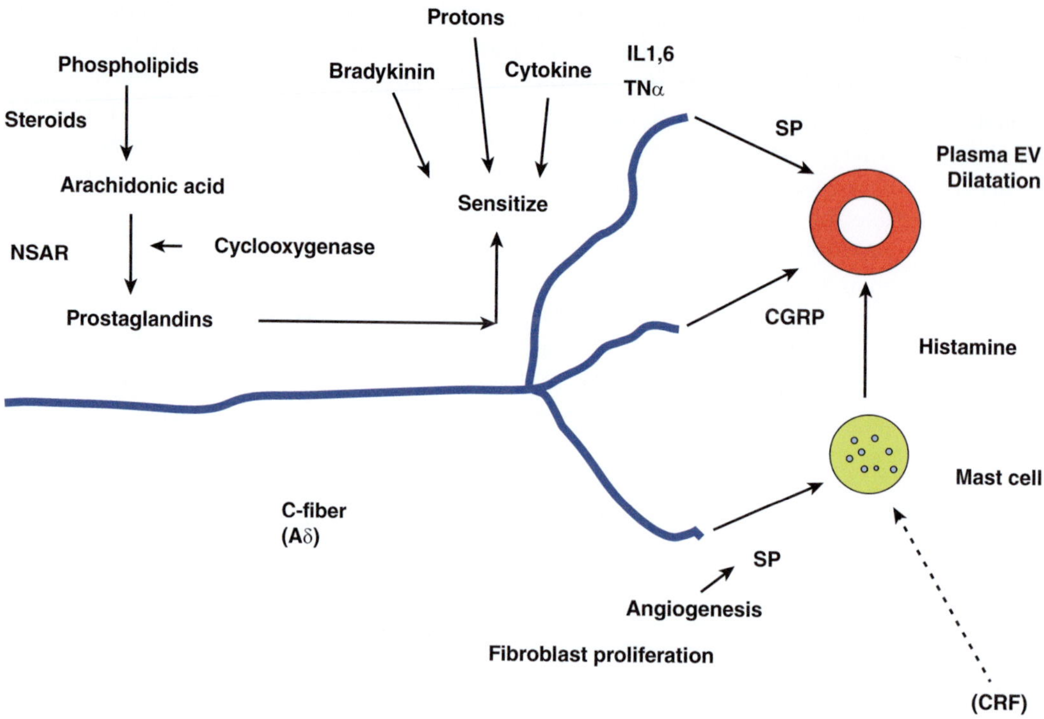

Fig. 2.11 Neurogenic inflammation

transported to the peripheral nerve terminals by fast axoplasmic flow at a rate of about 40 cm per day. There, they are stored in vesicles and released upon stimulation. Individual ganglion cells can contain two to four of these neuropeptides in various combinations (Yaksh and Di Nardo 2018) (Fig. 2.11).

According to current knowledge, the early phase of extravasation is triggered by the direct action of SP. In the late phase, secondarily released mediators such as histamine, serotonin, prostaglandins, and leukotrienes are also active. Rats and humans show different reactions when the skin is electrically stimulated (Sauerstein et al. 2000). In rats, for example, stimulation at 1 Hz, 0.5 ms, 80 mA, 30 min mainly releases CGRP and only a small amount of SP. Protein extravasation also occurs. In humans, 4 Hz stimulation (0.5 ms, 30 mA, 30 min) leads to the release of CGRP and SP and to a pronounced flare reaction. However, in humans, electrical stimulation does not cause protein extravasation. These different reactions show that experiments in rodents cannot be directly extrapolated to humans.

This neuropeptide release serves to maintain and protect tissue (Levine et al. 1993):

- Tachykinins (substance P, neurokinin A and B) stimulate fibroblast proliferation; SP and CGRP have a promoting effect on angiogenesis and accelerate wound healing (Scott et al. 2004). This is why trophic disorders occur in neuropathies, especially when the thin nerve fibers are damaged and neuropeptide secretion is therefore reduced—a well-known complication in diabetics (Oerstavik et al. 2006).
- The release of CGRP primarily causes dilation of terminal arterioles and thus increases blood flow.
- The release of SP directly and via the release of mediators from mast cells (including histamine) causes plasma extravasation from the venules, but only at relatively high doses (Weidner et al. 2000).

Release can be triggered in various ways: by H_3O^+, i.e., by a pH change in the tissue, by stimulation of the axon terminals with capsaicin, by mechanical and thermal stimuli and with UV light, and demonstrably by electrical stimulation with an intensity sufficient to stimulate C and Aδ fibers. Therefore, compensated TENS impulses can also trigger local hyperemia. If the C fibers have been sensitized in the case of inflammation, low TENS with its long pulses (250 μs or longer) can also induce neuropeptide release. Any redness after low TENS does not necessarily mean that the patient is allergic to the electrodes.

2.9.1 The Axon Reflex

Neuropeptides are not only released locally by direct stimulation of C and Aδ fibers. An *antidromic, i.e., opposite to the normal direction of conduction,* stimulus conducted via branches of the stimulated nerve to the terminals can also trigger release in the *innervation area of the stimulated nerve*. This is called the axon reflex (Chal 1988; Sorkin et al. 2018). This reaction presents as irregular redness around the actually stimulated area, the aforementioned flare.

2.9.2 The Dorsal Root Reflex

An important mechanism contributing to neurogenic inflammation is the dorsal root reflex (Willis 1999; Peng et al. 2001; Sorkin et al. 2018). Action potentials generated by stimulation of peripheral nociceptors are, after synapsing via interneurons at the spinal level, conducted back to the periphery through the dorsal roots via what are actually afferent neurons on the same side of the body. Neuropeptides are also released from the terminals of these neurons in the periphery, contributing to redness more or less *outside the innervation area of the primarily stimulated nerve fiber(s)*. In contrast, the axon reflex leads to redness in the innervation area of the stimulated nerve.

2.9.3 Crossed Neurogenic Inflammation, Reflex Neurogenic Inflammation

Neurogenic inflammation can also reflexively trigger the same reaction on the *contralateral* side of the body (Levine et al. 1985; Peng et al. 2001; Kelly et al. 2007; Sorkin et al. 2018). This second inflammatory reaction can occur within a few hours after the first inflammation at a symmetrical site. Levine demonstrated that this reaction is also neurogenically mediated via segmental connections and not via inflammatory mediators transported through the circulation (Levine et al. 1985). A centrally acting mechanism could not be ruled out (Gjerstad et al. 1999; Peng et al. 2001); sympathectomy reduces pain and swelling on both sides. Levine refers to the reaction as *reflex neurogenic inflammation*. To better distinguish it from the dorsal root reflex, the author prefers the term "crossed neurogenic inflammation." The dorsal root reflex is also a reflex phenomenon that occurs segmentally, and is therefore actually also a type of "reflex neurogenic inflammation" (Fig. 2.12).

Crossed neurogenic inflammation is a plausible explanation for the bilateral occurrence of certain musculoskeletal problems (Leis et al. 2004; Kelly et al. 2007). It could also explain why some patients sometimes experience mild symptoms on the contralateral (untreated!) side after a therapeutic intervention. This is usually explained by saying that the joint on the healthy side was also examined. However, a "normal" joint should not react to an examination with pain, whereas a sensitized joint, due to the mechanism described, will.

Neurogenic inflammation does not always occur with pain. However, mediators not primarily associated with neurogenic inflammation can intensify the symptoms. Inflammatory mediators produced by immune cells and mast cells (cytokines such as interleukin-1, tumor necrosis factor-α = TNF-α) interact with neuropeptides and sensitize the involved receptors on C and Aδ fibers. This can, for example, cause a receptor such as the TRPV1 receptor to respond not

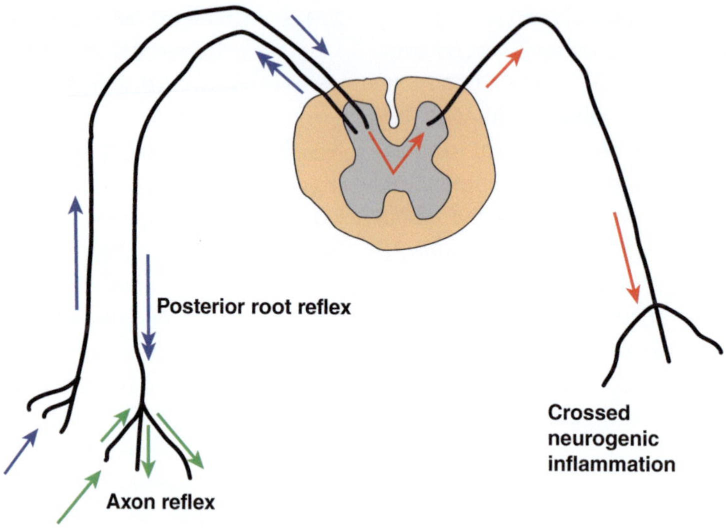

Fig. 2.12 Neurogenic inflammation can occur at various locations

as intended to temperatures above 43 °C, but already to fire at 37 °C. As a result, the patient experiences pain at body temperature—this is the well-known throbbing resting pain in inflammation.

Some authors (Herbert and Holzer 2002a, b) explain the poor efficacy of NSAIDs and glucocorticoids in some syndromes (including many chronic pain syndromes of the musculoskeletal system, such as periarthritis "PHS," epicondylopathies, tendinopathies, tenosynovitides, insertion tendinopathies, and spondyloarthropathies) by the fact that, in these cases, other mediators are also involved in the development of inflammatory signs and pain, in addition to those whose synthesis and action are inhibited by NSAIDs. This has been demonstrated several times in animal experiments and in humans. For example:

- In patients with so-called tennis elbow, immunohistochemical analyses of the extensor carpi radialis brevis muscle have demonstrated the involvement of substance P and CGRP (Ljung et al. 1999; Uchio et al. 2002).
- In patients with arthritis, in addition to CGRP and SP, interleukin-1, prostaglandins, and TNF-α have been detected in plasma, synovial fluid, and synovial tissue (Malone et al. 1986; Marshall et al. 1990; Balblanc et al. 1991; Westermark et al. 2001).
- In patients with chronic temporomandibular joint problems, elevated concentrations of TNF-α have been detected in the synovial fluid (Nordahl et al. 2000).
- SP- and CGRP-producing C and Aδ fibers have been found in the joint capsules of cervical zygapophyseal joints (Kallakuri et al. 2004).
- In the joints of patients with coxarthrosis, neurokinin-1 (NK1-R) receptors (which mediate the effects of SP) have been found on the walls of venous vessels, on Schwann cells of nerve bundles, and on nerve fibers (Saxler et al. 2005).
- In the joints of patients with gonarthrosis, many SP-producing nerve fibers were found, especially in the medial compartment (Tomoyuki 2003; Saito 2003).
- In general, the inflammatory process appears to underlie the development of osteoarthritis and tendinosis (Decaris et al. 1999; Niissalo et al. 2002; Konttinen et al. 2006; McDougall 2006; Fredberg and Stengaard-Pedersen 2008; Harden et al. 2013; Walsh et al. 2015; Raney et al. 2017; Dobson et al. 2018).

Mast cells play a special role in this context. It is known that mast cells in the joints of some patients with rheumatoid arthritis express receptors for corticotropin-releasing factor (CRF). In patients in whom this was the case, arthritis symptoms worsened under stress (Theoharides et al. 1998). The CRF released during a stress reaction triggers the release of vasoactive substances such as histamine, VIP, cytokines (including interleukins), and TNF-α from mast cells, and these substances in turn influence the inflammatory process. Comparable mechanisms occur in other pathologies in which mast cell involvement is suspected: migraine, asthma, fibromyalgia, irritable bowel syndrome, various skin diseases, even multiple sclerosis—all conditions in which symptoms can worsen under stress (Littlejohn and Guymer 2018; Kempuraj et al. 2019; Theoharides and Cochrane 2004).

An increase in pain could also be caused by sensitization of the nociceptors involved in the existing inflammation by cytokines. Animal experiments have shown that interleukin-1 enhances capsaicin-induced neurogenic vasodilation via sensitization of nociceptive afferents. This sensitization depends on the action of other inflammatory mediators such as prostaglandins. Depending on its concentration, bradykinin significantly lowers the excitability threshold of the TRPV1 receptor for heat stimuli below body temperature.

2.10 Capsaicin

Capsaicin (trans-8-methyl-N-vanillyl-6-nonenamide = (E)-N-(4-hydroxy-3-methoxybenzyl)-8-methylnon-6-enamide) is a compound found in many types of peppers (chilis) and is responsible for their pungent taste. In the laboratory, it is used in the standard procedure for inducing a neurogenic inflammation: the absence of a reaction to a specific stimulus after capsaicin pretreatment confirms the involvement of polymodal nociceptive C fibers and certain Aδ fibers in this reaction.

Capsaicin has a specific excitatory effect on these fibers, which is why they are sometimes referred to as "capsaicin-sensitive afferents." With prolonged or high-dose application of capsaicin to the skin, a reversible desensitization occurs first. With longer application or very high doses, a so-called defunctionalization of these fibers follows, more precisely of the TRPV1 receptor (Nolano et al. 1999; Simone et al. 1998; Anand and Bley 2011). This defunctionalization is due to a series of effects, including the temporary loss of membrane potential, the inability to transport neurotrophic factors, and the reversible retraction of epidermal and dermal nerve fiber endings—de facto a destruction of the fibers. These can regenerate over the course of days to weeks. This is why regular chili consumers tolerate spicier foods than people who are not accustomed to them. If capsaicin is applied directly to C fibers, a complete blockade of nerve conduction in these fibers occurs within a few minutes (Ainsworth et al. 1981; Fattori et al. 2016).

However: Not all C fibers are capsaicin-sensitive: about 20% of these fibers do not respond to capsaicin. Likewise, not all Aδ fibers are capsaicin-*in*sensitive. Of these Aδ fibers, about one third are capsaicin-sensitive, namely the type II AHM fibers (A for A fiber, H for Heat, and M for Mechanic): these Aδ fibers respond to heat stimuli below 50 °C. The HTM fibers (High Threshold Mechanic) and the type I AMH fibers (which respond to heat stimuli above 50 °C) are not desensitized by capsaicin. Therefore, not all burning pain disappears with the use of capsaicin cream, and one never fully adapts to spicy foods. For a detailed description, see Magerl et al. 2001.

The mechanism of action is quite well understood (Anand and Bley 2011):

- Capsaicin acts on the TRPV1 receptor (Transient Receptor Potential Vanilloid = Vanilloid receptor = VR1, a heat receptor, member of the large TRPV family) and triggers a strong influx of Ca and Na. The Ca influx triggers exocytosis (release) of neuropeptides and glutamate at the terminals and segmentally in the dorsal horn.

The so-called stimulated exocytosis proceeds as follows: the vesicles move toward the cell membrane in response to a specific stimulus, dock against the membrane, and fuse with it. The cell membrane opens and the contents of the vesicle are released from the cell into the extracellular space.

- Repeated release of these substances leads to depletion of neuropeptide stores and consequently to a decrease in the tissue response to the aforementioned release: local neurogenic inflammation is therefore less pronounced, and pain decreases. In addition, the segmental transmission of nociceptive information is reduced, which explains the analgesic effect in deeper pain (Fietz-Rubusch 2000). The fact that naloxone increases pain after capsaicin application in humans suggests activation of a central inhibitory mechanism (Anderson et al. 2002).
- Repeated activation of the TPRV1 receptor leads, via second messenger processes involving, among others, probably cAMP and certainly calcium, to inhibition of voltage-dependent Na channels and probably also of the receptor itself. This results in decreased excitability of the cell (the aforementioned defunctionalization). At higher capsaicin doses, K and Ca channels are also inhibited. The exact process is not yet known, but involvement of an intracellular "key protein" (probably calcineurin) or the receptor itself is suspected.
- The increased cation influx and the associated rise in intracellular Cl concentration lead to changes in osmotic conditions with consequent damage and destruction of the cell, including swelling of the mitochondria. The elevated Ca concentration can also cause cell damage via enzymatic reactions. This destruction is reversible.

The desensitizing/defunctionalizing effect is successfully used for pain relief in various pain syndromes. Capsaicin is applied as a cream (0.025–0.075%) 3 to 4 times daily over a longer period (2–6 weeks) to the skin (Rains and Bryson 1995; Dubner 1991). Adhesive pads with a higher concentration (8%) are also used, for example in the treatment of diabetic neuralgia (Simpson et al. 2017; Tenreiro Pinto et al. 2018). This then leads, via the process described above, to a reversible loss of function of the pain-conducting fibers (Malmberg et al. 2004). Unfortunately, only frequent repeated application of the cream produces the desired desensitization and thus pain relief. Initially, the unpleasant "irritant" effect of capsaicin is perceived, which is why many patients discontinue therapy prematurely. Therefore, the pharmaceutical industry is feverishly searching for alternatives that have the same effect as capsaicin without causing additional pain. The aforementioned pads are said not to have this irritant effect, and a single application can suppress pain for several months (Mankowski et al. 2016).

Capsaicin cream is used, for example, in postherpetic neuralgia, diabetic neuropathies, polyneuropathies, arthritis, rheumatoid arthritis, meralgia paresthetica, trigeminal neuralgia, fibromyalgia, insertional tendinosis, and myofascial pain. In principle, our daily bread.

The effectiveness of capsaicin treatment in these pain syndromes confirms the involvement of capsaicin-sensitive afferents and that neurogenic inflammation originating from these afferents plays a role in the pathogenesis of these syndromes.

By the way: The so-called chili high after extensive chili consumption is due to β-endorphin release. Our brain interprets the pain in the mouth as a burn and wants to suppress it. Stimulation of the TRPV1 receptors thus leads to the release of β-endorphin, which can result in an increased sense of well-being: a mild euphoria, which in a convivial setting is usually mistakenly attributed to the beer consumed with the chili. Experts refer to this state as a "pepper high." The whole thing is, of course, completely harmless and should not deter anyone from consuming chili. Since capsaicin is lipophilic, a glass of milk helps relieve the burning pain. It is also soluble in ethanol, so beer and wine also help.

2.10.1 Cutaneous Field Stimulation (CFS)

Cutaneous field stimulation is used for pain relief and for the treatment of chronic pruritus (Nilsson and Schouenborg 1999; Nilsson et al. 1997, 2003, 2004; Wallengren and Sundler 2001). Special electrodes are used in CFS. The indifferent electrode is a standard commercial one. The different electrode, however, consists of a flexible rubber compound with 16 small, sharp needle electrodes embedded in it, which penetrate the stratum corneum by about 0.3 mm, so the tips reach approximately to the dermis-epidermis junction. The electrodes are usually 8 × 8 cm and 8 × 2 cm in size. Stimulation is performed with monophasic (i.e., non-compensated) pulses with a phase duration of 1 ms, a fixed frequency of 4 Hz, and intensities up to 1 mA. Because the current density at the electrode tips is high, relatively unpleasant sensations (burning) occur in the first minutes of treatment. However, these sensations subside almost completely after a few minutes. It is recommended to increase the intensity in small steps during the first minutes so that the current is better tolerated. This method specifically stimulates Aδ and C fibers, resulting in erythema, which is accompanied by a flare around the stimulating electrode. This clearly indicates an axon reflex. Biopsies have shown that after a treatment series of 5 weeks, 20 min daily, 0.8 mA, the number of C fibers in the skin had decreased. After an unfortunately not precisely defined period, reinnervation occurred: thus, the destruction of nerve fibers, as with capsaicin application, is reversible.

Based on the findings regarding CFS, it is very likely that the attenuation of the direct current erythema and the pain relief can at least partially be explained by the destruction of the involved nerve fibers.

2.10.2 Consequences for Therapy

The author is aware that, apart from strong indications, there is no solid evidence for the following statements. The proposed treatment model applies not only to continuous direct current, but also to current forms with a more or less large direct current component, such as diadynamic current, high-intensity stimulation current, and non-compensated (monophasic) TENS currents.

The starting point (all references can be found above):

- Neurogenic inflammation is involved in many musculoskeletal disorders, especially tendinoses, insertional tendinopathies, and arthritis.
- These pathologies often do not respond, or only temporarily respond, to therapies with NSAIDs and glucocorticoids (cortisone). This means that other inflammatory mediators must be involved in the pathology in addition to those that respond to drugs from these groups.
- After repeated application of hyperemic current forms (direct current, monophasic pulsed current), there is a marked decrease in direct current erythema. This reversible decrease is very likely caused by depletion of the neuropeptides involved in erythema formation, defunctionalization of the involved nerve fibers, and their destruction. This effect is comparable to the reaction after repeated capsaicin application.
- Depletion, defunctionalization, and/or damage to the involved nerve fibers leads to anti-inflammatory effects and pain relief because there are not enough inflammatory mediators available. Damage to the terminals and desensitization of the receptors reduce excitability. This is confirmed by the results of treatment with capsaicin cream and cutaneous field stimulation.
- The inhibition of pain from deeper structures can be explained by activation of descending and central pain inhibition systems through stimulation of polymodal nociceptors. Feedback via the dorsal horn reflex may also play a role.
- The extent of erythema is determined by the current dose and not by high current intensity. This means that the total amount of charge transferred and the associated tissue

response determine erythema formation. With sufficiently long application, even a subthreshold intensity leads to erythema and pain relief. Specifically: ½ sensory threshold, 20–30 min treatment time. The longer current exposure probably results in more efficient depletion, as the vesicles need some time to empty.
- The decrease in erythema after repeated direct current application depends on treatment frequency. Multiple daily applications lead to rapid depletion of neuropeptide reserves in the nociceptors. Longer breaks between treatments allow for complete replenishment of neuropeptide stores in the nerve terminals. The rate of axonal transport of neuropeptides produced in the cell nucleus is about 40 cm per day. This means, for example, that after treatment at the knee, the depleted stores are probably replenished after about 2 days; at the foot, it takes up to 4 days. Depending on body size, of course.
- The analgesic effect depends on the extent of erythema. The more pronounced erythema occurs under the cathode. Under the anode, excitability is reduced, but only as long as the current is applied. Depletion of neuropeptides leads to longer-lasting pain relief. The claim that the stronger analgesic effect occurs under the anode is not correct in this case.

2.10.3 Proposal for a Treatment Protocol

The treatment goals are inhibition of the local inflammatory reaction and pain relief.

- The treatment should
  - deplete the neuropeptide stores in the terminals of the involved Aδ and C fibers,
  - defunctionalize the TRPV1 receptors, and
  - temporarily destroy the involved C and Aδ fiber terminals.
  - As a result, local (C and Aδ fiber) pain is reduced, and the neurogenic inflammatory reaction is suppressed.
  - Ultimately, the reduced inflammatory reaction and pain relief should lead to normalization of the local situation.
- Indications: All musculoskeletal disorders associated with neurogenic inflammation and/or C and Aδ fiber pain that can be addressed with this application—thus, rather superficially localized pathologies such as enthesopathies ("PHS," "tennis elbow," "golfer's elbow," "jumper's knee," etc.), arthritis as in chronic polyarthritis (cP), in activated osteoarthritis (in easily accessible joints such as the knee, finger and toe joints, ankle), trigger points, "tendovaginitis," chronic mal- and overuse problems, "RSI," neuralgias such as postherpetic neuralgia and meralgia paresthetica. A treatment attempt should be made in all chronic, so-called therapy-resistant problems.
- Schnizer (2003) achieved, in a simulated clinical situation, a 50–60% reduction in direct current erythema after 7 direct current applications (15 min, 0.1 mA/cm^2) in 2 weeks. In a clinical setting, more frequent treatments can be used to achieve more rapid depletion.
- Simultaneous use of capsaicin cream can support the treatment, as long as its application does not cause severe skin irritation.
- The intensity is set just below the sensory threshold (half the sensory threshold), with a treatment duration of 20–30 min. So: turn up the intensity until the patient just feels something, and then either set it just below this intensity (if the sensory threshold is very low) or halve the intensity (if the sensory threshold is high).
- The number of treatments is, of course, individual. Schnizer found a little over 50% reduction in direct current erythema after 7 treatments at 1- to 2-day intervals; after 12 treatments, the reduction was only slightly greater. Since a normal healing process certainly takes longer, a second series of treatments can be expected, which can then be considered a "maintenance dose." In my own experience, 2–3 treatments per week are

sufficient for this. Since the treatment is usually used in chronic patients, referring physicians are generally very cooperative when it comes to "extending" the treatment.

- A treatment break leads to replenishment of neuropeptide stores and recovery of defunctionalized nerve fibers. This does not correspond to the goals of this application.
- There are small, inexpensive devices for home treatment with iontophoresis. These devices can be used in suitable patients. Usually, the electrode connections need to be slightly modified—a small DIY task for the interested colleague or the technical service.
- Of course, patients must be extremely well instructed and monitored!

The following should be noted:

- All regulations for the use of hyperemic current forms must be observed, especially the contraindications and all measures to prevent burns.
- Direct current is aggressive. After a few treatments, the skin under both electrodes will temporarily change slightly, especially under the anode, where it will become somewhat dry over the course of treatment. Of course, the patient may care for the skin, but greasy creams must be thoroughly removed before therapy.
- Instead of direct current, diadynamic current can be used as a second choice; the DF Diphasé fixe, see Sect. 2.14.4, has the greatest direct current-like effect and is therefore the most effective. In my experience, high-intensity stimulation is the least effective in this case.
- The cathode produces the stronger erythema and is placed on the symptomatic area. If, for example, the entire knee is symptomatic in a knee patient, polarity can be reversed after 15 min or the polarity can be alternated per session.
- The electrodes should be as large as possible and, of course, very wet. Since the electrodes dry out somewhat during the long treatment time, they must be re-moistened. When fixing the electrodes, care must be taken to ensure even pressure distribution.
- For (fore-)arm, hand, lower leg, or foot problems, cell bath accessories can be usefully employed.
- Initially, there may be a usually mild exacerbation of existing symptoms after treatment. This can be explained by the forced release of neuropeptides. This reaction usually subsides after a few treatments.
- Mild symptoms may also sometimes occur on the contralateral side, especially if there are or have been problems there. This is probably due to crossed neurogenic inflammation. These symptoms also subside quickly. The patient must be informed about this in advance.
- Because of the long treatment time, it is advisable to give the comfortably positioned patient something to read. A cup of coffee or similar is usually greatly appreciated. Caffeine has no detectable effect on erythema formation.

A challenge for electrotherapy? An idea for a doctoral thesis? In any case, a motivation to take a closer look at the "good old" current forms again.

2.10.4 Analgesic Effect

The pain-relieving effect of direct current has been known for a long time and was widely used in the past, before the equally effective pulsed currents became available. Today, it is known that stimulation of C and Aδ fibers leads to descending and central pain inhibition, which is why pain relief persists even after application. While the current is flowing, hyperpolarization of the cell membrane of sensory nerves occurs under the anode; this raises the threshold for stimulation, which can result in pain relief. However, this has no lasting effect.

Today, the pain-relieving effect is mainly associated with the mechanisms described above and with erythema: the more pronounced the redness, the greater the pain relief. Because the more pronounced erythema occurs under the cathode, some authors now doubt the analgesic effect of the anode.

2.10.5 Trophic Effects

It has been shown that direct current treatments with very low intensities and long treatment times (several hours daily) can lead to improved wound healing in chronic skin ulcers. This topic is discussed in detail in Chap. 3.

2.10.6 Effects on CNS Excitability

When the stimulating pole (the cathode) is located near the head during a full bath treatment and the anode is at the other end (= so-called ascending current direction), interesting phenomena occur in animal experiments. Frogs, at sufficiently high intensities, go into an electroconvulsive state (electrotetanus), worms contract, and fish become restless and try to turn their heads toward the anode (Falkenbach and Wendt 1993). In humans, this electrode position is said to increase the patellar tendon reflexes. There is no explanation for these phenomena. If the anode is placed at the head end and the cathode at the other end (descending current direction), the aforementioned animals experience "galvanonarcosis." Fish are even said to fall completely asleep, and worms become longer due to relaxation, supposedly. Or because the circular muscles are stimulated, causing the worm to elongate (comment from a biologist). In humans, reduced reflex activity (PSR) was observed. This phenomenon also cannot be explained. Trnavsy found no effect on the H-reflex in 1984, and Falkenbach and Wendt did not confirm the various effects in humans. Nevertheless, these effects are cited as justification for the use of descending or ascending direct current applications. The terms "ascending" and "descending" are unfortunately chosen, since in the human body, ion flow always occurs in both directions.

2.10.7 Sensation of Warmth

A few seconds after the intensity has been turned up sufficiently, the patient feels a sensation of warmth under the electrodes. This sensation of warmth is caused by direct stimulation of certain receptors on C and Aδ fibers and not by an increase in temperature; the current is too weak for that. The stimulated TRPV1 receptors merely convey to the brain the impression of a temperature increase (cf. chili consumption). The temperature increase under the electrodes measured by Ulrich and Graßhoff (1994) after a TENS application is due to the hyperemic effect of long monophasic pulses (up to 750 μs) and is not a specific warming effect of TENS. In fact, the warming is negligible, as the following calculation example will illustrate.

Physicists and similarly educated specialists may forgive the simplification. The author is aware that certain factors are not taken into account: the capacitive resistance of the skin, the decrease in ohmic resistance due to improved blood flow, possible uneven pressure, etc. All of this would only result in *even* less heat being produced. Moreover, it would make the calculation too complicated.

So:

$$P = V \times I \ (P \ \textit{ist die Leistung in Watt})$$

$$\textit{und} \ V = I \times R$$

So, $P = I^2 \times R$

Let us assume an average skin resistance of 1000 Ω, an intensity of 0.2 mA/cm², and an electrode area of 50 cm² (i.e., 10 mA set on the device).

Then $P = 100 \times 1000 = 100\ \text{mW} = 0.1\ \text{W}$.

If this current runs for 15 min (900 s), the power output done in joules is $900 \times 0.1 = 90$ J.

To heat 1 kg of water by 1 K, about 4200 J are needed. So, with the 90 J generated, you do not get very far. Especially when you realize that the circulatory system acts as a cooling system and that electrotherapy is usually performed with pulsed currents, where the average current is much lower. Of course, it is a completely different story if, instead of 10 mA/50 V, you apply 2 A/2000 V to the tissue. Then about 4000 W are delivered, and if this happens several times for a few minutes, 100 kg of tissue (about 75 kg of water) will quickly become 20 °C warmer.

2.10.8 Electrotonus

Electrotonus refers to the change in membrane potential caused by the flow of current when a cell is stimulated with a constant current. Such subthreshold stimulations do not trigger an action potential; depending on the polarity, they influence the resting potential "anodically" or "cathodically." Under the anode, hyperpolarization (an-electrotonus) occurs. The threshold for stimulation is increased, and thus excitability is reduced. The reason is that K ions migrate away from the outer side of the membrane, thereby increasing the diffusion of K ions from inside the cell. This increases the resting membrane potential. Under the cathode, local depolarization (cat-electrotonus) occurs. The cathode lowers the resting potential and thus increases excitability. However, if this cat-electrotonus persists for a longer time, the Na^+/K^+-ATPase, the so-called sodium-potassium pump, is impaired. The Na carrier systems are deactivated by cat-electrotonus and are then no longer able to provide the Na^+ influx necessary for excitation. This ultimately also leads to a decrease in excitability.

2.11 General Treatment Guidelines

The following are general guidelines for the practical implementation of electrotherapy treatment for hyperemia or pain relief. These measures apply to all applications in the low- and medium-frequency range. Of course, treatment is always preceded by a thorough assessment.

Each type of electrical current application has its own specific characteristics. These are discussed in detail in the respective sections. The author asks for forgiveness if he is perhaps stating the obvious at times.

2.11.1 General Measures Before the First Treatment

- The required materials are prepared. The device is positioned so that the therapist can keep an eye on both the device and the patient at the same time. It does no harm if the patient can also see the device.
- You should be familiar with the device and, for credibility, know from personal experience how the type of current intended for treatment feels.
- The presence of any contraindications should already have been clarified, but the question should be asked at the latest now.
- The patient is informed about the treatment in an understandable way. Some clinics require a signed consent form from the patient. From a quality or risk management perspective, this is not at all unreasonable!
- The skin is inspected for any wounds. Small wounds and pustules can be covered with Vaseline. Lip balm will also do, but does not last as long. If available, special waterproof plasters can be used.
- Sensitivity in the treatment area is checked at the latest now: warm-cold (C and Aδ fibers) and dull-sharp (Aβ and Aδ fibers).
- Especially with older devices, make sure that the intensity is turned down to 0 mA before switching on.
- With (very) old devices, the capacitors may not have fully discharged, so the electrodes should be briefly held together; otherwise, the patient may receive a shock when connecting them.
- Patient cables must always be checked for insulation and breaks.
- Modern devices perform a self-test after being switched on: there are clicks and beeps for a few seconds. In the event of a malfunction, it is usually due to a defective power

cable, a broken patient cable, or a blown (device) fuse. It can also happen that the power cable is simply not plugged in, especially during exams.

- The correct electrode size is selected. Most adhesive electrodes can be cut to the appropriate size, but be sure to pay attention to the connector and cable!
- The patient must be positioned comfortably and covered to prevent cooling. Rule of thumb: those who are already lying down cannot fall over.
- Electrodes and uninsulated plugs or clamps must never touch the skin directly due to the risk of burns. Cables should be routed so that they are not under tension. Caution when raising or lowering the treatment table—cables are often pinched!
- Older, loosened plug connections can come apart during treatment even without much tension.
- The electrodes are either placed in a sponge pouch or padded with a sponge (about 1–1½ cm thick) or a sufficiently thick cloth (terrycloth, washcloth, usually folded 4 to 8 times). Such padding must extend at least 1–2 cm beyond the electrode on each side.
- The padding is thoroughly moistened with lukewarm tap water. Since the padding dries out during treatment, it may need to be remoistened. For this, a large syringe or laboratory squeeze bottles should be prepared. However, the padding must not be too wet, as depending on placement, dripping sponges could cause a short circuit.
- Standard electrodes are fixed with rubber or Velcro straps. The straps must not be too tight, as uneven pressure leads to uneven current distribution. With Velcro straps, the soft side goes against the skin.
- Lead or tin electrodes really should no longer be used, unless you intend to administer a heavy metal iontophoresis.
- If necessary, sandbags or weight cuffs can be used for fixation, especially on the back; these must not slip. If needed, adhesive tape or medical tape can be used, but these are usually not waterproof and do not hold well. Do not simply slap on cold weight cuffs.
- So-called vacuum electrodes (Vacotron®, Vaco Gymna®, Vacumed Bosch®, etc.) are practical. The suction force must not be set too high, as this quickly leads to unsightly hematomas. Due to poorer blood circulation under the suction cups, there is a higher risk of burns with hyperemic currents. The sponges also dry out very quickly, again increasing the risk of burns with the mentioned types of current! Please note the hygiene instructions regarding these devices in the chapter on medium frequency (3.10).
- Adhesive electrodes are **absolutely unsuitable** for hyperemic currents (direct current, monophasic non-compensated pulse currents) due to the risk of burns!
- The electrodes fixed to the body are connected to the device. When using monophasic and asymmetrically compensated pulse currents, polarity must be observed. The cathode, as it is the most stimulating, is placed on the most painful area.
- Note: Normally, the cathode is black and the anode is red (Mnemonic: **black CAT**; **KNAP**: Cathode Negative Anode Positive). In Germany, the cathode may also be blue. And if the technical service did not have black or red in stock, of course, other colors are possible as well.
- The current type and treatment time are set.
- The patient is informed about the sensations to be expected (hence the earlier comment about personal experience). Note: If the therapist dislikes a certain type of current, this does not mean the patient will feel the same!
- Dosage for a *conventional direct current application: maximum 0.1–0.3 mA/cm*^{2} for about 15 min of treatment; the patient should feel a slight to moderate tingling. Whether this method of dosing makes sense is debatable. In any case, with direct current, the dosage must never be so high that pain occurs.
- For such a hyperemic application, the author prefers first to determine the sensory threshold and then either halve the intensity or treat

just below the sensory threshold. The treatment time should be doubled if the intensity is halved. If you want to use DF as an alternative to treat neurogenic inflammation, proceed the same way: first determine the sensory threshold, then reduce the intensity accordingly and extend the treatment duration.

- There should never be a distinct burning sensation, as this indicates overdosing. Localized burning usually points to a pustule.
- Depending on the treatment goal, the patient should feel a distinct vibration or buzzing with diadynamic current, and a pressure sensation with ultra-stimulation therapy (Träbert, 2–5 current)—more on this later. The settings for various TENS applications are discussed in detail in Chap. 3. In pain treatment, (very) unpleasant sensations should generally be avoided.
- The intensity is increased quickly but carefully. While increasing the intensity, keep your eyes on the patient, not the device.
- Note that the patient's perception of current can vary greatly. Older people perceive current differently than younger ones. A patient who has just come in from the cold will have a different sensation due to increased skin resistance than if he had exercised on the ergometer in the warm practice before treatment. Sensation also depends on the time of day (between 2 and 3 p.m. people are said to be least sensitive) and, in women, on hormonal status. Pain perception seems to be highest during the menstrual cycle when estrogen levels are lowest. Other researchers claim the opposite. So don't count on it.
- Current perception also depends on the present state of the problem: If there is improvement, the pain-conducting fibers are less sensitized, and thus current perception is reduced. In such cases, a previously used intensity will be perceived as less strong. For the same reason, the therapist should be informed about the patient's (pain) medication use.
- The opposite occurs with worsening: Due to increased sensitization of nerve fibers, even a lower intensity than usual may be clearly felt. The same applies to phase duration. Very painful problems require a short phase duration due to increased excitability (e.g., High TENS 10–20 μs). Over the course of a treatment series, if improvement occurs, the phase duration will need to be increased to elicit the desired response.

2.11.2 Measures During Treatment

- The current strength is set. The intensity is determined subjectively based on the patient's feedback or according to the specific guidelines for the application.
- Note that with Träbert's 2–5 therapy, diadynamic current (DD current), and TENS applications, the intensity must be readjusted in the event of adaptation. After appropriate instruction and supervision, certain patients can be allowed to do this themselves. There are practical remote controls for this. If you do not have one, the device must be positioned within easy reach. If the patient is lying on their stomach for a back treatment, be aware that tensing the back muscles changes the pressure on the electrodes, which can unpleasantly affect the sensation of current.
- Regularly ask how and where the patient feels the current, and adjust the intensity if necessary. The therapist must never be out of earshot.
- For longer treatments, most patients appreciate being given something to read or being offered a drink.
- After the set treatment time has elapsed, modern devices automatically reduce the intensity. If not, the therapist does this quickly but cautious.
- The electrodes are removed from the body and the device is switched off.

2.11.3 Measures After Treatment

- The skin is checked and gently dried.
- If there is any irritation, the patient is instructed not to scratch under any circumstances, as the skin is especially softened after hyperemic applications.

- The patient is told that any redness that may have occurred can last for some time and may reappear with renewed irritation (such as showering, sun exposure, or emotional excitement). This is completely normal.
- The materials are thoroughly cleaned and put away. The padding must be rinsed well. Sponges should not be stacked on top of each other to dry.
- Adhesive electrodes must be stored in a sealed container after use, otherwise the adhesive layer will dry out. Good adhesive electrodes can be reused up to 20 times (or more). These electrodes must, of course, never be used for other patients and should therefore be labeled with the patient's name.
- The patient's response and the treatment parameters are documented.

2.11.4 Electrode Technique

- The electrode size should be adapted to the size of the area to be treated. Widespread pain should therefore be treated with large electrodes, possibly using the so-called two-channel or 2 + 2 technique. Almost all modern devices allow the use of two channels, so that two pairs of electrodes can be used simultaneously (Fig. 2.13). This application technique should not be confused with the outdated tetrapolar application of interferential current (see "Therapy with MF Currents" Sect. 3.10).

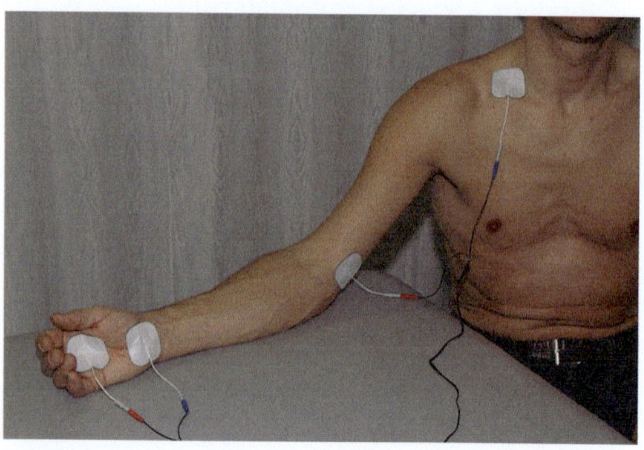

Fig. 2.13 2 + 2 application, here for CTS. One pair of electrodes locally (left in the image), one pair along the course of the median nerve

- The placement of the electrodes depends on the location of the problem (for a detailed description, see the section "Electrode Placement" Sect. 3.3.2). There are a variety of options: local, large-area or highly selective, transregional, "crosswise" or "lengthwise," etc., but it should be noted that nothing actually flows crosswise or lengthwise—the stimulation occurs under the electrodes.
- On the spine, electrodes can be placed to the left and right of the midline for symmetrical complaints, unilaterally for one-sided pain, or both electrodes can be placed centrally over the spine for midline pain. For unilateral pain radiating into the buttock or leg, one electrode can be placed on the back and one distally in the dermatome, or one pair of electrodes on the spine and a second pair distally in the corresponding dermatome (2 + 2). Joint pain can be treated locally "transregionally," with local treatment combined with segmental treatment. For example, in knee treatment, one pair of electrodes is placed medially and laterally to the knee joint, and the second pair unilaterally at the level of L3/4. Comparable applications are possible for all peripheral joints.
- Another option is to combine local treatment with a generally effective application such as Kaada stimulation.
- Any therapy, whether it is exercise therapy, mobilization, or electrotherapy, must always be as specific as possible. This means that if improvement occurs and the pain area becomes smaller, the electrode size should be adjusted. Instead of a large-area transregional placement, one should switch to stimulation of specific trigger points. Likewise, electrode placement should be adapted to changes in pain location. As long as an application is successful, all parameters should be maintained.
- The treatment method should also be adapted as improvement occurs. For example, if you initially had to use rather mild High TENS in a pain patient (see Sect. 1.16, "Stress

Reaction"), you should, over time, try to switch to a more aggressive but longer-lasting TENS application such as Burst TENS or Low TENS.

2.12 Application of Direct Current

Direct current can be applied in two ways:

- conventionally, using padded electrodes, directly on the patient ("dry," traditionally also called stable galvanization),
- via a partial or full bath, in so-called hydrogalvanization (cell bath, Stanger bath).

The aforementioned electrolytic phenomena mean that only relatively low current strengths can be used in conventional direct current treatment. This limits the effect to superficial structures, with the probable limit at 1–2 cm. Deeper muscle groups and joints such as the hip and shoulder joints are not directly accessible. Pain relief occurring in deeper tissues is probably related to the activation of descending and central pain inhibition mechanisms.

With direct current application in a full or partial bath (see below), theoretically higher intensities are possible, as the risk of burns is naturally much lower. However, due to unpleasant sensations, the tolerance threshold is still quickly reached. Therefore, a deeper effect is not to be expected even at higher settings, as in a full bath most of the current bypasses the patient.

Cell Bath, Stanger Bath

In the cell bath, one, two, or even all extremities are immersed in a water bath with large electrodes, and a large electrode (200–300 cm^2) may be placed on the lumbar or cervical region. Whether it makes sense to choose "descending" or "ascending" polarity is questionable. The more effective electrode is the cathode. Therefore, for example, in a patient with CRPS (Complex Regional Pain Syndrome, a pathology in which neurogenic inflammation is suspected; Cheshire and Snyder 1990; Bennett 2001; Weber et al. 2001; Birklein and Schmelz 2008), the bath for the affected extremity should be cathodically polarized (Fietz-Rubusch 2000). Applying a neck or back electrode is cumbersome. In the case mentioned, it is therefore easier to place the other extremity in a second, anodically polarized bath or to fix a large electrode to the ipsilateral upper arm.

The water should have a comfortable temperature of about 36–37 °C. Higher water temperatures allow for higher intensity, as the sensation of current is less pronounced in warm water. Whether higher intensity is useful is questionable. Fietz-Rubusch (2000) has shown that with direct current, it is the current dose that matters, not the intensity, and that a longer-lasting subthreshold application is more effective than a typical one. In simple terms: longer with less is better than short with more.

The risk of burns is significantly lower in the cell bath (except, of course, with a possible back or neck electrode!). However, the patient must be instructed to move their extremities slightly from time to time, otherwise unpleasant irritation may occur at the waterline. The electrodes must, of course, not be touched, and local jewelry must be removed.

The Stanger bath or hydroelectric full bath was first described in 1866. The tanner J.J. Stanger from Reutlingen used such a galvanic full bath with tanning liquor (a tanning agent) as a bath additive to treat his rheumatism. He had this bath patented as an "electric lohtannin bath." His son H. Stanger, an engineer, improved the design in the 1930s. That is why it is still commonly referred to as the Stanger bath today.

In this application, the patient lies in a full bath. The tub is equipped with 8 electrodes: one at the head and foot ends and 3 on each side. Sometimes a 9th, lumbar electrode is used. The electrodes can be polarized in different ways: so-called longitudinal flows (ascending: cathode at the head, supposedly more stimulating, or descending: anode at the head, supposedly more calming) or so-called transverse flows.

For example, on one side, 3 electrodes and on the other side, 1 electrode can be activated to achieve a (relative) local effect (for example, the hip region on one side).

This bath allows the use of high current strengths. If bath additives are used, the intensity can usually be set even higher, as the water then conducts better. However, since the current takes the path of least resistance, most of it unfortunately bypasses the patient.

The effect of such a bath is undoubtedly complex. The effects of the current occur alongside the relaxing effect of the warm water and any bath additives. The placebo effect of this elaborate therapy is probably very large. The influence on any existing neurogenic inflammation nevertheless seems plausible, but this problem can also be treated with less effort. Falkenbach and Wendt (1993) did not confirm the effects of the Stanger bath.

2.13 Iontophoresis

The application of direct current sets ions in motion. This ion movement can be utilized for introducing ionized medications through the skin. This is based on the principle that like poles repel each other. If a chemical substance dissolved in water is applied under the electrodes, for example on filter paper, the negatively charged ions are increasingly transported through the skin under the cathode, and the positively charged ions under the anode. Today, special electrodes are also used for this purpose. These consist of a type of chamber into which the dissolved medication is injected.

The method, sometimes also called ionophoresis, is not exactly new. Allegedly, a certain Pivati already treated arthritis with iontophoresis in 1747. Unfortunately, more precise information and references are lacking, but this would have had to take place pre-Volta with Leyden jars, which seems rather unlikely. The conclusive proof of efficacy was provided by the Breton Stéphane Leduc (1853–1939) in 1900 with his famous pair of rabbits (Fig. 2.14). He applied a strychnine solution (red in the image) under the cathode in one rabbit and under the anode in the other. The positively charged strychnine is repelled by the anode and migrates through the skin. The second rabbit (strychnine under the anode, left) met its demise (Edel 1977). Leduc was not the first to conduct this experiment; that honor goes to Herman Munk (1839–1912), who had already performed similar experiments around 1870.

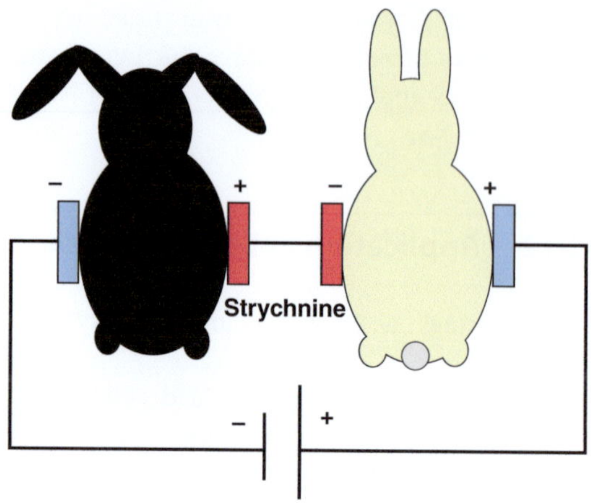

Fig. 2.14 Leduc's bunnies

This also demonstrated that the chemical substance used (the medication) does not act only locally, but also exerts a systemic effect. The substance is absorbed directly under the electrode into the bloodstream and transported further. The advantage of this method is that a medication can be applied locally without injuring the skin and does not pass through the liver very early, where it would be metabolized.

Part of the substance is said to remain in the tissue as a depot and could thus exert its effect over a longer period. However, a significant local deep effect is not to be expected. Panus et al. showed that with ketoprofen iontophoresis, the medication was detectable at a depth of 1–2 cm in (porcine) muscle tissue, which is at least the depth at which many musculoskeletal pathologies are localized (Panus et al.

1999). The amount delivered by iontophoresis at a depth of 1 cm was greater than when the ointment was used "passively," i.e., without ionto. Panus's parameters: 0.28 mA/cm^2, 40 min (4 mA total), ketoprofen under the anode. However, the agent was specially prepared for the study, so it did not correspond to a commercially available substance (300 mg/mL in a phosphate-buffered physiological saline solution with 20% ethanol, 2.5 mL in the applicator). The special preparations used in some studies are a problem, as it is impossible to transfer the study results to everyday therapeutic practice. The penetration ability of a medication depends greatly on its composition; any changes in the chemical components compared to commercial preparations can strongly influence this ability (Allen Jr 2002a, b).

A major disadvantage of iontophoresis in therapy is the difficulty of dosing. The most important parameter in everyday therapeutic dosing is the duration of treatment. The recommendations vary, but with most medications, no significant effect is to be expected in less than 30 min (Ammer 2001). Treatment times of 40–60 min are more realistic (Pratzel et al. 1986a, b, c; Ebel and Dittrich 1986).

The concentration of the medication in the solution plays a rather subordinate role, as only a certain amount of the medication can pass through the skin per unit of time. In addition, therapists cannot increase the concentration anyway.

The intensity (current strength) cannot be varied significantly, as too high an intensity not only greatly increases the risk of burns, but can also cause electrolysis of the medication, rendering it ineffective. As a general guideline, **0.03 to a maximum of 0.2 mA per cm^2** of electrode area is recommended, so Panus was quite generous with his pigs. With an electrode area of 5 cm^2, this means that a maximum of $5 \times 0.2 = 1$ mA can be set.

A general note: Many complex compounds are negatively charged, so these are applied under the cathode. If you are unsure about the polarity: call the manufacturer!

The following are applied under the cathode:

- Contractubex® for scar treatment
- Dexamethasone: anti-inflammatory, a corticosteroid
- Diclofenac (Voltaren®): anti-inflammatory, an NSAID
- Dolo-Arthrosenex®: anti-inflammatory, an NSAID (hydroxyethyl salicylate, caution in patients with an Aspirin® allergy)
- Forapin (bee venom): strongly hyperemic (ALLERGIC PATIENTS!!)
- Potassium iodide solution 1% for scar treatment
- Mobilat®: anti-inflammatory (contains salicylate, caution Aspirin® allergy)

The following are applied under the anode:

- Hyaluronidase for scar treatment
- Ketoprofen (an NSAID), anti-inflammatory
- Lidocaine, Novocaine, Procaine, Scandicain, Lignocaine, all 1–5% solutions for local anesthesia
- Prednisolone, hydrocortisone for anti-inflammatory purposes

2.13.1 Iontophoresis as Therapy

Iontophoresis is an established application in basic pharmacological research. It is used as a diagnostic test in cystic fibrosis, for assessing microcirculation in various diseases, and in neurophysiological experiments. The effect of lidocaine iontophoresis for rapid local anesthesia (Strout et al. 2004) and for the administration of analgesics such as fentanyl (Skledar et al. 2015) is considered proven. Cosmetic applications are not discussed here.

Therapeutically, the application is used in the musculoskeletal system, most commonly in patients with superficial insertional tendinopathies such as tennis and golfer's elbow, shoulder problems, and plantar fasciitis. Study results vary widely and are often contradictory. Tinnitus treatment does not fall within the scope of physical or occupational therapy, but is mentioned here nonetheless, as the study results for this treatment are also diametrically opposed, yet it is still promoted as successful.

The following is an overview. Studies in which medications were used at non-commercial concentrations or where treatment parameters could not be determined were not considered.

- Li et al. (1996) performed dexamethasone iontophoresis on 10 patients with rheumatoid arthritis of the knee (4 mA, 20 min, indifferent electrode 40 cm^2, 20 treatments). Compared to a "standard" direct current treatment, patients in the ionto group had significantly less resting pain. Pressure pain, range of motion, and movement pain were the same in both groups.
- Demirtaş and Oner (1998) found that diclofenac iontophoresis for treating tennis elbow was more effective than iontophoresis with salicylate. Pain during resisted wrist extension and local pressure pain were reduced after a maximum of 18 treatments. Parameters: diclofenac under the cathode, 6–11 mA, electrodes 4.5 × 8 cm (36 cm^2), 20 min, once daily, 5 times/week, maximum 18 treatments.
- Laffrée et al. (1989) found no improvement in 40 tinnitus patients after lignocaine iontophoresis. Neither lignocaine nor its metabolites were detectable in the patients' blood samples after application. In this application, the local anesthetic is applied directly to the eardrum in the ear canal. The electrode is then inserted. The indifferent electrode was placed on the contralateral arm. Their parameters: lignocaine 2% in the ear canal, anode in the ear, 0.7–2 mA, 10 min, once daily, 4 days.
- Zeuner et al. (1989) conducted a study with 51 tinnitus patients, comparing the effect of lidocaine iontophoresis with placebo iontophoresis and TENS at the mastoid process. In all groups, 8–9 patients reported a brief improvement. The authors attribute any effect to the direct current. Parameters: same as Laffrée et al. (1989), but once a week, 5 times.
- Japour et al. (1999) treated 35 patients with heel pain using acetic acid iontophoresis (ethanoic acid 5%). The pain had various causes, including superior and inferior heel spurs and bursitis. After an average of 5.7 sessions over 2.8 weeks, 94% of patients experienced significant improvement. The improvement persisted after 27 months. Parameters: acid under a self-made aluminium foil cathode (12 × 18 cm = 216 cm^2), 2–3 mA (0.01 mA/cm^2), 15–20 min, 2–3 times/week. The authors suspect some kind of interaction between the acid and local calcium. Note: Unfortunately, there was no control group.
- da Luz et al. (2019) performed dexamethasone iontophoresis on 12 patients with tennis elbow and compared this group with an equally sized group treated with direct current. Both groups showed improvement in several areas, with the ionto group having the edge. Parameters: dexamethasone (4%) under the 5 × 10 cm cathode, 5 mA (0.1 mA/cm^2), 15 min, 3 times/week, 4 weeks. If irritation occurred, the intensity was reduced to 3 mA and the duration extended to 20 min.
- García et al. (2016) divided 88 patients with shoulder impingement into three groups. All groups received the same exercise therapy for 15 consecutive days. One group additionally received placebo iontophoresis and placebo sonophoresis, one group received verum iontophoresis with sodium diclofenac (from the standard 75-mg ampoule) and placebo sono, and the third group received placebo ionto and verum sono with diclofenac gel. Parameters: verum ionto: electrodes 5 × 5 cm, 0.1–0.2 mA/cm^2, 10 min. Diclofenac under the cathode. Verum sono: ERA 5 cm^2, 1 MHz, continuous mode, 0.7 W/cm^2, BNR < 5, treatment area 4 times the ERA, 5 min. The sonophoresis group clearly outperformed the ionto group. The latter was as effective as the placebo group. Note: 10 min is definitely too short for iontophoresis.

There are publications on iontophoresis reporting clear successes in the treatment of muscle insertion problems. The studies were almost always conducted on small groups of around 10 people, but were often of good methodological quality. However, it is regrettable and incomprehensible that it is usually impossible to determine the exact treatment parameters. The size of the electrodes is almost never mentioned, making it impossible to provide precise dosing information. This is partly because specially designed electrodes are often used for iontophoresis, with the active electrode being a type of chamber filled with the medication. These electrodes come in different sizes, and this is where the guessing begins. Manufacturer size specifications range from 7 × 7 cm (49 cm^2) to 10 × 10 cm (100 cm^2), and it is often unclear whether this refers to the chamber or the total electrode area. Nevertheless, based on the available publications, the following statements can be made:

- Iontophoresis with analgesic and/or anti-inflammatory medications such as dexamethasone and diclofenac can be used successfully for superficial musculoskeletal problems.
- A maximum current density of about 0.2 mA/cm^2 should be observed.
- Treatment times of 40 min or longer should be used.
- For local anesthesia with lidocaine and similar agents, treatment times of 10–15 min are sufficient.

The previously quite commonly prescribed histamine iontophoresis has fallen somewhat out of fashion and is not discussed here in detail. Older electrotherapy books explain this method extensively. The method is suitable only for inducing a pronounced local superficial hyperemia, which might trigger a reflex effect. There are no studies on this. Harris et al. (1955) demonstrated in 37 healthy subjects using isotope clearance measurement that after histamine iontophoresis, there was no improvement in blood flow at a depth of 1.5 cm in the brachioradialis muscle; in fact, blood flow in the muscle even decreased. Only in three subjects who had a generalized allergic reaction, including collapse, did blood flow increase. Their parameters: histamine gel 1% under the anode, 3.75 × 5 cm (18.75 cm^2), cathode 75 cm^2, 5–7.5 mA, 10–20 min.

Before iontophoresis, the skin should be thoroughly cleaned with alcohol or soap and checked for injuries. Sometimes the callus is gently abraded with very fine sandpaper, but caution is needed to avoid injury! Cleaning is important because otherwise contaminants present on the skin could displace the ions of the medication to be introduced, especially if these so-called parasitic ions are smaller and more mobile. This results in even less medication being delivered. Sensation must not be impaired due to the risk of burns. The patient must be specifically asked about allergies (salicylate in, e.g., Sportusal®: Aspirin® allergy).

Consideration
What is somewhat puzzling is the fact that immediately after lidocaine iontophoresis, local anesthesia of the skin occurs (Irsfeld et al. 1993), and that after ketoprofen iontophoresis, the medication is detectable at a depth of 1 cm (Panus et al. 1999), but that almost no patient, for example after diclofenac iontophoresis, experiences pain relief; it almost always takes several applications. This, even though it is a very potent analgesic. Almost everyone who has taken it as a tablet can confirm that the pain usually subsides after 15–20 min. So why not just as quickly after ionto? Shouldn't it also work immediately here? The idea that a sufficiently high concentration builds up over a certain number of treatments is unlikely: by the next treatment, the agent has been transported away and metabolized.

One could, of course, ask whether an improvement that occurs after 5–6 treatments is causally related to the medication used, or whether C fibers have been successfully desensitized. For example, if a so-called tennis elbow is treated over a period of 3–4 weeks, three times a week, with a treatment time of 30–40 min and an intensity that is barely or just perceptible, an effect on these fibers is quite plausible (Nilsson and Schouenborg 1999; Fietz-Rubusch 2000; Wallengren and Sundler 2001). The improvement can be explained by the defunctionalization of the involved nerve fibers, depletion of neuropeptide stores, and destruction of nerve terminals. That would be a good topic for a physiotherapy dissertation, wouldn't it?

2.13.2 Tap Water Iontophoresis

The term is actually nonsensical. It is not iontophoresis, but a direct current application like the cell bath, since no medications are "iontophoresed." Unless one accepts the introduction of dissociated water molecules (H_3O^+, "protons") as a mechanism of action (Sato et al. 1985), in which case the treatment should be called proton iontophoresis. Sato and colleagues suspect that the H_3O^+ molecules block certain ion channels and thus reduce sweat secretion. The theory is quite plausible. The anode is the effective electrode in this application and, as we have seen, H_3O^+ is produced here. Of course, one could also use the term "cell bath." The application is used successfully in the treatment of hyperhidrosis palmaris and pedis, i.e., pathologically increased sweating of the hands and/or feet or in the armpits, and in eczema of the hands and feet (Reinauer et al. 1993; Schauf et al. 1994; Wollina et al. 1998; Ammer 2001; Sonntag and Ruzicka 2004).

For application:

- The palms or soles, of course without jewelry, are immersed in separate shallow plastic trays (pre-digital photo accessories), without wetting the back of the fingers/hands or toes/feet. There are special electrodes for the armpits.
- The intensity is increased up to the tolerance limit. Small skin cracks, etc., are not a problem, as the intensity is set subjectively.
- The treatment duration is, depending on the author, 10–30 min.
- Treatment is performed, depending on the author, once a week up to daily.
- Results may be seen after as few as 4 treatments.

In a study by Reinauer (1993), the method was successful in 90% of subjects. Since the anode is most effective in this application, it makes sense to switch polarity. The use of medium-frequency alternating current (5.1 kHz) is ineffective (Reinauer et al. 1993). In addition to normal direct current and the aforementioned ineffective alternating current, Reinauer et al. used a somewhat special pulsed current with a frequency of 4.3 kHz. They refer to this current as alternating current with a direct current component (AC with DC offset); in fact, it was a monophasic (uncompensated) pulsed current. In a later study (1995), Reinauer et al. compared the effect of normal direct current, a monophasic pulsed current with a frequency of 4.3 kHz, and a similarly monophasic one with 10 kHz. Normal direct current was the most effective, and the 10 kHz pulsed current was more effective than the 4.3 kHz one. Since the 10 kHz current was less unpleasant, the authors recommend it for "pulsed direct current iontophoresis."

The following treatment protocol has proven effective (Schauf et al. 1994):

- Initially, treatment is performed 3 times a week, duration 10–15 min. It makes sense to start with the dominant hand.
- The anode remains on the same side until a clear improvement occurs. Only then is the other hand (foot) treated anodically until improvement is also achieved there.
- In the subsequent "maintenance phase," patients are treated about once a week for 10–15 min (every 6–8 days). Polarity is changed each week, but not during the session (i.e., one week the left hand anodic, the next week the right hand).
- Normal, non-demineralized tap water is used.

The German Dermatological Society and the Professional Association of German Dermatologists e. V. provide detailed information about this interesting application on the internet, see https://dgdc.de/hyperhidrose.html.

There are small, relatively inexpensive battery-operated devices for iontophoresis, as well as medications in similar packaging, such as nicotine or hormone patches. Some even have integrated electrodes, so the patient does not have to deal with cables. These devices allow patients to conveniently perform iontophoresis at home, for example for chronic pain (fentanyl ionto in terminal cancer patients) or other chronic conditions (Ashburn et al. 1995; Fanelli et al. 2016). The same devices are used for home treatment of hyperhidrosis.

2.14 Pulsed Current

In electrotherapy, a pulse is a surge of current generated by a change in current strength or voltage, affecting those structures specialized in excitation generation and conduction. The effect of electrical charges in tissue depends on the speed at which a change in current strength occurs. If the change is rapid and the pulse duration is sufficiently long and the intensity high enough, the ionic equilibrium along excitable membranes is disturbed, triggering action potentials. Uncompensated (unbalanced) pulses also trigger chemical processes, but these are less pronounced with shorter pulses. In other words: the shorter the pulse, the smaller the ion flow and the fewer chemical changes in the tissue. With compensated (balanced) pulses, the chemical changes of one phase are offset by the second phase. In low-frequency stimulation with uncompensated or asymmetrically compensated pulses, the cathode has the stronger effect.

2.14.1 Chronaxie, Rheobase

Current strength and pulse duration are directly related in triggering an action potential: at a certain intensity, a certain minimum pulse duration is required to trigger an action potential. At a certain pulse duration, a certain minimum intensity must be exceeded.

The *rheobase* is the minimum intensity required to trigger an action potential in a nerve or a minimal contraction (twitch) in a muscle at a pulse duration of 1000 ms. The *chronaxie* is the minimum phase duration (pulse duration) that, at twice the rheobase value, triggers an action potential in a nerve or a minimal contraction in a muscle. The main utilization time is the minimum time a current at single rheobase strength must flow to trigger an action potential in a nerve or a minimal contraction in a muscle.

The relationship between phase duration and amplitude is shown in the SD curve (strength-duration curve). Creating SD curves enables the therapist to (very) roughly assess the condition of the musculature in a peripheral nerve lesion and to determine the correct parameters for muscle stimulation. A detailed description of this stimulation can be found under "muscle stimulation" (Sect. 4.9.2).

2.14.2 The Pulse

A pulse is characterized by various parameters (Table 2.1, Fig. 2.15):

Amplitude, rise and fall time, and pulse duration determine the *amount of charge* that is moved. Pulse trains can be modulated in terms of amplitude, frequency, and polarity.

If all pulses have the same polarity, they are called monophasic. With currents of this pulse form, an ion current flows and chemical changes occur in the tissue; therefore, the pulses are referred to as *non-compensated or unbalanced*. Examples: Träbert's ultrastimulation current (= 2–5 current) and Bernard's diadynamic current (Fig. 2.16).

When the polarity alternates, these are called *biphasic* pulses. These can be shaped so that the ion current generated during the positive part of the pulse is immediately balanced by the subsequent negative part. As a result, the net ion current is zero, and chemical changes are neutralized. These pulses are referred to as *compensated* or balanced. This compensation can be symmetric or asymmetric. With symmetric compensation, the positive and negative pulse parts

Table 2.1 Pulse parameters

Current intensity I = amplitude of the current, the intensity	This determines whether and to what extent the stimulation threshold is exceeded. The unit of current intensity is 1 ampere (A) or milliampere (mA). This is what the patient feels
Rise and fall time	Describes the time it takes for the pulse to reach its maximum strength or to return to zero. These times depend on the *geometry* (shape) of the pulse, e.g., triangular, rectangular, trapezoidal- or exponential pulse
Phase duration T (= pulse duration, pulse width), T = time	The duration during which current actually flows. The phase duration determines the so-called direct current component of the current's effect. The longer the pulse at the same frequency, the greater the ion flow and the chemical load on the tissue. Unit: s, ms, or µs
Phase interval R (= pause duration), R = rest	The time between pulses. Together with the phase duration, it determines the pulse frequency, i.e., the number of pulses per second. Phase duration and phase interval together make up the duration of the actual pulse (period duration). Unit: s, ms, or µs
Frequency f	This is defined as the number of pulses per second or the reciprocal of the period duration $f = 1/(T + R)$. The unit of frequency is 1 Hz (1 Hz = 1/s). Also pps: pulses per second
Direct current component (galvanic component)	This component of the physiological effect of a pulse determines the hyperemic effect of a pulsed current. The direct current component of the current *effect* should not be confused with the (in electrotherapy otherwise irrelevant) direct current component of the current when a direct current is superimposed on an alternating current. "DC component" is more general, i.e., for current, voltage, etc. Direct current component is a specific term for the offset of current
Compensated, non-compensated = balanced, unbalanced	When using alternating current pulses, there is no net current flow. The chemical reactions from the first part of the pulse are counteracted by the second part. Compensation can be symmetric or asymmetric; this is also referred to as zero-line symmetric (= bidirectional) or zero-line asymmetric (= unidirectional). Monophasic and biphasic usually mean the same, but (unfortunately) there are also biphasic asymmetric (i.e., NOT compensated) pulses

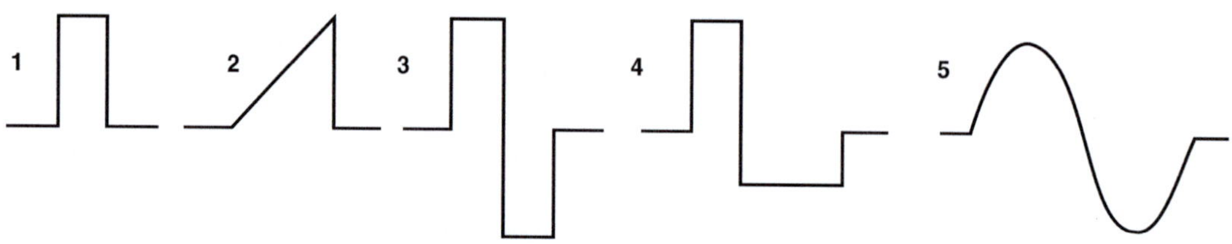

Fig. 2.15 Various pulse shapes. 1 = monophasic rectangular (non-compensated); 2 = monophasic triangular; 3 = biphasic rectangular, symmetrically compensated; 4 = biphasic rectangular, asymmetrically compensated; 5 = sine, biphasic, compensated

look the same. With asymmetric compensation, the shape of the compensating pulse part differs from the preceding one. The shape of a pulse has no effect on its efficacy (Hingne and Sluka 2007). Theoretically, a symmetrically compensated pulse can be considered a "double pulse." Such symmetrically compensated rectangular pulses elicit the strongest contractions when stimulating innervated muscles at the same intensity and are therefore preferred in NMES.

The intensity setting for pulsed currents can be classified as follows:

- Sensory subthreshold = subsensory: no sensations are perceived.
- Sensory threshold = sensory: sensations are perceived.
- Motor threshold: a muscle contraction is elicited.

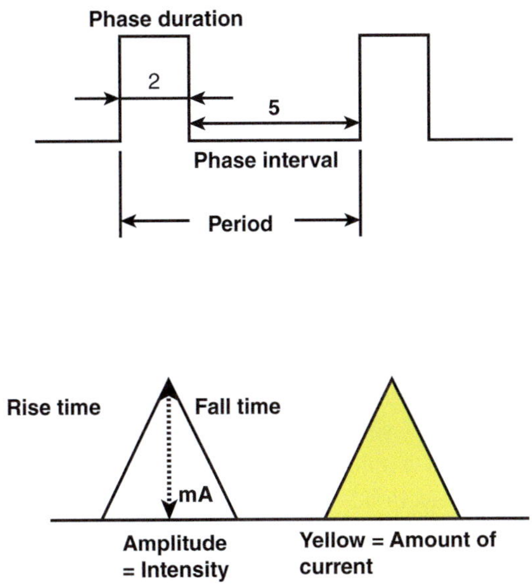

Fig. 2.16 Pulse parameters, above: 2–5 current according to Träbert

- Tolerance limit: very clearly perceptible, but not yet painful application.
- Pain threshold: the application becomes painful.

In pathological cases, the order may change, for example, the tolerance limit may be reached before a contraction is visible.

For motor criteria, the following distinctions are made:

- Motor subthreshold: no visible contraction
- Motor threshold: just visible contraction ("waves")
- Motor suprathreshold: clearly wave-like contractions ("kneading".)

The low-frequency range (LF) is defined as the frequency range between 0 and 1000 Hz. Here, the principle of *period-synchronous* (= cycle-synchronous) stimulation applies. This means that each pulse, provided phase duration and amplitude are sufficient, triggers an excitation (an action potential). The action potentials are triggered at the same rhythm as the frequency of the current. The 1000 Hz limit, as explained elsewhere, is rather arbitrarily chosen.

The so-called classic LF includes the old *faradization*, an alternating current with irregular frequencies between 50 Hz and 100 Hz, which was used for muscle stimulation at the end of the 19th century. The frequency fluctuated due to the lack of technical equipment at the time and was replaced in the 1950s by "neofaradization," an alternating current with a steady 50 Hz frequency (phase duration = 1 ms, phase interval = 19 ms). Today, we have much more comfortable current forms available for eliciting muscle contraction, so this current form will not be discussed further. However, the long pulse (1 ms = 1000 μs), combined with a frequency of 100 Hz, elicits different reactions in muscle stimulation than the usual NMES parameters. These so-called wide pulse NMES are discussed in the relevant chapter (Sect. 4.6.1).

Other classics are the *diadynamic currents according to Bernard* and the *ultrastimulation current according to Träbert*. When used and applied correctly, these two current forms repeatedly yield good results. The following sections will discuss these two current forms in more detail.

For a better understanding of the mechanisms of action of hyperemic current forms, refer to the section on *neurogenic inflammation* (Sect. 2.9).

The different types of nerve fibers can, due to their varying excitability, be selectively stimulated with certain phase durations. This is utilized in TENS applications. Very short pulses, up to about 100 μs, stimulate the most sensitive, fast-conducting nerve fibers of type Aα and Aβ, without—depending on intensity and any sensitization—stimulating the Aδ and C fibers. Slightly longer pulses, 100 μs to about 300 μs, are used to stimulate Aδ fibers (and simultaneously stimulate Aα and Aβ fibers). C fibers are stimulated with phase durations from about 500 μs to 1 ms. Of course, with longer phase durations, the faster-conducting Aα, Aβ, and Aδ fibers are also co-stimulated.

It should be noted that, if inflammation is present, the nerve fibers are sensitized by inflammatory mediators. This means that the fibers can fire at very low intensities and short pulses.

2.14.3 Ultrastimulation Current According to Träbert (UR, 2–5 Current)

In 1957, the physician H. Träbert published his experiences with a current form with a 2 ms phase duration and a 5 ms phase interval (Fig. 2.17, top). This resulted in a frequency of about 143 Hz ($F = 1000/R + T = 1000/2 + 5 = 1000/7 = 143$ Hz). This current is very effective as a pain-relieving measure in certain cases, and the parameters can, if not already pre-programmed, be conveniently set on most electrotherapy devices; for this reason, the method became quite well known.

Compared to the diadynamic currents discussed below, this current form has a significantly lower direct current component, which greatly reduces the risk of burns. For the same reason, one would expect a less pronounced erythema. However, the current is much more comfortable than DD, and one can (and should) therefore set the intensity much higher. For lumbar applications, settings up to 70–80 mA with electrode sizes of 8 × 12 cm are not uncommon! For this reason, despite the low direct current component, UR application usually results in a very pronounced erythema.

With this current form, habituation almost always occurs very quickly. Therefore, the intensity must be continuously readjusted during treatment.

The patient should perceive a distinct pressure sensation; a possible, not too strong muscle contraction ("waves") is desirable due to the detoning effect. It is possible that deep Aδ fibers are additionally stimulated, resulting in an effect comparable to low TENS.

A variant of the UR according to Träbert is the modified UR with unipolar rectangular pulses of 0.5 ms phase duration and 5 ms phase interval (frequency 182 Hz). The shorter pulses stimulate the pain fibers of the skin less and are perceived as more comfortable. The hyperemia and thus the influence on neurogenic inflammation are correspondingly less pronounced due to the much shorter phase duration, and the typical pressure sensation is less prominent. Colleagues report better efficacy with the 2–5 form, which also matches the author's experience. There are no studies on this.

The following should be observed during application.

- Usually, two equally sized, well-padded electrodes are used. Electrode size ranges from 3 × 4 cm (cervical spine) to 8 × 12 cm (lumbar spine).
- The electrodes should be about 3 cm apart. On the spine, the electrodes are usually placed cranio-caudally; on peripheral joints, the electrodes are placed ventro-dorsally or medio-laterally.
- The cathode, the differential electrode, is placed on the most painful spot. For EL4, Träbert recommends placing the cathode distally.
- Treatment should be performed daily. If there is no improvement after 3 to a maximum of 6 sessions, another method should be used. If the method is successful, a series of 6 sessions is usually sufficient.
- Applications to the cervical and thoracic spine are often perceived as (very) unpleasant due to the high intensity required. Therefore, the method is mainly used on the lumbar spine (evidence level IV and V).
- When the current is first increased, the patient feels a slight tingling (probably Aβ, see MacKenzie et al. 1975; Beissner et al. 2010), then a prickling (probably Aδ) under the electrodes, usually first under the cathode, as this is the most stimulating. However, this also depends on the location and skin sensitivity.
- Then the intensity is further increased relatively quickly but carefully, and after the tingling or prickling becomes stronger, a burning sensation usually occurs. *This is a normal C-fiber burning and does not usually indicate damage*. With further increase, the patient feels a pressure or a peculiar vibration ("buzzing, humming") instead of burning, which overrides the burning sensation. Mild

to moderate muscle contractions may occur, which are desirable, but strong sustained contractions are not.

If the burning occurs at a specific point, it may be a small skin lesion, a pustule. These should be covered with Vaseline or lip balm. The problem is that the intensity must be reduced for this, and the treatment must then be restarted. In practice, it is usually impossible to achieve the desired pressure sensation again. In this case, it is better to discontinue the treatment.

- For lumbar application, the patient may feel as if someone is pressing very firmly on their back. This pressure sensation quickly subsides, sometimes within the first minute. Now the current must be carefully readjusted, often by only 1 mA, until the typical pressure sensation reappears. *Caution with devices that do not allow stepless adjustment!* The small intensity jumps can be very unpleasant.
- Usually, the current only needs to be readjusted during the first 7–8 min; after that, the pressure sensation usually remains constant. Treatment lasts about 15 min. If, despite correct application, no pressure sensation occurs or if burning remains too prominent, the treatment should be discontinued.

Pre-existing pain often disappears abruptly. The pain relief can last for several hours, after which the pain may return, though less intense (Long Term Depression?).

This description makes it clear that patient information and feedback are of utmost importance for successful treatment. The treatment is absolutely unsuitable for anxious patients or those with communication problems. It is also clear that the therapist must remain with the patient to continuously increase the current. Suitable patients can, over time, be instructed to do this themselves.

The pain relief can be explained by the gate control theory; the pressure sensation indicates involvement of the Aβ fibers, and it is possible that the pressure receptors themselves are stimulated at high intensities. In addition, long term depression probably plays a role. Due to the relatively strong erythema, as with DD current, an effect on the TRPV1 receptor is quite plausible.

Notes on Ultrastimulation Current

Strictly speaking, ultrastimulation is a TENS application, namely a monophasic variant of high TENS or high frequency high intensity TENS (Hifi-TENS). The direct current component in UR is about 30% of a continuous direct current application, so caution: risk of burns! Interestingly, with the mentioned TENS forms, the typical pressure sensation that occurs with UR is not felt. Very good effects have been observed in acute lumbar pain and, interestingly, in knee osteoarthritis pain (evidence level V). It is possible that, as with DD, defunctionalization of the nerve fibers involved in the inflammatory process occurs.

The application only makes sense if communication with the patient works. If the feedback is limited to "Yeah, yeah, it's fine ... it's okay," the success will not be overwhelming. Note: There are no specific scientific studies on ultrastimulation application. However, the effect of the application is confirmed by studies on TENS.

2.14.4 Diadynamic Currents According to Bernard

In 1950, the French dentist P. D. Bernard published a study on the effects he discovered from various variations of a unidirectional 50 Hz alternating current. Rectification ensures that only half of a sinusoidal current flows, resulting in a current of sinusoidal half-waves. The rise and fall time of these half-waves is 5 ms each, resulting in a pulse duration of 10 ms. The pause after such a half-wave is also 10 ms (period duration = 20 ms).

These relatively long impulses have a large direct current component, so all measures to prevent burns should be observed. However, it is this direct current component that gives the current its very pronounced superficial hyperemic effect. The direct current component is about 70% for DF and about 35% for MF compared to a normal direct current (mean value of the current = maximum value ÷ √2).

In addition to the impulse currents, Bernard used a galvanic "base current" dosed below the sensory threshold, which was intended to increase the effectiveness of the impulses (Table 2.2, Fig. 2.17).

In his publication (Bernard 1950), Bernard himself does not make any treatment recommendations, but instead presents a large number of case reports of various pathologies. Many "recipes" were later developed from these by other authors. His method of treating herpes zoster (shingles) with DD was popular for a time (Vossen and de Wijer 2019). However, the treatment effect is difficult to assess in this self-limiting pathology. After van Ree (1977) was unable to detect any effect in a small study and Lanting et al. in 1996, despite finding three positive studies, gave a negative assessment, the method was

Table 2.2 Current forms distinguished by Bernard

Monophasé fixe (MF)	50 Hz, a 10 ms pulse is followed by a 10 ms pause
Diphasé fixe (DF)	100 Hz, the 10 ms impulses run continuously
Courant modulé en courtes périodes (CP)	1 s of 50 Hz (MF) and 1 s of 100 Hz (DF) alternate abruptly
Courant modulé en longues periods (LP)	As with CP, MF and DF alternate, but now in longer periods and gradually (every 12–16 s according to Bernard). The periods vary in rhythm depending on the device manufacturer
Courant modulé en moyenne périodes (MP)	Like LP, but with 5 s DF and 5 s MF; no longer found on more modern devices
Rhythme syncopé 50 (RS50)	After 1 s MF, 1 s pause follows
Rhythme syncopé 100 (RS100)	After 1 s DF, 1 s pause follows; no longer found on more modern devices
The base current	Direct current just below the threshold of perception, which is superimposed on the impulses so that these impulses are fully raised into the sensory range. Not useful

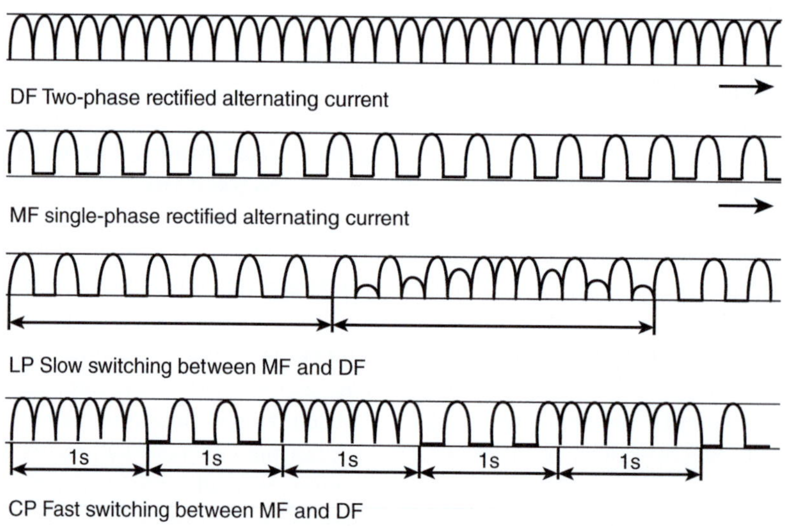

Fig. 2.17 Diadynamic current according to Bernard, the most commonly used modulations. The current forms may vary depending on the manufacturer. © Enraf-Nonius, Delft, Netherlands, with kind permission

at least abandoned in the Netherlands (Ree and Lanting are mentioned in Vossen and de Wijer 2019). Due to modern (and cheaper!) pharmacological options, the method has been completely forgotten. Since expensive capsaicin patches are used successfully, among other things, in the treatment of postherpetic neuralgia, the use of DD could well be worthwhile. Perhaps someone will take up this method as the basis for a study and provide the treatment with a scientific foundation.

2.14.4.1 Treating Herpes Zoster with DD Current

Treatment should begin as early as possible, ideally before the blisters have fully erupted.

- Treatment is performed with two cup electrodes about 5 cm in size, as known from the "head-phone-like" electrode.
- The patient lies on their side, with the affected side up. The two electrodes are placed unilaterally paravertebrally on the thorax, cranially and caudally to the affected nerve (held in place by hand, not fixed), with about 5 cm between the electrodes.
- Optionally, start with 1 min DF, then reverse polarity and apply another 1 min DF. Intensity: very clearly perceptible, at the tolerance limit (Bernard's original wording: "au maximum supportable par le malade").
- Then, as Bernard did, use CP: 2 min, then reverse polarity, another 2 min at the same intensity as above.
- The patient then holds one electrode ventrally on the thorax, where the pain or blisters end. The other electrode is held by the therapist dorsally, paravertebrally over the exit point of the affected intercostal nerve.
- Procedure: optionally again 1 min DF, then reverse polarity, another 1 min DF. Then 2 min CP, reverse polarity, 2 min CP. Intensity as above.
- Due to the risk of infection, the sponges should be used only for this one patient and discarded after treatment is completed.
- In cases of severe pain, treatment can also be performed with DF or LP only.

Bernard originally treated only with CP, without prior DF. However, patients often find this preparation very pleasant.

For larger skin defects and for herpes zoster on the face, the electrodes are placed directly on the blisters. Allegedly, the blisters disappear very quickly (within days) and, in particular, the dreaded persistent postherpetic neuralgia occurs—also allegedly—much less frequently (statement by Dr. Bernard during a lecture). Bernard explained the effect of this application by the improved trophic state due to the current. However, an effect comparable to cutaneous field stimulation is also conceivable: defunctionalization of the involved nerve fibers.

Bernard attributed different effects to his current forms; see his 1950 publication or, for example, Edel (1977). There is no reason to assume that these effects actually occur; the modulations differ only in their direct current component due to the different frequencies.

CP is traditionally used for swellings and effusions, possibly after pretreatment with DF. There is neither evidence nor rationale for its effectiveness. DF, due to its higher direct current component, would be more hyperemic; the supposed "pumping effect" of CP only occurs if CP is dosed to produce a motor response, and even then it is much less pronounced and certainly much more unpleasant than a swelling current application.

DD can be used for pain relief. However, TENS is certainly more pleasant and less risky. If the goal is to influence both neurogenic inflammation and pain simultaneously, the following method is worth a try. The method is not described here for historical reasons, but because there is evidence for its effectiveness (Heggannavar et al. 2015; Sayilir and Yildizgoren 2017; Senthilkumar et al. 2019).

2.14.4.2 DF-LP-CP

There is no evidence or meaningful physiological rationale for the "recipes" described by Bernard and his followers, such as "so many minutes DF, reverse polarity, again so many minutes, and so on." Nevertheless, it can be assumed that the application stimulates Aβ, Aδ, and C fibers, with all the described consequences. If you want to use DD according to more modern insights, you can do so in two ways:

- You can use the application as an alternative to direct current and force neuropeptide depletion in the relevant nerve fibers and induce their defunctionalization. DF, compared to "normal" direct current, has the highest direct current component (70%) and is therefore most effective for this purpose. Determine the sensory threshold, halve it or go slightly below this threshold, and treat for 20–30 min. Since the direct current component is 70% of a normal direct current, the treatment duration must be extended by about two thirds, i.e., 30–40 min. Continue as described under direct current (Sect. 2.10.3).
- The second method is based on the fact that stimulation of Aβ, Aδ, and C fibers simultaneously activates several pain inhibition mechanisms. Additionally, provoking neuropeptide depletion is a useful side effect. The following method is used:
  - As the first and mildest current form, choose DF. Increase the intensity until the patient perceives a distinct vibration (involvement of Aβ fibers). Some patients describe this as a "vise-like feeling." Patients sometimes think the electrode has slipped. Before the vibration occurs, the patient usually feels a C-fiber burning sensation. This usually disappears abruptly as soon as the vibration is perceived. Please note that it is only a sensation of vibration; nothing is actually vibrating.
  - When the patient has become accustomed to the current, i.e., when adaptation occurs, there are two options. You can increase the intensity slightly until the pressure sensation returns. This is what you would do in a TENS application, and it is also possible in this case. Some colleagues do this once or twice if a patient adapts very quickly to the current, instead of immediately switching the modulation. However, the disadvantage of repeatedly increasing the intensity is that with DD current there is a risk of burns, and the higher you turn it up, the greater this risk becomes. However, with DD, various modulations are available to prevent adaptation. Therefore, after possibly increasing the current once or twice, reduce it and switch to the somewhat less mild LP. Increase again until a changing vibration sensation occurs. The required intensity is usually only 1–2 mA above the previous setting. If the current sensation changes again after some time, use CP as the final modulation.
  - The application traditionally lasts about 15 min, but can certainly last longer.
  - MF and RS are clearly too unpleasant for pain treatments.

The aim of this method is to bypass adaptation without having to greatly increase the intensity, as with Träberts ultra-high stimulation current. The modulations do not have different effects; the sequence is only intended to prevent adaptation. Pain relief can be explained on the one hand by the gate control theory via stimulation of Aβ fibers. On the other hand, stimulation of Aδ and C fibers will very likely activate descending and central pain inhibition. Locally, a capsaicin-like effect can be assumed, with desensitization and reversible destruction of the involved nerve terminals.

In this context, it is interesting that Bernard, in his list of case reports, mentions some diagnoses in which some authors today suspect a neurogenic inflammation in the background (Herbert and Holzer 2002a, b): neuralgias, PHS, epicondylitis, and similar conditions.

2.14.4.3 Base Current

A major point of criticism concerns the use of the *base current*. According to Bernard, this was supposed to make the treatment method more effective by "raising" the impulse. The raising was intended to ensure that the entire impulse was in the sensory range and could fully exert its effect, and to prevent part of the impulse from remaining subthreshold. However, with prolonged, subthreshold, cathodic stimulation

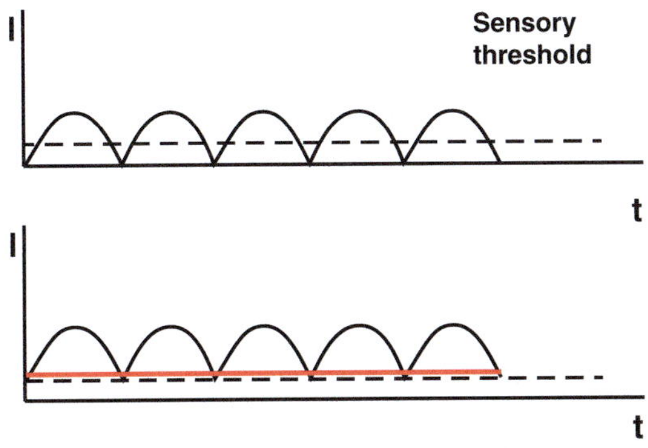

Fig. 2.18 The base current. The impulse series is "raised" so that the entire impulse lies within the sensory range

currents, instead of increased excitability, there is a decrease in excitability or, in extreme cases, a block of excitation. The Na carrier systems are inactivated by catelectrotonus and are then no longer able to allow the Na influx necessary for excitation. Consequently, the effect of incoming impulses is reduced. Therefore, the author definitely advises against the use of the base current (Fig. 2.18).

2.14.4.4 Notes on Diadynamic Current

The clinical significance of DD should not be overestimated. Apart from their respective direct current component, the individual modulations have no specific effects. DD is indeed an effective method when it comes to inducing local superficial hyperemia and influencing local trophic state; however, this can also be achieved with a simple direct current application. In addition to the direct current effect, the method also has an analgesic effect. This is explained by Aβ fiber stimulation via a gate control mechanism; stimulation of Aδ and C fibers will activate descending and central pain inhibition. In addition, long-term depression probably also plays a role due to Aδ fiber stimulation. The strong hyperemic effect due to the large direct current component makes a capsaicin-like effect likely. All of these are arguments for its use in appropriate cases. As a pain treatment, it is certainly useful, especially when neurogenic inflammation is suspected, as in enthesopathies and chronic arthritis.

2.15 Contraindications

The contraindications are the same as for all low-frequency applications; see the list in Ch. 3. There are no publications on the occurrence of disturbances in pacemakers and implanted cardioverter-defibrillators (ICDs) in connection with direct current, but it still seems sensible to maintain a minimum safety distance of 50 cm and, if necessary, consult a cardiologist. In any case, these patients should be particularly well monitored. That a Stanger bath and a two-cell bath of the upper extremities are absolutely contraindicated for these patients is self-evident. This also applies to tap water iontophoresis. Metal in the treatment area is an absolute contraindication for the reasons given above, not because of possible heating, but because of local chemical changes. Deep-seated metal-containing intrauterine contraceptives (IUDs) are very likely not a contraindication for treatment on the back or abdomen. There are no studies on this. Heating of the IUD can be excluded due to the low current strengths.

References

Ainsworth A, Hall P, Wall PD, Allt G, MacKenzie L, Gibson S, Polak JM (1981) Effects of Capsaicin applied locally to adult peripheral nerve. 2. Anatomy and enzyme and peptide chemistry of peripheral nerve and spinal cord. Pain 11:379–388

Allen LV Jr (2002a) Basics of compounding: iontophoresis. Int J Pharm Compd 6(3):194–197

Allen LV Jr (2002b) Basics of compounding: iontophoresis, part 2. Int J Pharm Compd 6(4):288–292

Ammer K (2001) Iontophorese – ein Überblick. Österr Z Phys Med Rehabil 11:25–31

Anand P, Bley K (2011) Topical capsaicin for pain management: therapeutic potential and mechanisms of action of the new high-concentration capsaicin 8% patch. Br J Anaesth 107(4):490–502

Anderson W, Sheth R, Bencherif B, Frost J, Campbell J (2002) Naloxone increases pain induced by topical capsaicin in healthy human volunteers. Pain 99:207–216

Ashburn MA, Streisand J, Zhang J, Love G, Rowin M, Niu S, Kievit JK, Kroep JR, Mertens MJ (1995) The iontophoresis of fentanyl citrate in humans. Anesthesiology 82(5):1146–1153

Balblanc JC, Vignon E, Mathieu P, Broquet P, Conrozier T, Richard M (1991) Cytokines, prostaglandin E2, phospholipase A and metalloproteases in synovial

fluid in osteoarthritis. Rev Rheum Mal Osteoartic 58(5):343–347
Bayliss WM (1901) On the origin from the spinal cord of vasodilator fibres of the hind limb and on the nature of these fibres. J Physiol 26:173–209
Beissner F, Brandau A, Henke C, Felden L, Baumgärtner U, Treede RD, Oertel BG, Lötsch J (2010) Quick discrimination of A(delta) and C fiber mediated pain based on three verbal descriptors. PLoS One 5(9):e12944
Bennett GJ (2001) Are the complex regional pain syndromes due to neurogenic inflammation? Neurology 57:2161–2162
Berliner MN (1997) Reduced skin hyperemia during tap water iontophoresis after intake of acetylsalicylic acid. Am J Phys Med Rehabil 76(6):482–487
Bernard PD (1950) La thérapie dia-dynamique. Éditions „Physio", 34, Avenue A.-Briand – B.P. No 11, 94114 Arceuil Cédex
Birklein F, Schmelz M (2008) Neuropeptides, neurogenic inflammation and complex regional pain syndrome (CRPS). Neurosci Lett 437(3):199–202
Chal LA (1988) Antidromic vasodilatation and neurogenic inflammation. Pharmac Ther 37:275–300
Cheshire WP, Snyder CR (1990) Treatment of reflex sympathetic dystrophy with topical capsaicin, Case report. Pain 42:307–311
Decaris E, Guingamp C, Chat M, Philippe L, Grillasca JP, Abid A, Minn A, Gillet P, Netter P, Terlain B (1999) Evidence for neurogenic transmission inducing degenerative cartilage damage distant from local inflammation. Arthritis Rheum 42(9):1951–1960
Demirtaş RN, Oner C (1998) The treatment of lateral epicondylitis by iontophoresis of sodium salicylate and sodium diclofenac. Clin Rehabil Feb 12(1):23–29
Dobson GP, Letson HL, Grant A, McEwen P, Hazratwala K, Wilkinson M, Morris JL (2018) Defining the osteoarthritis patient: back to the future. Osteoarthr Cartil 26(8):1003–1007
Dubner R (1991) Topical capsaicin therapy for neuropathic pain. Pain 47:247–248
Durand S, Fromy B, Bouyé P, Saumet JL, Abraham P (2002a) Vasodilatation in response to repeated anodal current application in the human skin relies on aspirin-sensitive mechanisms. J Physiol 540(Pt 1):261–269
Durand S, Fromy B, Koïtka A, Tartas M, Saumet JL, Abraham P (2002b) Oral single high-dose aspirin results in a long-lived inhibition of anodal current-induced vasodilatation. Br J Pharmacol 137(3):384–390
Ebel R, Dittrich P (1986) Indometacin-Spiegel nach Applikation von Amuno Gel unter Iontophorese. Akt Rheumatol 11:23–24
Edel H (1977) Fibel der Elektrodiagnostik und Elektrotherapie, 4. Aufl. Verlag Theodor Steinkopff, Dresden
Falkenbach A, Wendt T (1993) The effect of „ascending" and „descending" Stanger-baths on the autonomous cardiac innervation and on mental relaxation. Clin Invest Med 16:B110
Fanelli A, Sorella MC, Chelly JE (2016) Iontophoretic transdermal fentanyl for the management of acute perioperative pain in hospitalized patients. Expert Opin Pharmacother 17(4):571–577
Fattori V, Hohmann MS, Rossaneis AC, Pinho-Ribeiro FA, Verri WA (2016) Capsaicin: current understanding of its mechanisms and therapy of pain and other pre-clinical and clinical uses. Molecules 21(7):844
Fietz-Rubusch S (2000) Vergleichende Untersuchung zweier verschiedener Dosisanordnungen der Galvanisation auf das Modell des experimentell erzeugten ischämischen Muskelschmerzes am Menschen. Inaugural-Dissertation, Justus-Liebig-Universität Giessen. http://geb.uni-giessen.de/geb/volltexte/2001/514/. Zugegriffen am 14.06.2012
Fredberg U, Stengaard-Pedersen K (2008) Chronic tendinopathy tissue pathology, pain mechanisms, and etiology with a special focus on inflammation. Scand J Med Sci Sports 18(1):3–15
García I, Lobo C, López E, Serván JL, Tenías JM (2016) Comparative effectiveness of ultrasonophoresis and iontophoresis in impingement syndrome: a double-blind, randomized, placebo controlled trial. Clin Rehabil 30(4):347–358
Gjerstad J, Tjölsen A, Svendsen F, Hole K (1999) Inhibition of evoked C-fibre responses in the dorsal horn after contralateral intramuscular injection of capsaicin involves activation of descending pathways. Pain 80:413–418
Handwerker HO (1999) Einführung in die Pathophysiologie des Schmerzes. Springer, Berlin/Heidelberg, ISBN 3-540-62798-7
Harden RN, Wallach G, Gagnon CM, Zereshki A, Mukai A, Saracoglu M, Kuroda MM, Graciosa JR, Bruehl S (2013) The osteoarthritis knee model: psychophysical characteristics and putative outcomes. J Pain 14(3):281–289
Harris R, Williams HS, Buckler WSJ (1955) Local vascular effects of histamine iontophoresis and the direct current. A comparative study. Ann Phys Med. January 2(5):153–163
Heggannavar AB, Ramannavar PR, Bhodaji SS (2015) Effectiveness of diadynamic current and MENS in heel pain: a randomized clinical trial. Int J Physiother Res 2:992–998
Herbert MK, Holzer P (2002a) Die neurogene Entzündung 1. Grundlegende Mechanismen. Anaesth Intensivmed Notfallmed Schmerzther 37:314–325
Herbert MK, Holzer P (2002b) Die neurogene Entzündung 2. Pathophysiologie und klinische Implikationen. Anaesth Intensivmed Notfallmed Schmerzther 37:386–394
Hingne PM, Sluka KA (2007) Differences in waveform characteristics have no effect on the anti-hyperalgesia produced by Transcutaneous Electrical Nerve

Stimulation (TENS) in rats with joint inflammation. J Pain 8(3):251–255
Irsfeld S, Klement W, Lipfert P (1993) Dermal anaesthesia: comparison of EMLA cream with iontophoretic local anaesthesia. Br J Anaesth 71(3):375–378
Japour CJ, Vohra R, Vohra PK, Garfunkel L, Chin N (1999) Management of heel pain syndrome with acetic acid iontophoresis. J Am Podiatr Med Assoc 89(5):251–257
Kallakuri S, Singh A, Chen C, Cavanaugh JM (2004) Demonstration of substance P, calcitonin gene-related peptide, and protein gene product 9.5 containing nerve fibers in human cervical facet joint capsules. Spine 29(11):1182–1186
Kelly S, Dunham JP, Donaldson LF (2007) Sensory nerves have altered function contralateral to a monoarthritis and may contribute to the symmetrical spread of inflammation. Eur J Neurosci 26(4):935–942
Kempuraj D, Mentor S, Thangavel R, Ahmed ME, Selvakumar GP, Raikwar SP, Dubova I, Zaheer S, Iyer SS, Zaheer A (2019) Mast cells in stress, pain, blood-brain barrier, neuroinflammation and Alzheimer's disease. Front Cell Neurosci 13:54
Koltzenburg M, Handwerker HO (1994) Differential ability of human cutaneous nociceptors to signal mechanical pain and to produce vasodilatation. J Neurosci 14(3):1756–1765
Konttinen YT, Tiainen VM, Gomez-Barrena E, Hukkanen M, Salo J (2006) Innervation of the joint and role of neuropeptides. Ann N Y Acad Sci 1069:149–154
Kowalski M, Kaliner M (1988) Neurogenic inflammation, vascular permeability and mast cells. J Immunol 140:3905–3911
Laffrée JB, Vermeij P, Hulshof JH (1989) The effect of iontophoresis of lignocaine in the treatment of tinnitus. Clin Otolaryngol Allied Sci 14(5):401–404
Leis S, Weber M, Schmelz M, Birklein F (2004) Facilitated neurogenic inflammation in unaffected limbs of patients with complex regional pain syndrome. Neurosci Lett 359(3):163–166
Levine JD, Dardick SJ, Basbaum AI, Scipio E (1985) Reflex neurogenic inflammation. I. Contribution of the peripheral nervous system to spatially remote inflammatory responses that follow injury. J Neurosci 5(5):1380–1386
Levine JD, Fields HL, Basbaum AI (1993) Peptides and the primary afferent nociceptor. J Neurosci 13(6):2273–2286
Li LC, Scudds RA, Heck CS, Harth M (1996) The efficacy of dexamethasone iontophoresis for the treatment of rheumatoid arthritic knees: a pilot study. Arthritis Care Res 9(2):126–132
Lissner S (1963) Pulsoszillographische Messungen mit dem Infratonsystem nach Brecht und Boucke nach stabiler Galvanisation. Inauguraldissertation, Medizinische Akademie „Carl Gustav Carus", Dresden
Littlejohn G, Guymer E (2018) Neurogenic inflammation in fibromyalgia. Semin Immunopathol 40(3):291–300
Ljung BO, Forsgren S, Friden J (1999) Substance P and calcitonin gene-related peptide expression at the extensor carpi radialis brevis muscle origin: implications for the etiology of tennis elbow. J Orthop Res 17(4):554–559
da Luz DC, de Borba Y, Ravanello EM, Daitx RB, Döhnert MB (2019) Iontophoresis in lateral epicondylitis: a randomized, double-blind clinical trial. J Shoulder Elb Surg 28(9):1743–1749
Mackenzie RA, Burke D, Skuse NF, Lethlean AK (1975) Fibre function and perception during cutaneous nerve block. J Neurol Neurosurg Psychiatry 38(9):865–873
Magerl W, Fuchs PN, Meyer RA, Treede RD (2001) Roles of capsaicin-insensitive nociceptors in cutaneous pain and secondary hyperalgesia. Brain 124(Pt 9):1754–1764
Malmberg AB, Mizisin AP, Calcutt NA, von Stein T, Robbins WR, Bley KR (2004) Reduced heat sensitivity and epidermal nerve fiber immunostaining following single applications of a high-concentration capsaicin patch. Pain 111:360–367
Malone DG, Irani AM, Schwartz LB, Barrett KE, Metcalfe DD (1986) Mast cell numbers and histamine levels in synovial fluids from patients with diverse arthritides. Arthritis Rheum 29(8):956–963
Mankowski C, Patel S, Trueman D, Bentley A, Poole C (2016) Cost-effectiveness of capsaicin 8% patch compared with pregabalin for the treatment of patients with peripheral neuropathic pain in Scotland. PLoS One 11(3):e0150973
Marshall KW, Chiu B, Inman RD (1990) Substance P and arthritis: analysis of plasma and synovial fluid levels. Arthritis Rheum 33(1):87–90
McDougall JJ (2006) Arthritis and pain. Neurogenic origin of joint pain. Arthritis Res Ther 8(6):220
Niissalo S, Hukkanen M, Imai S, Törnwall J, Konttinen YT (2002) Neuropeptides in experimental and degenerative arthritis. Ann N Y Acad Sci 966:384–399
Nilsson HJ, Schouenborg J (1999) Differential inhibitory effect on human nociceptive skin senses induced by local stimulation of thin cutaneous fibers. Pain 80:103–112
Nilsson HJ, Levinsson A, Schouenborg J (1997) Cutaneous field stimulation (CFS): a new powerful method to combat itch. Pain 71(1):49–55
Nilsson HJ, Psouni E, Schouenborg J (2003) Long term depression of human nociceptive skin senses induced by thin fibre stimulation. Eur J Pain 7(3):225–233
Nilsson HJ, Psouni E, Carstam R, Schouenborg J (2004) Profound inhibition of chronic itch induced by stimulation of thin cutaneous nerve fibres. J Eur Acad Dermatol Venereol 18(1):37–43
Nolano M, Simone DA, Wendelschafer-Crabb G, Johnson T, Hazen E, Kennedy WR (1999) Topical capsaicin in humans: parallel loss of epidermal nerve fibers and pain sensation. Pain 81:135–145

Nordahl S, Alstergren P, Kopp S (2000) Tumor necrosis factor-alpha in synovial fluid and plasma from patients with chronic connective tissue disease and its relation to temporomandibular joint pain. J Oral Maxillofac Surg 58(5):525–530

Oerstavik K, Namer B, Schmidt R, Schmelz M, Hilliges M, Weidner C, Carr RW, Handwerker HO, Jörum E, Torebjork HE (2006) Abnormal function of C-fibers in patients with diabetic neuropathy. J Neurosci 26(44):11287–11294

Panus PC, Ferslew KE, Tober-Meyer B, Kao RL (1999) Ketoprofen tissue permeation in swine following cathodic iontophoresis. Phys Ther 79(1):40–49

Pape HC, Kurtz A, Silbernagl S (2019) Physiologie. Thieme, Stuttgart, ISBN-13: 978-3132423916

Peng YB, Wu J, Willis WD, Kenshalo DR (2001) GABA(A) and 5-HT(3) receptors are involved in dorsal root reflexes: possible role in periaqueductal gray descending inhibition. J Neurophysiol 86(1):49–58

Pierau F, Szolcsányi J (1989) Neurogenic inflammation: axon reflex in pigs. Agents Actions 26:231–232

Pratzel H, Dittrich P, Kukovetz W (1986a) Spontaneous and forced cutaneous absorption of Indomethacin in pigs and humans. J Rheumatol 13(6):1122–1125

Pratzel H, Machens R, Dittrich P (1986b) Iontophorese zur forcierten Hautresorption von Indometazin und Salizylsäure. Z Rheumatol 45:74–78

Pratzel H, Seemüller U, Dodt J, Gemmerli R (1986c) Forcierte und spontane Hautresorption von Hirudin bei Schweinen und am Menschen. Z Phys Med Baln Med Klim 15:129–142

Rains C, Bryson HM (1995) Topical capsaicin. A review of its pharmacological properties and therapeutic potential in post-herpetic neuralgia, diabetic neuropathy and osteoarthritis. Drugs Aging 7(4):317–328

Raney EB, Thankam FG, Dilisio MF, Agrawal DK (2017) Pain and the pathogenesis of biceps tendinopathy. Am J Transl Res 9(6):2668–2683

Reinauer S, Neusser A, Schauf G, Holzle E (1993) Iontophoresis with alternating current and direct current offset (AC/DC iontophoresis): a new approach for the treatment of hyperhidrosis. Br J Dermatol 129(2):166–169

Richardson JD, Vasko MR (2002) Cellular mechanisms of neurogenic inflammation. J Pharmacol Exp Ther 302(3):839–845

Ringkamp M, Peng YB, Wu G, Hartke TV, Campbell JN, Meyer RA (2001) Capsaicin responses in heat-sensitive and heat-insensitive a-fiber nociceptors. J Neurosci 21(12):4460–4468

Rusch D, Neeck G, Schmidt KL (1988) Galvanisches Erythem und Capsaicin. Z Phys Med Baln Med Klim 17:286

Saito T (2003) Neurogenic inflammation in osteoarthritis of the knee. Mod Rheumatol 13(4):301–304

Sasamura T, Kuraishi Y (1999) Peripheral and central actions of capsaicin and VR1 receptor. Jpn J Pharmacol 80(4):275–280

Sato K, Timm DE, Sato F, Templeton EA, Meletiou DS, Toyomoto T, Soos G (1985) Sato SK (1993) Generation and transit pathway of H+ is critical for inhibition of palmar sweating by iontophoresis in water. J Appl Physiol 75(5):2258–2264

Sauerstein K, Klede M, Hilliges M, Schmelz M (2000) Electrically evoked neuropeptide release and neurogenic inflammation differ between rat and human skin. J Physiol 529(Pt 3):803–810

Saxler G, Löer F, von Knoch M, von Knoch F, Hanesch U (2005) Die Lokalisation des Neurokinin 1-Rezeptors im Hüftgelenk von Patienten mit schmerzhafter Osteoarthrose. Z Orthop Ihre Grenzgeb 143:424–430

Sayilir S, Yildizgoren MT (2017) The medium-term effects of diadynamic currents in chronic low back pain; TENS versus diadynamic currents: a randomised, follow-up study. Complement Ther Clin Pract 29:16–19

Schauf G, Hubert M, Reinauer S, Holze E (1994) Modification and optimization of tap water iontophoresis. Hautarzt 45(11):756–761

Schmidt RF, Lang F, Heckmann M (2011) Physiologie des Menschen, mit Pathophysiologie. Springer, Berlin/Heidelberg, Print ISBN-13: 978-3-642-01650-9

Schnizer W, Kröling P (2001) Ist das anodische galvanische Erythem pH-abhängig? Phys Med Rehab Kuror 11(2):68–70

Schnizer W, Manert W (1980) Untersuchung zur Frage der transkutanen Wirkung des elektrischen Stromes auf das periphere Gefässsystem des Menschen. Z F Phys Med Baln Med Klim 9:238–244

Schnizer W, Knorr H, Lindner J, Magyarosy J, Wenemoser A (1993) Die Untersuchung physikalisch-medizinischer und balneotherapeutischer Erytheme (Wärme, Gleichstrom, CO2, H2S) am Capsaicinmodell. Phys Rehab Kur Med 03(5):125–129

Schnizer W, Kröling P, Claußen A, Magyarosy I (2003) Die Abschwächung (Desensibilisierung) des galvanischen Erythems durch wiederholte Gleichstromreizung. Phys Med Rehab Kuror 13(3):145–148

Schöps P, Kröling P, El-Tahlaoui E, Schnizer W (1998a) Das galvanische Erythem besitzt eine neurogene Komponente. Phys Rehab Kur Med 08(2):52–53

Schöps P, Kröling P, El-Tahlaoui E, Schnizer W (1998b) Die unterschiedliche Ausprägung des galvanischen Erythems an Kathode und Anode ist auf die unterschiedliche Bedeutung der Stromflußzeit zurückzuführen. Phys Rehab Kur Med 8:25–26

Scott A, Khan KM, Roberts CR, Cook JL, Duronio V (2004) What do we mean by the term „inflammation“? A contemporary basic science update for sports medicine. Br J Sports Med 38(3):372–380

Senthilkumar S, Afrose Fathima A, Nivedha S (2019) A study on effectiveness of diadynamic current in Osgood Schlatters disease among young athletes. Int J Recent Sci Res 10(10):35564–35567

Serra J, Campero M, Ochoa J (1998) Flare and hyperalgesia after intradermal capsaicin injection in human skin. J Neurophysiol 80(6):2801–2810

Simone DA, Nolano M, Johnson T, Wendelschafer-Crabb G, Kennedy WA (1998) Intradermal injection of capsaicin in humans produces degeneration and subsequent reinnervation of epidermal nerve fibers: correlation with sensory function. J Neurosci 18(21):8947–8959

Simpson DM, Robinson-Papp J, Van J, Stoker M, Jacobs H, Snijder RJ, Schregardus DS, Long SK, Lambourg B, Katz N (2017) Capsaicin 8% patch in painful diabetic peripheral neuropathy: a randomized, double-blind, placebo-controlled study. J Pain 18(1):42–53

Skledar SJ, Lachell CM, Chelly JE (2015) Pharmacodynamics and clinical efficacy of fentanyl iontophoretic transdermal system for post-operative pain in hospitalized patients. Expert Opin Drug Metab Toxicol 11(12):1925–1935

Sonntag M, Ruzicka T (2004) Hyperhidrose – Ursachen und aktuelle Behandlungsmöglichkeiten. Z Allg Med 80:289–294

Sorkin LS, Eddinger KA, Woller SA, Yaksh TL (2018) Origins of antidromic activity in sensory afferent fibers and neurogenic inflammation. Semin Immunopathol 40(3):237–247

Strout TD, Schultz AA, Baumann MR, Jordan PJ, Worthing B, Burton JH (2004) Reducing pain in ED patients during lumbar puncture: the efficacy and feasibility of iontophoresis, collaborative approach. J Emerg Nurs 30(5):423–430

Tenreiro Pinto J, Pereira FC, Loureiro MC, Gama R, Fernandes HL (2018) Efficacy analysis of Capsaicin 8% patch in neuropathic peripheral pain treatment. Pharmacology 101(5–6):290–297

Theoharides TC, Cochrane D (2004) Critical role of mast cells in inflammatory diseases and the effect of acute Sress. J Neuroimmunol 146:1–12

Theoharides TC, Singh LK, Boucher W, Pang X, Letourneau R, Webster E, Chrousos G (1998) Corticotropin-releasing hormone induces skin mast cell degranulation and increased vascular permeability, a possible explanation for its proinflammatory effects. Endocrinology 139(1):403–413

Tomoyuki S (2003) Neurogenic inflammation in osteoarthritis of the knee. Mod Rheumatol 13:301–304

Träbert H (1957) „Ultra-Reizstrom" ein neues therapeutisches Phänomen. Biomed Eng/Biomed Tech 2(7):197–206

Trnavsky G (1984) Überprüfung des Hoffmann-Reflexes bei absteigender Galvanisation. Phys Med Rehab Kuror 36(4):257–259

Uchio Y, Ochi M, Ryoke K, Sakai Y, Ito Y, Kuwata S (2002) Expression of neuropeptides and cytokines at the extensor carpi radialis brevis muscle origin. Shoulder Elbow Surg 11(6):570–575

Ulrich H, Graßhoff H (1994) Der thermische Effekt der TENS. Phys Rehab Kur Med 4:79–82

Urry L, Cain M, Wasserman S, Minorsky P, Reece J (2016) Campbell biology, Campbell biology series, 11. Aufl. Pearson, New York, ISBN-13: 978-0134093413

Vossen H, de Wijer A (2019) Diadynamische stroom bij Herpes Zoster, verdwenen behandeling. Stichting Geschiedenis Fysiotherapie. http://www.sgfinfo.nl/wp-content/uploads/2019/09/SGF_fysiotherapie-inperspectief_column_september_2019_online_FysioPraxis.pdf. Zugegriffen am 13.04.2020

Wagner J (1995) Vergleichende Untersuchung zur analgetischen Wirkung einer Gleichstrombehandlung mit unterschiedlicher Polung auf den experimentell erzeugten, ischämischen Muskelschmerz beim Menschen. Medizinische Dissertation, Justus-Liebig Universität, Gießen

Wall PD, Fitzgerald M (1981) Effects of capsaicin applied locally to adult peripheral nerve. 1. Physiology of peripheral nerve and spinal cord. Pain 11:363–378

Wallengren J, Sundler F (2001) Cutaneous field stimulation in the treatment of severe itch. Arch Dermatol 137(10):1323–1325

Walsh DA, Mapp PI, Kelly S (2015) Calcitonin gene-related peptide in the joint: contributions to pain and inflammation. Br J Clin Pharmacol 80(5):965–978

Weber M, Birklein F, Neundorfer B, Schmelz M (2001) Facilitated neurogenic inflammation in complex regional pain syndrome. Pain 91:251–257

Weidner C, Klede M, Rukwied R, Lischetzki G, Neisius U, Skov PS, Petersen LJ, Schmelz M (2000) Acute effects of substance P and calcitonin gene-related peptide in human skin – a microdialysis study. J Invest Dermatol 115(6):1015–1020

Westermark T, Rantapaa-Dahlqvist S, Wallberg-Jonsson S, Kjorell U, Forsgren S (2001) Increased content of bombesin/CGRP in human synovial fluid in early arthritis: different pattern compared with substance P. Clin Exp Rheumatol 19(6):715–720

Willis WD Jr (1999) Dorsal root potentials and dorsal root reflexes: a double-edged sword. Exp Brain Res 124(4):395–421

Wollina U, Uhlemann C, Elstermann D, Köber L, Barta U (1998) Therapie der Hyperhidrosis mittels Leitungswasseriontophorese. Positive Effekte auf Abheilungszeit und Rezidivfreiheit bei Hand-Fuß-Ekzemen. Hautarzt 49(2):109–113

Yaksh TL, Di Nardo A (2018) Complexity of systems and actions underlying neurogenic inflammation. Semin Immunopathol 40(3):225–228

Zeuner HA, Lenarz T, Trost HE (1989) Wirkungsweise und Stellenwert der Lidocain-Iontophorese bei Tinnitus aurium. Audiol Akustik 3:84–95

3 Transcutaneous Electrical Nerve Stimulation (TENS)

3.1 Classical Classification of Electrotherapy Methods

Electrotherapy methods can, if you like be grouped (Table 3.1). Every German electrotherapy textbook refers to Heinrich Edel (1977), who in turn refers to Josef Kowarschik (1957). Table 3.2 explains the technical terms used in the text.

The goal of TENS (or TNS) is the stimulation of afferent nerve fibers for pain relief or improvement of trophism. In principle, any form of electrical stimulation therapy in which the skin is not penetrated is a transcutaneous nerve stimulation; otherwise, it would be a PENS: a percutaneous-and-so-on. Direct current, UR, DD, and interference currents are also included. Today, unfortunately, the term is mainly used to refer to small battery-operated electrotherapy devices for home treatment. But TENS is not a device, it is an application. This application enables the activation of various pain inhibition mechanisms in the nervous system, and does so in a cost-effective manner with virtually no side effects.

There are two major criticisms regarding TENS that keep coming up: First, that it is all just a placebo effect, and second, that TENS is not a remedy but only suitable for symptom control.

In the following, the multitude of presented studies will show readers that a great deal of serious research has been and is being conducted on the topic of TENS, and that today we can not only confirm the effectiveness of TENS with certainty, but we even know quite precisely how TENS works (and why it sometimes does not). Regarding the second point, it should be emphasized here that in most cases TENS indeed "only" combats symptoms. Just like pain medications. The "only" is completely misplaced. If a patient can reduce their dose of pain medication thanks to TENS, this is not only a cost issue (Toroski et al. 2018), but it also means a reduction in side effects, a not insignificant advantage for chronic pain patients.

P. van Kerkhof, *Evidence-Based Electrotherapy*, https://doi.org/10.1007/978-3-662-73019-5_3

Table 3.1 Classification of Electrotherapy Methods

Range	Goal	Application
Low frequency 0–1000 Hz	Diagnostics, pain relief, improvement of trophism improvement of muscle function	SD curve Direct current, iontophoresis, diadynamic currents, ultra-stimulation current, TENS, stimulation of denervated muscles, neuromuscular electrical stimulation, functional muscle stimulation
Medium frequency 1000 Hz–300 kHz	Pain relief, improvement of trophism improvement of muscle function	Amplitude-modulated IF current, frequency-modulated IF current
High frequency > 300 kHz	Pain relief, improvement of trophism	SWD (11.06 m, 27.12 MHz) 69 cm wave therapy (69 cm, 433.92 MHz), microwave therapy (12.5 cm, 2450 MHz)
Other	Pain relief, improvement of trophism	Ultrasound, photobiostimulation (LLLT)

This overview refers to the applications discussed in this book.

Table 3.2 Glossary

Phase duration, also T (Time)	Pulse duration, pulse width
Phase interval, also R (Rest)	Pause between two phases
Duty cycle	Ratio between phase duration and phase interval; duty ratio
Frequency	Number of pulses per second. Also "pps": pulses per second
Burst	Short series of pulses, also called salve or train
Monophasic	Pulse is either positive or negative, as for example with ultra-stimulation (Trabert's) current
Biphasic	Pulse has a positive and a negative component
Compensated or balanced	Balanced current flow in biphasic pulses, can be symmetric or asymmetric; this is the case with almost all TENS currents
Cathode	Negative electrode, usually marked black, sometimes blue
Anode	Positive electrode, usually marked red
Intensity or amplitude	Current strength in milliamperes
Dosage	Total of intensity, treatment duration, number of treatments, and treatment frequency

3.2 Types of TENS

Although there are device manufacturers who offer their own, sometimes rather exotic "specific" type of TENS, the demonstrably effective TENS applications can be divided into two groups, which differ in their effects:

- High Frequency TENS

and

- Low Frequency TENS

In German-speaking countries, High Frequency TENS is usually referred to as "conventional TENS," while Low TENS is usually, and incorrectly, referred to as only as "Burst TENS." To avoid confusion, the English terms will be used in the following. This is intended to make literature searches easier for interested readers.

3.2.1 Terminology: Confusion

There are types of TENS that appear in the literature under various names, which does not exactly make the interpretation of study results easier. When these terms are then also imaginatively translated into German, chaos is complete.

- High Frequency TENS is exactly what the name says: a TENS application with a high frequency. More on this in the relevant section (Sect. 3.3).

- Low Frequency TENS likewise delivers exactly what it says: a TENS application with a low frequency. Low Frequency TENS also gets its own chapter.
- High Frequency-High Intensity TENS is now usually referred to as (Brief) Intense TENS, and sometimes the term HiFi-TENS is encountered. Intense TENS is a form of TENS in which high frequencies are combined with an intensity at or just above the pain threshold. For "proper" Intense TENS, the electrodes are placed over the peripheral nerve that innervates the painful area. This type of TENS is therefore genuinely painful, and its effect can best be explained by the DNIC mechanism (see Sect. 1.12). The method is sometimes used for a painful dressing change or a problematic venipuncture. Some colleagues report successful use in trigger point therapy or on the sports field; more on this later. The term High Frequency HIGH Intensity TENS is intended to make clear that the method differs in the intensity used from High Frequency LOW Intensity TENS. The latter, until not so long ago, was dosed as "just perceptible." The "High Intensity" version is set to a very clearly perceptible level, really just barely tolerable. Today, much higher intensities are recommended for High Frequency TENS anyway; the version with low intensity is almost ineffective. The difference between conventional (High) TENS and Intense TENS therefore lies in the few milliamperes between "just about tolerable" and "almost painful," and in the localization. More on the localization of High TENS later.
- For further clarification of terms, Brief Intense Transcutaneous Somatic Stimulation should also be mentioned here. This term occasionally appears in cases where Intense TENS is actually meant. The application was used by Melzack as a kind of hyperstimulation therapy with success in therapy-refractory patients. The parameters are similar to those of Low TENS, 3 or 10 Hz, phase duration unfortunately unknown, 20 min application, intensity at the tolerance limit but not painful (Melzack 1975); here too, DNIC very likely plays the main role. The electrodes are placed near the painful site, i.e., not over the relevant innervating nerve as in Intense TENS.
- There is great confusion regarding the terms Acu-TENS and AL-TENS (also called APL-TENS). Acu-TENS (also: Aku-TENS) refers to a form of TENS that is applied exclusively to acupuncture points. This can involve Low, High, or Dense Disperse TENS (see below), and either electrodes or needles are used. AL-TENS stands for Acupuncture-like TENS. This form of TENS was proposed in the 1970s by Sjölund and Erikson as an alternative to Low TENS. AL-TENS has an effect comparable to acupuncture, hence the name. However, AL-TENS is not applied to acupuncture points, but to nerve stimulation points of the nerves that innervate the muscles innervated by the same segment where the pain is localized (Sjölund and Eriksson 1979). More on this below. Interestingly, many nerve stimulation points are located at the same sites as many acupuncture points (Melzack et al. 1977; Melzack 1981; Hong 2000; Dorsher 2008).
- Even more chaos? Then TEAS should be mentioned: Transcutaneous Electrical Acupoint Stimulation. In this application, only acupuncture points are stimulated, just as with Acu-TENS. However, with TEAS, the frequencies are repeatedly set differently.
- Next up is IMES: Intramuscular Electrical Stimulation. An allegedly new technology. Trigger point therapists who practice dry needling sometimes use TENS, with the needles placed in a trigger point serving as electrodes. Sounds like PENS: Percutaneous Electrical Nerve Stimulation. Or, indeed, like EAP: Electroacupuncture.
- The last form is MM-TENS (Mickey Mouse TENS). This form of TENS is more intended to influence the manufacturer's sales than the pain of our patients.

With TENS, almost always compensated pulses are used, sometimes symmetrically compensated, sometimes asymmetrically, whereby the shape of the pulses has no demonstrable influence on the effect of TENS (Hingne and Sluka 2007). So if a patient prefers a particular pulse shape, it can be used with a clear conscience. With these pulses, no ion current flows and there are no net chemical changes in the tissue, so the risk of burns is practically negligible. Therefore, standard adhesive electrodes can be used. If redness occurs, it is usually due to an allergic reaction to the electrode material, the most common side effect of TENS. If very long pulses are used (> 250–400 µs), it can happen that sensitized C fibers release their neuropeptides. This then leads to neurogenic inflammation with corresponding redness. More on this under "Neurogenic Inflammation" in Chap. 2.

However, it would be a mistake to believe that all TENS devices *only* use compensated pulses! There is an older, indestructible clinical TENS device with a pleasingly large number of setting options, which produces uncompensated pulses, so beware: risk of burns, always read the instructions for use carefully!

For home treatment devices, in addition to intensity, one should also be able to set the frequency, phase duration, and burst frequencies, providing a wide range of options. There are already very good devices available for around €200; for a little more, you can get a device that is also suitable for stimulating innervated musculature. The simpler and correspondingly cheaper devices, with their manufacturer-preferred programs and fixed pre-programmed standard settings, only allow treatments for standard problems. And who actually has those. Incidentally, with cheap devices, it is not always guaranteed that no net current flows, and this can lead to very unpleasant skin injuries.

Since with modern electrotherapy devices for clinical use, almost all parameters can (still) be set more or less laboriously by hand, it makes sense to use these devices to find the optimal setting for the patient. This setting can then be used for about 2 weeks under supervision (i.e., in the clinic or practice) so that its effect can be assessed. If the result is positive after this time, the setting found can be used on the small TENS device (Fig. 3.1).

It is a major mistake to give a device to a patient without such a trial phase. It goes without saying that the patient must be extremely well informed about the use of the device provided and that the application must be regularly monitored. It is truly incredible what some patients do with their device. Nevertheless, patients should be encouraged to experiment

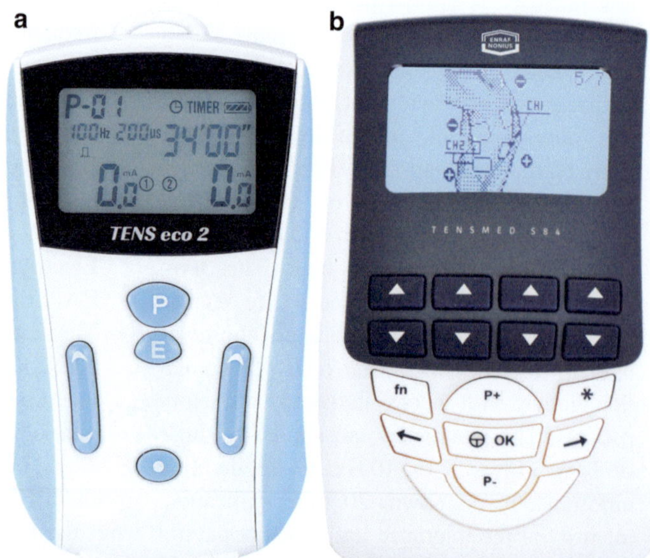

Fig. 3.1 (**a**,**b**) (**a**) Stimulation according to Prof. Han is a type of TENS. © Schwa-Medico AG, Ehringshausen, with kind permission. (**b**) A TENS device with many options. © Enraf-Nonius B.V. Delft, Netherlands, with kind permission

with the parameters, including electrode positioning, to optimize the treatment (Johnson 2014)! The author would be very pleased if manufacturers would equip their devices with a function for "application evaluation."

3.2.2 Stimulation Parameters of Different Nerve Fiber Types

The TENS types mentioned above act on different types of nerve fibers due to their stimulation parameters, because these nerve fibers have different properties regarding their excitability. Depending on the type of fiber stimulated, different pain inhibition mechanisms are activated, and this gives us the opportunity to use TENS in a differentiated manner. Figure 3.2 shows a SD curve of the saphenous nerve of a cat. The composition of the nerve is comparable to that of a human. The graph shows the response of the individual nerve fiber types to current pulses of different durations. The shorter the pulse, the higher the intensity (in mA) required to trigger an action potential. The graph shows that fast-conducting Aβ fibers can be selectively stimulated with pulses up to about 10 µs, without stimulating Aδ or even C fibers. As long as the intensity remains low, pulses up to about 100 µs can be used. Aδ fibers are stimulated, at sufficiently high intensity, with pulses longer than 10 µs, and from about 500 µs phase duration, C fibers are additionally stimulated. Note that it is impossible to stimulate Aδ or C fibers without also stimulating Aβ fibers. The stimulation of different nerve fibers thus depends on the phase duration and the intensity. According to Lullies, with medium-frequency currents, frequency also plays a role in the differentiated stimulation of fast and slow-conducting nerve fibers. Slow-conducting nerve fibers respond less to high frequencies and require higher intensities for depolarization. This is not surprising, since with increasing frequency the phase duration becomes shorter, and Aδ and C fibers only respond to longer pulses (Lullies and Trincker 1974).

Which fiber type is being stimulated is reported by the patient (MacKenzie et al. 1975; Beissner et al. 2010). The investigators have teased apart how subjective perception of current and the nerve fiber type involved are related. A sensation similar to light touch is conducted by Aβ fibers. Aδ fibers conduct a tingling pain sensation, C fibers conduct a sensation of heat or a burning pain. We will see later that these exact sensations occur, for example, when the intensity is increased during an ultra-stimulation application (Träbert's 2–5 current).

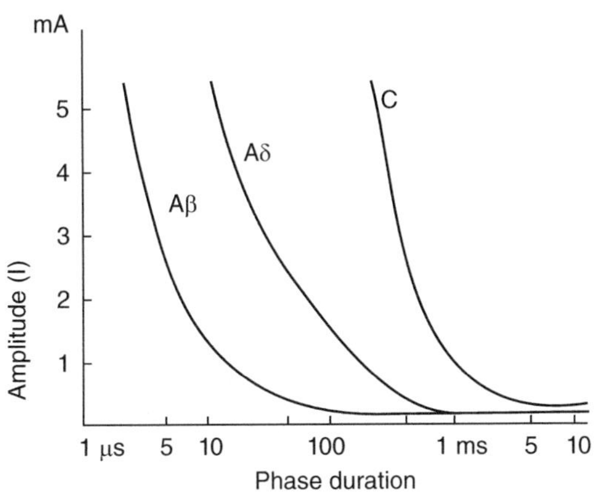

Fig. 3.2 SD curve of the saphenous nerve of a cat. After Howson 1978 and Li and Bak 1976, with kind permission

3.3 High Frequency TENS

Also called conventional TENS, High Frequency Low Intensity TENS, or Sensory TENS. Or simply TENS. Today, in the specialized literature, the term High TENS is almost exclusively used. The method became very popular after the formulation of the gate control theory, because it is based on non-painful stimulation of Aβ fibers and is thus intended to activate the gate control mechanism (Sluka and Walsh 2003). Due to this popularity, High TENS is unfortunately often regarded as the only TENS application. As already explained above, the label "Low Intensity" should no longer be used, as this form of TENS is now applied with much higher intensities than was previously customary; "Low Intensity" is almost ineffective (Chesterton et al. 2002, 2003; Claydon et al. 2011; Wang et al. 1997).

Frequencies between 50 and 150 Hz are most effective, phase duration 10–100 μs, but sometimes up to 250 μs. Thus, clinicians have a considerable range at their disposal. Most studies are conducted with 80–100 Hz, which at least leads to comparable results. During the application, the patient should feel a very distinct, but just not painful, tolerable current sensation, which ideally spreads into the pain area. The sensation can hardly be described as mere "tingling" or "pins and needles." Some patients perceive pressure, pinching, tearing, or pulling. The highest possible intensity that is still tolerated by the patient should be used (Chesterton et al. 2002, 2003; Aarskog et al. 2007; Lazarou et al. 2009; Claydon et al. 2011; Moran et al. 2011; Pantaleão et al. 2011; Sluka et al. 2013; Vance et al. 2015).

When we, as we should, try out the devices on ourselves, we find that applications with phase durations between 10 and 30 μs are almost imperceptible or only at very high intensities. When practicing (on each other), we therefore tend to use longer pulses, around 50–100 μs and longer. However, patients perceive the current quite differently! Their pain-conducting nerves and CNS are, unlike "ours," sensitized and therefore react to much shorter pulses! So be careful.

3.3.1 Intensity

Because it is so important, it is mentioned again: The intensity should be "very clearly perceptible, but just shy of being unpleasant." Note the nuance: "Not unpleasant" is not the same as "pleasant." Due to adaptation, the sensation of the current usually decreases after a few minutes, so the intensity must then be carefully readjusted (Pantaleão et al. 2011). Defrin et al. (2005) claimed this was unimportant, but the majority of researchers seem to disagree. Some devices allow the use of a so-called spectrum or frequency modulation to prevent such adaptation. Here, the stimulation frequency is automatically varied over a previously selected range in a certain rhythm. Stochastic currents, in which the frequency is automatically changed "randomly," are intended to achieve the same effect. It took until 2019 for a group of researchers to seriously address this topic. The result: With the spectrum enabled, during a 30-min session in healthy subjects, the intensity had to be readjusted one time less: 3 times instead of 4. The parameters: one group 6 s, 80 Hz, gradually up to 120 Hz over 6 s and back down in 6 s (6/\6), second group 80–100 Hz "randomly," third group continuously 100 Hz, fourth group placebo. Pulse duration 200 μs, intensity in all groups equally "clearly perceptible, but tolerable, no muscle contractions." The effect of the applications, measured by the pressure pain threshold, was the same, except in the placebo group, which showed no change. Whether this is also the case in patients is not known (Avendaño-Coy et al. 2019). A gradual modulation of the frequency from 20 to 100 Hz and back over 8 s does not change the pressure pain threshold in healthy subjects (Chen and Johnson 2009).

3.3.1.1 Practical Implementation

The following method works quite well for setting the intensity, but unfortunately is not possible with all TENS devices:

- First, set the pulse duration on the device to the lower limit, for example 20 μs, then carefully increase the intensity. When the patient perceives the current as "clearly perceptible, but just tolerable," carefully increase the pulse duration stepwise by 10–20 μs (but keep the amplitude the same!). If the patient perceives the tingling as *deeper* ("Oh yes, now it really goes into the joint!") or *spreading over a larger area* ("Now it's going towards the thumb!"), this phase duration is maintained. If the stimulus only becomes more intense, but not deeper or spreading, stick with the initial setting. Reference: Apart from my teacher from way back when: none. Sorry.
- Ideally, the patient should feel paresthesias in the symptomatic area.

- Treatment duration: 20–30 min. Some patients use High TENS for hours as needed and leave the electrodes on all day.
- Treatment frequency: once a day to several times daily.
- If habituation occurs during treatment, the intensity must be readjusted.

If the method described above does not work, you can proceed as follows:

- First, set the phase duration to the upper limit of the device, usually around 100 μs, depending on the device. Then turn up the intensity, again to "clearly perceptible, but just tolerable." If the current is perceived as too unpleasant, shorten the phase duration until the sensation improves.
- Otherwise, proceed as above.

For anxious patients, it is worthwhile to perform the "SIT test," see under "Anxiety and Intensity" below.

3.3.1.2 Habituation

It is known that about 30% of High and Low TENS users show a habituation effect after daily use with exactly the same parameters and electrode placement after just 4–5 days, with μ-opioid receptors likely playing a role (Johnson et al. 1991; Liebano et al. 2011). This habituation can be avoided by varying the electrode placement slightly each day, increasing the intensity by about 10%, or changing the frequency—but please, not all at once. The use of spectra and stochastic currents has never been studied in patients, but their use to prevent long-term habituation is certainly worth a try. The use of a kind of mix-TENS with rhythmic 2–150 Hz alternation every 3 s delays habituation from 5 to 10 days (DeSantana et al. 2008). Daily alternation between 4 Hz Low TENS and 100 Hz High TENS has the same effect.

3.3.1.3 Summation Effect?

Marchand et al. (1993) found a significant improvement in patients with nonspecific back pain treated with High TENS compared to the control group (100 Hz, 125 μs, 30 min, paresthesias clearly perceptible in the dermatome, 20 treatments in 10 weeks). The improvement concerned pain intensity, not the unpleasant aspect of pain (unpleasantness). In addition, their High TENS patients showed a kind of summation effect: the improvement increased stepwise. It is unclear whether this was caused by central desensitization, a kind of rebooting effect known from animal experiments (e.g., Kalra et al. 2001; DeSantana et al. 2009). The cumulative improvement did not occur in the placebo group. Simon et al. (2015) could not detect any summation with comparable parameters, but they only treated 4 to 5 times over 2–3 weeks.

In some publications, the designation "T" for threshold is used. For example, it is mentioned that the intensity was increased up to 4 T. This means: the intensity is carefully increased until the patient just perceives something, which is their sensory threshold (= Threshold = T). For a certain electrode size, this might be, for example, 5 mA. If you want to reach 4 T, you carefully increase further up to $4 \times 5 = 20$ mA. This method can only be used as a rough dosing guide, as our perception is very variable! Sometimes "4 T motor" is written. In this case, T stands for the motor threshold, the intensity that just triggers a contraction; 4 T would then be 4 times this value in mA.

3.3.1.4 Anxiety and Intensity

In anxious patients, it is often difficult to achieve an adequate intensity. Rakel et al. (2014) found in a study of postoperative knee patients that anxious patients responded less well to High TENS than those who scored lower on the psychological tests used. It is very likely that the intensity could not be set adequately in the anxious patients. We know that fear of pain affects the pain threshold, but not pain tolerance (Lee et al. 2013; George et al. 2006). Vance et al. (2018) investigated this in a study with 143 patients with fibromyalgia (FM). TENS was applied to the lumbar region and the participants had to indicate when the sensation of current was "clearly perceptible, but just shy of being painful." This value was defined as SC1

(Strong but Comfortable 1). Then, as previously agreed with the participants, the intensity was increased until the participant rated it as "noxious, unhealthy." The intensity was then immediately reduced again to a level that the participant now rated as "clearly perceptible, but just shy of being painful." This was now SC2. The intensity of SC2 was significantly higher in almost all participants than SC1. In particular, the more anxious and older participants (aged 40 to 60) showed the greatest increase in tolerated intensity. The investigators point out that up to a good 60% of all FM patients exhibit anxiety behavior and that it is therefore understandable that these patients initially view TENS skeptically and therefore indicate relatively early that the intensity is sufficient. The investigators call this the SIT test: Setting of Intensity of TENS Test. The method may function as a kind of exposure therapy, helping patients to modify their expectations (Hofmann 2008; Vlaeyen and Linton 2012). It can be used in anxious patients to demonstrate a non-harmful effect, so that the patient can have a positive experience. Incidentally, the variation in older participants is explained by the fact that older people have a different perception of current, probably related to the reduced number of C fibers in the skin (Namer et al. 2009) and the changed structure of the dermis and epidermis (Calleja-Agius et al. 2013). It is unclear whether TENS is as effective in older people as in younger ones. There are studies showing that older patients respond less well, others contradict this (Bergeron-Vézina et al. 2015; Simon et al. 2015; Daguet et al. 2018). Perhaps this is also a question of the intensity used.

3.3.2 Electrode Placement

Traditionally, High TENS is used to stimulate structures that are embryologically related (Aarskog et al. 2007; Claydon et al. 2008; Buonocore and Camuzzini 2007; Tong et al. 2007). If a patient has radiating pain in the C4 dermatome on the left, it is supposedly pointless to treat the C7 dermatome on the right, since High TENS activates an inhibitory system that acts in the segment where the stimulus is applied. However, there is increasing evidence that High TENS, like Low TENS, also activates a central pain inhibition that suppresses non-segmental pain. Non-segmental here means that pain inhibition occurs in a segment that is not embryologically related to the segment where the stimulus was applied. This has been observed not only, as usual, in Rattus norvegicus (Somers and Clemente 2006, 2009), but also in humans (Kawamura et al. 1997; Dailey et al. 2013; Vance et al. 2012; Buonocore et al. 2015). For the clinician, this means that a wide range of options for electrode placement is available.

- The simplest and often most effective electrode placement for High TENS is on the location where it hurts. The electrodes should be placed so that the sensation of current spreads in the painful area (which is not always possible). This means that during the first treatment, you usually have to reposition several times. It is therefore practical in this case to use carbon rubber electrodes, either with contact gel or in wet sponge pouches. This makes repositioning easier than with adhesive electrodes. Most of the time, but not always, the cathode is proximal, of course only with asymmetrically compensated pulses. The reason for this placement is that a proximally placed anode could inhibit afferent conduction, and you want to stimulate, not inhibit. You stimulate because inhibition is to occur elsewhere. With symmetrically compensated pulses, anode and cathode alternate, so the location of the anode or cathode does not matter, unless the patient prefers a particular placement. As already mentioned, the pulse shape has no influence on the treatment outcome.
- Placement on acupuncture points, trigger points, tender points, or over the peripheral nerve that innervates the painful area works

very well. Here, the cathode is placed on the stimulation point. The debate as to whether trigger points and acupuncture points are the same is still ongoing, but that is actually irrelevant (Melzack et al. 1977; Hong 2000; Dorsher 2008). The fact is that these points are well suited as "attack points" for TENS treatment (Chen et al. 1998; Chesterton et al. 2002, 2003; Cheing and Chan 2009; Lang et al. 2010; Wang et al. 1997). Chesterton and Wang have shown that both a high-frequency high-intensity TENS and a low-frequency high-intensity TENS on GB34 or LI4 (Hegu) significantly reduce pressure pain sensitivity on the contralateral side (back of the hand). The increase in pain threshold occurred after about 20 min and lasted about 20–30 min after the 30-min application.

- In segmental treatment, if possible, both electrodes are placed in the segment where the pain is localized. Here too, the cathode is usually proximal. In the English-language literature, placement over the innervating nerve is also considered segmental. The electrodes can also be placed on the corresponding spinal segments. The 2 + 2 treatment is very effective: 2 electrodes local or regional and 2 segmental; with this method, strong afferent stimuli can be applied (Fig. 3.3). Simultaneous treatment with High TENS from the contralateral acupuncture point GB34 and the ipsilateral segment (radial nerve) leads to a significant increase in the pressure pain threshold on the back of the hand, but only lasts a few minutes (Chesterton et al. 2003); parameters: 110 Hz, 200 µ, 30 min, tolerance level. Treating pain in areas with reduced sensitivity is probably pointless (Pantaleão et al. 2011). Nevertheless, a small study in MS patients showed that hand sensitivity in these patients improved long-term after several TENS treatments in the affected area (where sensitivity was impaired) (Cuypers et al. 2010); parameters: 100 Hz, 250 µs, 60 min, once daily for 3 weeks; electrodes over the median nerve, submotoric intensity. To prevent habituation, frequency and phase duration were automatically varied. The improvement in sensitivity was in the area of the median and ulnar nerves and at a normal level.
- If the electrodes cannot be applied to the painful area, the contralateral side can be treated. The effectiveness of such an application was already demonstrated in a clinical study by Kawamura et al. in 1997 in the treatment of phantom pain and has been confirmed several times in laboratory animals (Ainsworth et al. 2006; Sabino et al. 2008; Somers and Clemente 2006). Buonocore et al. (2015) showed in healthy subjects that a High TENS application over the superficial branch of the left radial nerve (10 min, 100 Hz, 100 µs, intensity strong but tolerable) significantly reduced sensitivity to a painful heat stimulus on both sides. The effect lasted about 15 min after the application.

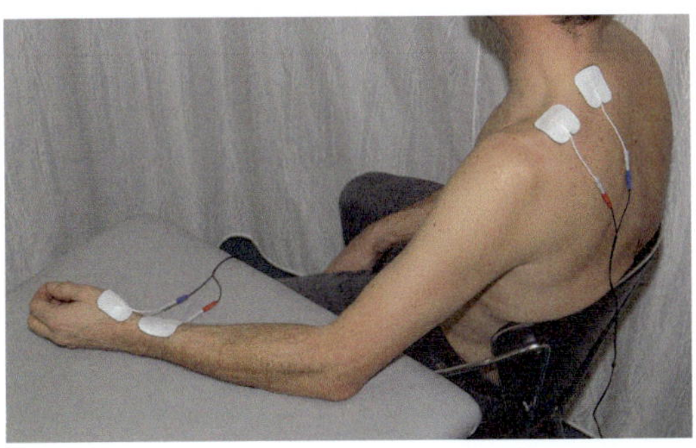

Fig. 3.3 2 + 2 method for pain at the base of the thumb. One pair of electrodes local, one pair segmental, cathode blue

3.3.3 Efficacy

To assess the efficacy of TENS, Vance et al. (2015) took the trouble to analyze a large number of systematic reviews on TENS regarding efficacy and intensity used. Their result: Low intensity makes TENS ineffective (Aarskog et al. 2007; Chesterton et al. 2002, 2003;

Claydon et al. 2008; Pantaleão et al. 2011). Where the intensity was set to "clearly perceptible, but just tolerable," TENS was effective. An updated overview of publications by authors who used adequate intensity with comprehensible parameters can be found in Table 3.3.

Large reviews such as those by Cochrane are, as so often in our field, very contradictory in their results. However, they all have one thing in common: the conclusion that the quality of the studies leaves much to be desired. This does not always concern the conduct of the studies regarding patient selection, randomization, blinding, etc.—methodologically, many investigators have now got the hang of it. It concerns, and this is very important, the precise description of the application. What was the electrode placement, their size, what was the stimulation frequency, the phase duration, the treatment duration? And most importantly: what was the intensity? In addition, it is not uncommon for an application to be performed and the result to be asked about several weeks later. That would be like giving a patient paracetamol (acetaminophen) today and asking about their symptoms a month later.

The area of application for High TENS is the treatment of acute and chronic pain due to inflammatory processes, peripheral nerve lesions, phantom pain, neuropathic pain, scar pain, and postoperative pain. Interestingly, High TENS seems to work better for movement pain than for resting pain (Rakel and Frantz 2003; Dailey et al. 2013; Elboim-Gabyzon et al. 2019). Of course, TENS is also used in patients with back pain, and there are numerous clinical studies that aim to demonstrate its efficacy. Due to various factors such as the heterogeneity of the groups studied, the timing of follow-up, incomprehensible parameters, and much more, unfortunately nothing more precise can be said about the actual efficacy of TENS in these patients. In patients in the "alarm phase" (Chap. 1, stress reaction), this method should be used, as the information necessary for pain inhibition is conducted via Aβ fibers and not via Aδ and C fibers.

High TENS is also used to improve wound healing, more on this later (Sect. 3.5). In addition, TENS is used in neurology. Since its use in this area partly overlaps with the application of

Table 3.3 Clinical studies on the effectiveness of TENS, sorted by adequate dosing

Pain	Author	Result
Postoperative	Bjordal et al. (2003) Gardner et al. (2014) Johnson (2017) Mahure et al. (2017) Wang et al. (1997)	Significantly less need for pain medication
Postpartum (C-section)	Kayman-Kose et al. (2014)	Significantly less pain, less need for pain medication
Osteoarthritis (knee)	Bjordal et al. (2007)	Clearly effective
Knee arthroplasty	Zhu et al. (2017)	Significantly better
Diabetic neuropathy	Jin et al. (2010) Kumar and Marshall (1997) Julka et al. (1998)	Better than placebo
Neuropathy	Celik et al. (2013)	Significantly better
Trigger points	Gemmell and Hilland (2011) Rodríguez-Fernández et al. (2011)	Better than placebo
Head, face	Antony et al. (2019)	Promising
Fibromyalgia	Dailey et al. (2013) Lauretti et al. (2013) Carbonario et al. (2013)	Significant improvement
Spasticity in spinal cord injury	Sivaramakrishnan et al. (2018)	Spasticity significantly reduced, comparable to FES
Phantom (arm, leg)	Kawamura et al. (1997)	Very good result
LBP		Nothing useful

neuromuscular electrical stimulation, this topic is discussed in the relevant chapter (Chap. 3).

Considerations in Treatment

A patient sprained her wrist in a fall while skiing. The X-ray is unremarkable. She comes to therapy after 10 days. The whole hand is swollen, bluish, and sweaty. All active movements are about half restricted and painful. She does not use the hand and is very worried. She has a friend who had the same thing happen. That friend had a fracture and underwent surgery. Something went wrong during the operation and she had to have another operation after 3 months. The healing process took over a year. The patient fears that the same fate awaits her.

It is obvious that the patient is still in the alarm phase. The inflammatory reaction should have subsided long ago. Her CNS is not working selectively, her central inhibitory mechanisms are not functioning, healing is impaired. It is pointless and probably counterproductive to use a therapy here that addresses the central inhibitory mechanisms via stimulation of Aδ and C fibers. Her "central" would probably interpret the afferent information as a further attack on the organism, no matter how eloquent the therapist is. High TENS is the method of choice here. Since it is the first session, a short phase duration and a high frequency are chosen, and the intensity is deliberately kept low. This is because the treatment is introduced cautiously in this way. For example, you choose 10–20 μs phase duration and 150–200 Hz, intensity perceptible but definitely not unpleasant. The electrodes are placed transregionally. If the situation improves, the phase duration can be extended.

3.4 Low Frequency TENS

Also called motor, motoric, Lo-, Low Frequency High Intensity TENS. Low TENS has its roots in electroacupuncture (EAP). Acupuncture-like TENS is something different, more on that below. All these terms refer to the same type of TENS. Today, the term Low TENS or AL-TENS is most commonly used. In this effective but rather intense method, low frequencies between 0.5 and 10 Hz are used, with 2–4 Hz being optimal. The impulses are longer, usually between 200 and 500 μs, and it is dosed motorically, meaning that muscle contractions *must* be elicited. This form of TENS was used in China with EAP for electroanalgesia. Manually stimulating the needles is very tiring for the anesthetist/acupuncturist in the long run, especially when caring for several patients; therefore, electrical stimulation was adopted. The 2–4 Hz stimulation frequency corresponds to the frequency with which the needles are manually stimulated. In therapy, in addition to needles, of course, normal electrodes are also used. The effects of High TENS and Low TENS are quite comparable, except that the effect of Low TENS usually lasts significantly longer.

3.4.1 AL-TENS, APL-TENS, Burst TENS

With Low TENS, visible contractions must necessarily occur in the muscles that are innervated by the same segment in which the pain is localized. The contractions are usually triggered by single pulses, and this is not exactly pleasant. That is why AL-TENS was developed. Here, the impulses are delivered in so-called bursts (groups of impulses, volleys, trains, Fig. 3.4), hence the name Burst TENS (Eriksson and Sjölund 1976). For this, tetanizing frequencies (80–100 Hz) are broken down into groups of impulses, and these short volleys then trigger contractions 2 to 4 times per second. According to studies by Eriksson and Sjölund (1976) and Sjölund et al. (1977) (Sjölund 1985, 1988), these frequencies, just like the single pulses used in Low TENS, release β-endorphins: the analgesia is reversed by naloxone. According to Pomeranz, the De-Qi sensation is difficult or impossible to elicit with Burst TENS, which is why he prefers Low TENS (Pomeranz in Stux et al. 2003, p. 318). Andersson et al. (1973) found EAP with standard electrodes to be more

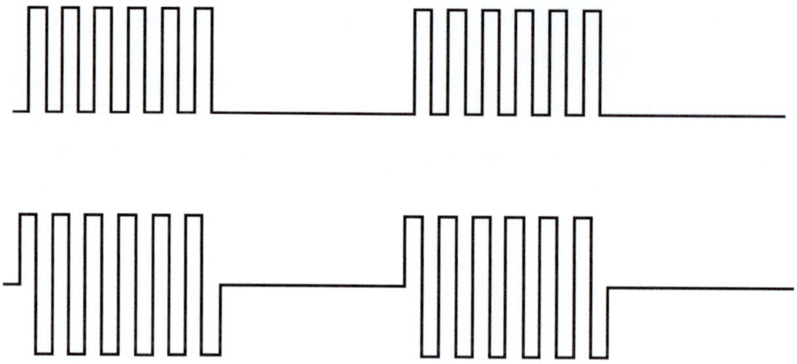

Fig. 3.4 Bursts or volleys. Top: rectangular, monophasic (not compensated); bottom: biphasic, symmetrically compensated

effective than with needles, probably because stronger stimuli can be applied.

A question that comes up again and again is this: "With a 2 Hz burst, I have 2 bursts per second. So one burst lasts less than half a second. The intra-burst frequency is 100 Hz. If each pulse lasts 200 μs, how do I fit 100 pulses into the burst?" Answer: The base frequency is 100 Hz. These 100 Hz are regularly interrupted, creating "pulse packets," i.e., bursts. Each individual packet (burst) contains, depending on the phase duration, 5–10 pulses, so it fits. If you did not include interruptions, 100 Hz would run continuously. All clear?

3.4.2 Intensity of Low TENS, AP-TENS

With Low TENS, the intensity is set clearly at the motor threshold, hence the term "Motor TENS." This form of TENS aims to stimulate deep Aδ fibers, and for this, the intensity must be set significantly higher depending on the location than with High TENS. The Aδ fibers are only stimulated at intensities more than twice the motor threshold (Radhakrishnan and Sluka 2005). The impulses used are therefore also significantly longer than with High TENS: between 200 and 500 μs (Bouhassira et al. 1987; Radhakrishnan and Sluka 2005; Hugosdottir et al. 2019). Traditionally, this application attempts, as with conventional acupuncture, to elicit the so-called De-Qi sensation (sometimes also written as "Teh Chi" or "Deqi"). This sensation is associated with the stimulation of deep Aδ pain afferents in the musculature (Chiang 1974). The De-Qi sensation is difficult to describe (Hui et al. 2007). Some patients describe it as "like a bruise," "cramp," or "pinching," or as "dull, heavy aching" (English: "ache," not "pain"), sometimes as "numbness" or "swelling," "ballooning," "throbbing." It is not exactly pleasant. As a rule, the De-Qi phenomenon only occurs at intensities around 5 to 10 times the *motor* threshold. If the ipsilateral side cannot be treated, Low TENS can be used contralaterally. This seems to be particularly the case when stimulating acupuncture points GB36 and LI4 (Hegu).

3.4.3 Mechanism of Action of High TENS and Low TENS

The effect of High TENS and Low TENS is based on several mechanisms. Today, a local, a segmental, a descending, and a central mechanism are assumed (Vance et al. 2015).

3.4.3.1 Local Effect

Walsh et al. (1998) and Nardone and Schieppati (1989) have demonstrated that in Aβ fibers, the impulses triggered by High TENS block the propagation of action potentials that were triggered further distally on the nerve. Put simply:

the line is busy. Normally, no noxious information is transmitted via Aβ fibers, except in neuropathic pain, where miswiring can occur due to nerve damage. However, if it is possible to stimulate Aδ and C fibers as well, as Ignelzi and Nyquist 1976 did, this mechanism could nevertheless trigger a kind of conduction block that actually prevents the transmission of pain-related information. This is particularly plausible in a situation where the pain-conducting fibers have been sensitized due to pathology and can be stimulated with much lower intensities than in healthy individuals. However, Janko and Trontelj (1980) and Lee et al. (1985) were able to show that pain conduction in the periphery remains intact during and after a TENS application. Moreover, a local conduction block would not explain why the effect of TENS sometimes lasts up to 24 h. These facts suggest the involvement of other mechanisms. Nevertheless, a lot happens locally, but this has not yet been demonstrated in humans. Studies in rodents have shown that those lacking the α2-adrenoreceptor (AR) respond less to High and Low TENS than their non-genetically modified siblings. When, in normal mice, an antagonist for the α2-receptor was injected into an inflamed joint after a TENS application, the TENS effect decreased. If the antagonist was injected intrathecally or intracerebroventricularly in the same mice, nothing changed (King et al. 2005). This supports a local effect of TENS. In addition, local opioid receptors very likely play a role in Low TENS. Sabino et al. (2008) were able to show that local blockade of μ-opioid receptors prevents the effect of Low TENS, but not that of High TENS. So a lot is probably happening in the periphery, but it is not yet entirely clear what exactly that is.

3.4.3.2 Segmental Effect

Stimulation of Aβ fibers by vibration has an inhibitory effect on nociceptive neurons in the spinal cord (Salter and Henry 1987; Salter et al. 1993). This inhibition is not reversed by administration of a GABA antagonist (bicuculline), an opioid antagonist (naloxone), or a glycine antagonist (strychnine). However, the inhibition is completely suppressed by methyltheobromine (yes, plain old caffeine), an antagonist for adenosine. Since High TENS mainly stimulates the fast-conducting Aβ fibers, this not only confirms a segmental effect of High TENS, but also explains why (excessive) coffee consumption can impair the effect of TENS (Marchand et al. 1995).

3.4.3.3 Central and Descending Effect

High and Low TENS increase the concentration of β-endorphin in the blood and in the cerebrospinal fluid in humans, as well as the met-enkephalin concentration in the CSF (Salar et al. 1981; Hughes et al. 1984; Han et al. 1991). High and Low TENS also increase the cerebrospinal dynorphin level in humans (Han et al. 1991; Han 2003; Léonard et al. 2010, 2011). Analgesia is prevented by blockade of opioid receptors in the nucleus raphe magnus and in the adjacent ventral reticular formation of the nucleus gigantocellularis reticularis and in the spinal cord (Kalra et al. 2001; Sluka et al. 1999; DeSantana et al. 2009) and by GABA and muscarinic (M1 and M3) receptors (Radhakrishnan and Sluka 2003; Maeda et al. 2007). It is now generally accepted that opioids activate the connection between the periaqueductal gray (PAG) and the raphe nuclei. On the one hand, this activation acts centrally directly on the PAG (DeSantana et al. 2009) and causes a global increase in pain threshold. This explains the inhibition of pain in a segment other than the one where TENS was applied (Dailey et al. 2013; Buonocore et al. 2015). On the other hand, activation of the receptors in the raphe nuclei has an antinociceptive effect on a descending inhibitory system (Radhakrishnan and Sluka 2003), with serotonin identified as the neurotransmitter. Administration of a serotonin precursor (L-hydroxytryptophan) enhances the effect of TENS; methysergide, a serotonin antagonist, abolishes the effect (Shimizu et al. 1981; Woolf et al. 1980). This descending system consists of pathways projecting segmentally from the raphe nuclei onto GABAergic and enkephalinergic inhibitory interneurons in the substantia gelatinosa, which trigger the gate control mechanism. The system inhibits the transmission of noxious information in the segment where the information entered the spinal cord.

The pain-inhibiting effect of High TENS is suppressed by administration of naltrindole, an antagonist for the Aδ opioid receptors; enkephalins bind here. In animal experiments, where certain substances can usually be administered in larger doses, naloxone also blocks the effect of High TENS. Naloxone occupies the μ-opioid receptor, where β-endorphin binds. Naloxone also occupies the κ-opioid receptor, where dynorphin binds. Thus, several opioid receptors are apparently involved in the effect of High TENS (Han et al. 1991; Woolf et al. 1980).

The pain-inhibiting effect of Low TENS is suppressed by blockade of μ-opioid receptors in the PAG, in the raphe nucleus, and in the spinal cord with naloxone. In addition, blockade of GABA, serotonin, and muscarinic M1 and M3 receptors in the spinal cord prevents pain inhibition by Low TENS. Sjölund and Eriksson demonstrated the involvement of β-endorphin in the effect of Low TENS in humans in 1979. Low TENS is less effective in patients treated with opioids; this is in contrast to High TENS (Liebano et al. 2011; Léonard et al. 2011). In direct comparison, Low TENS and High TENS are equally effective, but the effect of Low TENS lasts longer (Francis et al. 2011a, b).

3.4.4 Electrode Placement

With Low TENS, electrodes are traditionally placed over acupuncture points. If desired, these points can also include nerve stimulation points, trigger points, or motor stimulation points (in the same segment). Since contractions must be triggered with this application, the latter are particularly suitable. If local treatment is too painful or, for example, a dressing or open wound makes electrode placement impossible, it is perfectly acceptable to perform the treatment contralaterally, since Low TENS has a clearly central pain-inhibiting effect and therefore also works non-segmentally. Triggering contractions via the stimulation point for the motor nerve is not ideal, as this usually activates entire muscle groups. This is not always pleasant, especially if it hurts exactly there or if tendons have been repaired.

This type of TENS is particularly effective for deep, myopathic pain (myofascial pain syndrome) and for chronic pain. If High TENS does not produce satisfactory results, Low TENS should definitely be tried, either with single pulses or with bursts, depending on which is more effective.

The treatment should last at least 30–40 min, as otherwise the pain-relieving effect is only short-lived. In healthy subjects in the laboratory, an increase in pain threshold usually occurs only after about 20 min (Salar et al. 1981), when β-endorphin production begins. In patients, it often takes only a few minutes for pain relief to occur.

Because of the slight pain, muscle fatigue, and the fact that endorphin production decreases anyway, treatment is usually not performed for longer than 45 min, although it can be carried out several times a day. Pain relief can last for hours to days.

The methods are very effective, but also intense. Therefore, they cannot be used on every patient. It is advisable to introduce the therapy gradually, especially if the patient is unfamiliar with the treatment: For the first TENS application, the intensity can be increased from "slightly to clearly perceptible" to "motor threshold" (slight contractions). During the second session, it is usually possible to gradually reach a therapeutically effective intensity. The "SIT test" can also be used with Low TENS.

Problems in which the triggered contractions are too painful or even contraindicated cannot be treated locally with Low and Burst TENS. In such cases, it is worth trying the contralateral side. Adjusting the intensity so that contractions are not allowed renders the method ineffective (Fig. 3.5).

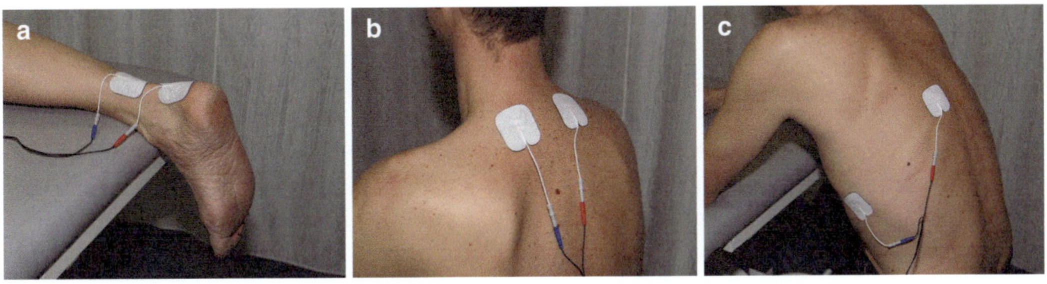

Fig. 3.5 (**a**–**c**) (**a**) Local application, (**b**) paravertebral application, (**c**) segmental application

3.4.4.1 Case Examples

- A patient has lumbar back pain and high muscle tension. The patient is familiar with the problem; it is not the first time he has experienced this. He does his exercises, but it is simply not enough. He is confident that the problem will be resolved with just a few therapy sessions. His CNS (and he himself) is in the adaptation phase, his CNS is working selectively. The pain inhibition mechanisms can be activated by a somewhat more aggressive approach. The options are Low Frequency TENS and Burst TENS. If you want to address the tension with repeated muscle contractions, Burst TENS is more suitable, as the series of impulses are more pleasant and more effective for triggering muscle contractions. Since this is the first session, a relatively short pulse duration can be chosen: these impulses are less unpleasant. If the contractions are too weak, the phase duration can be extended. The large electrodes are placed paravertebrally over the lumbar extensor muscles. Settings: 200 μs phase duration, 100 Hz, 2 Hz burst, at least 25–30 min treatment time, maximum 45 min. Increase intensity to the tolerance limit until clear muscle contractions are observed. If the contractions decrease, the intensity must be readjusted. After appropriate instruction, this can often be left to the patient, and the device positioned within reach.
- A patient has a knee joint effusion after a fall. To support the reduction of swelling using the muscle pump and stimulation of lymphatic drainage, 2-channel Burst TENS is chosen. The 4 large electrodes are placed to cover as much of the quadriceps muscle as possible. Placement "crosswise" as in 4-pole interference is pointless. A burst frequency of 1 or 2 Hz is set and a phase duration of 200–400 μs, so that a strong contraction is triggered; this works best with symmetrically compensated rectangular pulses. The treatment time is up to 30 min. If the contractions decrease, the intensity must be readjusted. This therapy can be applied before conventional therapy to prepare the tissue for subsequent active exercise therapy.
- A 24-year-old man had his left forearm amputated after a traffic accident. Several weeks after the operation, he developed severe phantom pain in the left, amputated hand, radiating to the thumb. He was treated with High TENS on the right arm and hand, with 4 electrodes placed on the areas that were most painful in the left arm. Parameters: once daily for 3 months, 60 min, 80 Hz, phase duration 50 μs, intensity very clearly perceptible but still tolerable. After 3 months under supervision, the patient continued the therapy independently for another 3 months. According to the Cambridge Phantom Limb Profile (CPLP), the Groningen Questionnaire: Problems after Arm Amputation (GQPAA), and the Visual Analog Scale, the patient was clearly better at follow-up after one year than before treatment (Giuffrida et al. 2010).

- Not a real case, but still interesting (Katz et al. 1989): A 23-year-old man had his right leg amputated above the knee after an accident. Immediately after the operation, he complained of phantom pain in the right amputated foot, cramps in the right calf, and stabbing pain in the knee. He compared the pain to "growing pains" as he had experienced at age 8. The phenomenon of the recurrence of past somatosensory experiences occurs more frequently after amputations (Katz and Melzack 1990). The patient had successfully participated in a study on therapy for phantom pain (High TENS contralateral), and was now selected for a special study. His phantom pain had significantly decreased after the TENS treatment, but he repeatedly experienced strange sensations in the right leg, as if the leg was being pressed through something. Electrode placement: over the left calf muscles, phase duration 80 μs, 100 Hz, intensity clearly perceptible but tolerable. The session lasted 60 min, with TENS applied several times for 10 min. Result: During the TENS application, the skin temperature at the stump steadily increased from 31°C to about 35°C, and the phantom sensation was significantly reduced during stimulation. Long-term results are not known.
- A 19-year-old patient with severe burns suffered from very severe itching in some areas, a complication that occurs very frequently with burns. When patients scratch themselves, this can lead to injury and infection in fresh skin grafts. Histamine is involved in the development of such pruritus. The release of histamine triggers a neurogenic reaction that initiates a mechanism in the spinal cord similar to that described in the gate control theory. However, itching is not a kind of subsensory pain, but a distinct modality (Sun et al. 2017). In the patient, where the itching was worst, about 15 cm left and right of L2, two lead rubber electrodes with contact gel were applied at 10 a.m. These remained in place until the patient went to bed in the evening. Parameters: probably > 180 Hz, phase duration < 150 μs – unfortunately, the dosage details were not recorded precisely – intensity "tolerable." The itching decreased gradually each day. From the third day, there was no itching for up to 4 h after treatment. On day 5, the VAS score before treatment was about 50% of the VAS score on day 1 at the same time. The patient continued the treatment at home, but had difficulty attaching the electrodes by himself (Whitaker 2001; Hettrick et al. 2004).

3.4.4.2 Attention: Medications

Patients treated with opiates such as tramadol (Tramal®) will not benefit, or will benefit only minimally, from Low and Burst TENS (Sluka et al. 2000; Léonard et al. 2011). The β-endorphins responsible for pain inhibition and tramadol bind to the same μ-opioid receptors. If these receptors, as can occur in neuropathic pain, are downregulated due to increased cholecystokinin production (Back et al. 2006), the method is also less effective or even ineffective. Cholecystokinin can also prevent the expression of δ-opioid receptors for enkephalins. For this reason, the pain-relieving effect of Low TENS and Burst TENS in these patients is sometimes less pronounced than hoped.

In pain patients who have been unsuccessfully treated with SSRIs (Selective Serotonin Reuptake Inhibitors, a group of antidepressants), the effect of Low and Burst TENS can also be disappointing, because descending pain inhibition partly depends on serotonin production. If this is impaired, this inhibitory system is not, or only partially, available. In these and the above-mentioned patients, the use of High TENS may still be successful.

Note that Low and Burst TENS, due to their intensity, are not suitable for anxious patients if they cannot always process the relatively mild pain that occurs during treatment in a differentiated manner. These methods stimulate Aδ and C fibers, and this "aggressive" stimulation is transmitted unfiltered in a fight-or-flight situation (ergotropic orientation, alarm phase) in the ARAS. In these patients, High Frequency TENS should be used: Aβ stimulation is not interpreted by the CNS as an attack (see Ch. 2, "Stress Reaction").

3.4.5 Non-segmental Stimulation according to B. Kaada

(Birger Kaada, MD, PhD, neurophysiologist, Norway)

Kaada stimulation is an AL-TENS treatment in which, regardless of the pain diagnosis, the same stimulation point on the hand is always used: the acupuncture point LI4 (Large Intestine 4, also known as Hegu). This point is also the trigger point for the first dorsal interosseous muscle. The cathode is placed dorsally on the hand at LI4 between metacarpals I and II, and the anode is placed on the ulnar edge of the hand opposite. Incidentally, SI4, -5, and -6 are located here over the ulnar nerve, but these are not relevant for this treatment. Often, the anode is placed on the back of the hand between metacarpals III and IV. Wang et al. (1997) also stimulated the Hegu point in their study, placing one electrode dorsally on the point and another electrode opposite on the opponens pollicis muscle. This stimulation leads to a general increase in pain threshold and results in significant improvement of blood flow in the lower extremities (Kaada 1982; Kaada and Eielsen 1983; Kaada and Melesse 1988; Kaada et al. 1989). In Traditional Chinese Medicine (TCM), LI4 is one of the most important analgesic acupuncture points (Stux et al. 2003), and there is hardly any acupuncture treatment in which Hegu is not stimulated (Fig. 3.6).

Kaada used

- *Low Frequency TENS* with compensated (balanced) rectangular pulses, phase duration 200 μs, frequency 2–5 Hz (single pulses)

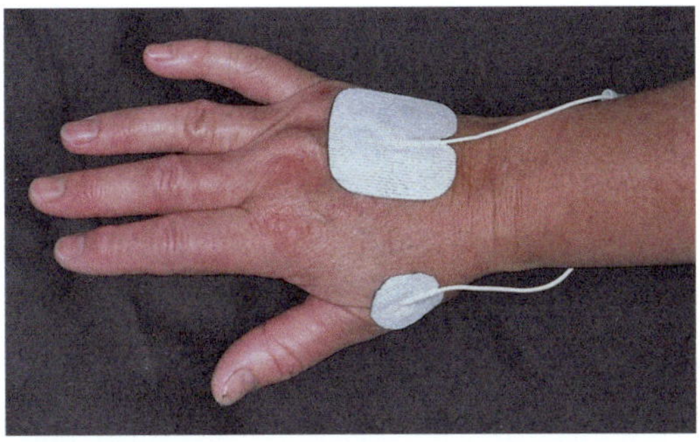

Fig. 3.6 Stimulation according to Kaada. Small, trimmed cathode on LI4

and

- *AP-TENS* with 2 Hz bursts, internal burst frequency 100 Hz (5 pulses per burst, phase duration 200 μs).

The intensity is set to a non-painful, just motor threshold, specifically 20–40 mA with "usual" electrode sizes (12 cm^2, conductive rubber, coupling with gel). The intensity corresponds to 2–4 T (sensory). The application becomes significantly more comfortable if the cathode is smaller than the anode. Adhesive electrodes can be trimmed, but care must be taken not to cut any relevant wires. As a reminder: the cathode is usually black (or blue …) and the anode is red. Mnemonic: "black **cat**hode." With symmetrically compensated pulses, cathode and anode alternate, so color choice does not matter here.

The intensity must be readjusted in the event of adaptation, when contractions become weaker. Treatments are performed up to 3 times daily and last 30–45 min. Kaada does not mention whether the different applications led to different results.

Pain conditions of all kinds, circulatory disorders (Raynaud's disease, CRPS I), diabetic neuropathies, poorly healing wounds and ulcers (leprosy), and even, for example, tinnitus and calcific peritendinitis can be successfully treated.

Kaada explains the effect of his method as follows:

- Central inhibition of the sympathetic nervous system. Kaada demonstrated that vasodilation is abolished by administration of a serotonin antagonist (cyproheptadine) and not by – albeit low-dose – administration of an opioid antagonist (naloxone).
- Release of VIP (vasoactive intestinal polypeptide, which has a vasodilatory effect, stimulates cAMP formation, and improves the binding of serotonin to its receptors).
- Release of ACTH. When ACTH is released, β-endorphins must also be produced. Both substances share the same precursor: pro-opiomelanocortin = POMC.

In measurements of a cold fifth toe (24° C) in patients with Raynaud's disease, Kaada was able to detect temperature increases of up to 10° C. This temperature increase lasted up to 4 h and then decreased rapidly, within about an hour. During this time, patients' pain was significantly reduced. The temperature at body sites with normal temperature (forehead) increased only slightly (0.5–2 °C).

Kaada has shown that his stimulation can be used successfully for a variety of problems, namely in various pain syndromes of the upper extremities (cervicobrachialgia, CRPS, shoulder-arm syndrome, tennis elbow, calcific tendinitis, postoperative pain, and many more) and in problems associated with circulatory disorders in the extremities (Raynaud's, CRPS, autonomic symptoms accompanying pain syndromes, postoperative and posttraumatic swelling). There is anecdotal evidence from course participants of good results in headache patients, hand patients with postoperative cold intolerance, patients after jaw surgery, thoracic surgery, and in women after mastectomy.

The treatment is very easy to apply and can be performed well, for example, when the patient is well "wrapped up" after shoulder surgery. If biphasic, compensated pulses are used, metal in the treatment field is a relative contraindication if the patient experiences unpleasant sensations. Patients should be closely monitored.

However, caution is advised in patients with pacemakers and those with an implanted defibrillator (ICD), as these devices may react to TENS treatment on the upper extremities. More on this below (Sect. 3.12.3).

3.4.6 Han Stimulation (= Dense-Disperse Stimulation)

Sometimes the term "2/100 Hz EAS stimulation" is used (Wang et al. 2005). "Mixed Frequency Stimulation" also appears occasionally, but this term is very confusing, as some manufacturers have their own interpretation. The method was developed by Prof. Ji-Sheng Han and his research group at the Neuroscience Research Institute of Peking University (Han et al. 1991, Han 2003; Wang et al. 2005). Han stimulation combines the effects of High TENS and Low TENS. In this type of stimulation, a 100 Hz and a 2 Hz stimulation alternate abruptly every 3 s. In this way, the effects of High TENS and Low TENS are combined, resulting in more pronounced pain relief. In this method, as with AP-TENS, acupuncture points are stimulated with standard electrodes. If such acupuncture points happen to be located at the same site as muscle trigger zones, nerve stimulation points, or tender points, this should not deter their use. By the way: Treating one site with Low TENS and another simultaneously with High TENS does not produce the same result. Most likely because "centrally" 102 Hz are received, which does not trigger the desired differentiated response (Wang et al. 2005).

When High TENS is used, dynorphin is released, which occupies the κ-opioid receptors, and met-enkephalin, which binds to δ-opioid receptors. Stimulation with Low TENS releases endomorphin (occupies the μ-opioid receptors) and β-endorphin (also occupies the μ-opioid receptors). Thus, all currently known opioid receptors would be occupied. When these stimulations alternate in a 3-s rhythm, there is an "overlap" of these two effects; Han refers to this as synergy. If the two types of TENS alternate at a slower rhythm, for example every 6 s, this overlap is reduced and the method becomes less effective.

- Wang et al. (1997) found in a placebo-controlled study with 101 women after gynecological surgery that their TEAS application with Han parameters led to a 65% reduction in postoperative analgesic use. As a result, the usual side effects of the analgesic, an opioid, also occurred significantly less frequently. The investigators stimulated the Hegu acupuncture point on the non-dominant hand and, depending on the incision, left and right or caudal and cranial to the surgical wound.
- Hamza et al. (1999) divided 100 women after gynecological surgery into 4 groups: placebo, low, high, and DD-TENS. The DD-TENS group required 50% less analgesic postoperatively than the placebo group, and Low and High TENS 30% less. In addition, the three active TENS groups experienced less nausea and dizziness. The electrodes were applied locally: for a vertical incision, two electrodes each left and right of the wound; for a horizontal incision, two each proximal and distal to the wound, without regard to any acupuncture points. Parameters: electrode size 5 × 5 cm, phase duration: spectrum from 200 to 600 µs, duration 30 min, application every 2 h or with longer intervals, intensity: tolerance threshold. About 20% of patients complained of sleep problems due to the cables, 75% of the active treatment patients would have been willing to pay extra for the treatment.
- Tong et al. (2007) compared High TENS and DD-TENS with a placebo group in healthy subjects. They found that High TENS (100 Hz) reduced sensitivity to a heat pain stimulus, while DD-TENS did so for both a heat pain stimulus and a pressure pain stimulus. Combined with the result from DeSantana (who reported reduced tolerance behavior, 2008), this should be reason enough to seriously consider Dense Disperse TENS.

It should be noted that during the 2 Hz phase—just as with "normal" Low TENS—muscle contractions must occur. During the 100 Hz phase, however, no contractions should occur, but the patient must, as with High TENS, feel a strong but just tolerable current sensation. As usual, the intensity should be readjusted if the current sensation diminishes. DD-TENS is applied like Low TENS for 30–45 min, possibly several times a day.

3.4.7 Brief Intense TENS

This application is sometimes also referred to as High Frequency High Intensity TENS (colloquially HiFi-TENS). The method should not be confused with an application that Melzack 1975 used in a study with therapy-resistant pain patients. Melzack used TENS with fixed frequencies of 3 or 10 Hz at intensities at and even above the tolerance threshold, similar to Low TENS parameters but more painful. The aim of this study was to find out whether a short, intense TENS application produces the same effect as a longer-lasting High TENS. He referred to the application as "Brief Intense Transcutaneous Somatic Stimulation." In Intense TENS, pulses with a phase duration of 150–250 µs and frequencies of 60–100 Hz are used. The amplitude is turned up to the tolerance threshold, sometimes just before or even above the pain threshold, and held there for 15–20 min (3–6 T or much more). Pain relief lasts for about the same length of time. The electrodes are placed over trigger points, acupuncture points, or the nerve innervating the painful area, proximal to the painful site.

There are different explanatory models for the effect. It is very likely based on the DNIC

Table 3.4 Low TENS and Burst TENS Parameters

	Phase duration	Frequency	Intensity	Duration
High	10–150 µs	50–200 Hz	Tolerance threshold, not motor	30 min to several hours
Low	200–400 µs	1–10 Hz, optimal 2–3 Hz	Tolerance threshold, motor stimulation level, 3–6 T	20–45 min
Burst	200–400 µs	80–100 Hz, bursts: 0.5–10 Hz, optimal 2 Hz	Tolerance threshold, motor stimulation level, 3–6 T	20–45 min
DD (Han)	Like High and Low TENS, switch every 3 s	Like High and Low TENS, switch every 3 s	Like High and Low TENS, switch every 3 s	20–45 min
HiFi	100–400 µs	60–100 Hz	Tolerance threshold, motor stimulation level, 3–6 T or much higher	15–20 min

The values vary depending on the author. T = Threshold = here: sensory threshold value

mechanism. Ignelzi and Nyquist (1976, 1979) also propose other mechanisms, such as hyperpolarization of the membrane due to strong potassium efflux or exhaustion of the Na-K pump because no ATP is available after strong stimulation. A high frequency electrical conduction block cannot be ruled out either (see under medium frequency/interferential current 3.10.3).

The method is used in motivated patients as a pretreatment, for example before painful mobilization or during trigger point therapy. The method can be combined with ultrasound here; see "High Power Pain Threshold Ultrasound, HPPTUS" in the ultrasound chapter (5.9.2). Athletes in particular appreciate this intense method, and there are colleagues who report successful use during halftime. If pain inhibition actually occurs due to the DNIC mechanism, both local and general pain perception would theoretically be reduced. This would theoretically increase the risk of injury. So be careful.

For trigger point treatment, a point electrode or a conductive rubber electrode can be used. The larger indifferent electrode is placed anywhere. If simultaneous therapy with ultrasound is chosen, the ultrasound head is negatively polarized with asymmetrically compensated pulses. Of course, an electrically conductive coupling gel is used.

The point is located and treated for about 3–5 min or longer if necessary. Normally, the current intensity must be readjusted several times. Afterwards, the point is treated manually as usual. Due to the pain relief, it may happen that the trigger point can no longer be found afterwards.

Low TENS and Burst TENS, Intensity

The parameters are summarized in Table 3.4.

- Normally, a clearly motor threshold dose must be used, but the intensity can, if necessary, be gradually increased over 1–2 sessions.
- 2–4 Hz single pulses are the most effective, but also the most intense.
- If the patient cannot tolerate these, bursts can be used, base frequency 80–100 Hz, 2–4 Hz bursts, with 2 Hz/100 Hz bursts usually perceived as more pleasant. Many colleagues have found that patients find Low TENS more comfortable than Burst TENS. So try it out.
- The goal is a feeling of heaviness, tension ("like swollen") or numbness and a mild, tolerable pain, the already mentioned De-Qi sensation from acupuncture. This feeling usually does not occur or only mildly with the burst variant.
- Treatment duration at least 25–30 min, maximum 45 min.
- Initially, treatment is daily; after 1–2 weeks, in some patients it can be reduced to 2–3 times per week. Some patients eventually find a certain "maintenance rhythm" to keep their pain under control.

3.5 TENS in Wound Healing

After an injury occurs, the process of wound healing normally begins immediately. This process includes a primary inflammatory reaction, followed by the formation of granulation tissue, re-epithelialization, angiogenesis, matrix formation, and so-called remodeling (Kordestani 2019). Various cells and substances are involved in these processes. Neutrophil granulocytes and macrophages clean the wound and, together with mast cells, produce fibroblasts and endothelial cells, as well as proinflammatory cytokines such as interleukin-1β, interleukin-6, and tumor necrosis factor-α. Cytokines play a role in preparing the tissue for repair, infection control, fibroblast growth, migration of keratinocytes into the wound, and much more.

Electrostimulation in various forms has been shown in vitro to influence the activity of cells involved in wound healing, such as macrophages (Hoare et al. 2016), fibroblasts (Rouabhia et al. 2016), epidermal cells (Li et al. 2012), endothelial cells (Bai et al. 2011), and bacteria (Asadi and Torkaman 2014). The list of in vitro studies is long; an overview can be found in Hunckler and De Mel (2017).

Translating the in vitro results into practice is somewhat challenging. A review of reviews—a true Herculean task—led Pamela Houghton (2017) to conclude that electrostimulation can clearly improve impaired wound healing. This applies to various types of poorly healing wounds of venous and arterial origin and pressure ulcers. Good, but how exactly? The studies cited used very different methods: High and Low TENS, microcurrent, galvanic current, and various variations of high voltage (High Voltage Pulsed Current, Biphasic Pulsed Current). All these methods, with different parameters, were successful compared to placebo applications. This is somewhat frustrating when trying to distill a common denominator. Nevertheless, here is an attempt:

- Liebano et al. 2008 found that transplanted skin flaps in rats had the best survival rates with Low TENS, 200 µs, daily, treatment duration unknown.
- Cosmo et al. (2000) found that blood flow in chronic ulcers in humans increased by 35% after 60 min of Low TENS (2 Hz, 10–45 mA, electrodes 5 cm proximal and 5 cm distal to the wound).
- Cramp et al. (2000) observed in healthy subjects a significant improvement in skin blood flow in the area between the electrodes after 15 min of Low TENS on the forearm (4 Hz, 200 µs).
- Wikström et al. (1999) found in healthy subjects that Low TENS on the lower leg resulted in a 40% improvement in skin blood flow (2 Hz, 60 min, clearly perceptible), while High TENS resulted in 12%.
- Kaada (1982) found that stimulation with Low TENS at the acupuncture point LI4 in patients with Raynaud's disease led to a temperature increase of 10 °C at the little toe.
- The same Kaada and Melesse (1988) successfully treated leprosy ulcers on the foot, this time locally with Low TENS (2 Hz bursts, 200 µs, 100 Hz burst internal frequency, 2 times daily 30 min, slight muscle contractions).
- Burssens et al. (2003) studied in 20 people after surgery for ruptured Achilles tendon the healing tendency with and without Low TENS (2 Hz bursts, 100 Hz burst internal frequency, phase duration 300 µs, 30 min, treatment in the 2nd and 3rd postoperative week, electrodes proximal and distal to the wound, intensity as high as possible without contractions—about 38 mA—3 times per week). 10 subjects received TENS, 10 did not. After 6 weeks, a needle biopsy in the TENS group showed about 30% more fibroblasts in the operated area.
- Lundeberg et al. (1988) successfully used High TENS in women after breast reconstruction with a skin graft. Their parameters: 80 Hz, 400 µs, electrodes "at the base of the skin graft," intensity 3 T, 2 h per day.
- The same Lundeberg (1992) successfully used High TENS (80 Hz, 1 ms [sic], 20 min, 2 times daily, clearly perceptible, 2 weeks, electrodes "just outside the wound") in patients with diabetic ulcers on the lower leg. Whether the mentioned phase duration of 1 ms is a misprint is unclear.

Conclusion: Low TENS apparently has the edge in wound treatment, but High TENS is also effective. This matches Houghton's result: many roads lead to Rome.

What does this tell us regarding the treatment of poorly healing wounds of various origins with TENS?

- The use of TENS is definitely justified.
- Both Low TENS and High TENS can be used successfully.
- Intensity: muscle contractions with Low TENS, clearly perceptible with High TENS.
- Duration: 1–2 h, 1–2 times daily.
- Electrode placement: near the wound, if possible proximal and distal. The location of the cathode is not mentioned by the authors cited; with biphasic, symmetrical pulses, this is irrelevant. Author's suggestion for asymmetrical pulses: cathode proximal.
- Martínez-Rodríguez et al. (2013) recommend the use of biphasic pulses for wound treatment, as these tend to produce better results, especially in skin grafts. This comes with the usual caveat that there are too few good studies and more research is needed.
- Do not forget Kaada stimulation at LI4.
- Be sure to document the course photographically and record the parameters precisely!

3.6 Wound Healing: General Principles

Currents of low current density accelerate wound healing. This applies to skin wounds and fractures. Bones under load produce an electrical potential (piezoelectric effect: see under Ultrasound 5.2.7), and there is also a voltage gradient across the skin between the stratum corneum (negative) and the dermis (positive) of about 23 mV. One could say that the skin acts as a kind of battery. The skin is naturally negatively charged. In skin injuries, the damaged area carries a relatively positive charge compared to the undamaged surroundings. The use of an anode on/in the wound promotes the ingrowth of granulation tissue, increased collagen formation is observed, and epithelialization occurs more rapidly. Thus, wound healing is accelerated and the scar tissue is also more tear-resistant. At the same time, however, any existing bacterial infection may worsen. The use of a cathode in/on the wound delays the ingrowth of granulation tissue, but at the same time significantly counteracts a bacterial infection.

Skin injuries cause a cation flow into the wound bed, probably through activation of the sodium pumps in epidermal cells. Apparently, wound healing is partially regulated by electrical signals. However, the exact mechanism of action is still not fully understood.

Substance P is suspected to play a role in this process. This substance is released upon injury and triggers the release of histamine. The resulting hyperemia induces an inflammatory reaction, which constitutes the first stage of wound healing. A second function of substance P (SP) is to stimulate fibroblasts to initiate a myofibroblastic effect, leading to contraction of the wound surface. In addition, SP induces vasodilation, and the resulting improvement in blood flow further benefits wound healing. It can therefore be assumed that SP has a tissue-regenerating effect. Apparently, in cases of impaired wound healing, there is no release of SP.

Electrostimulation influences the impaired wound healing process in two ways:

- Electrostimulation leads to antidromic (i.e., opposite to the natural direction) stimulation of polymodal nociceptors, which are thereby induced to release substance P and CGRP at their peripheral endings (axon reflex, dorsal root reflex).
- Electric current affects the vascular bed in the wound base. Through so-called sprouting of capillaries in the wound base, the granulation tissue is adequately supplied with nutrients, which in turn promotes the growth of granulation tissue.

The following rules should be observed.

- During the first 3 days, the cathode is placed on or in the immediate vicinity of the skin defect.
- The treatment duration is 2 h and is performed 2 to 6 times daily.
- After 3 days, the anode is placed on or in the immediate vicinity of the aseptic wound.
- For the treatment of deep wounds, a sterile compress soaked in distilled water or physiological saline is placed on the wound. The active electrode is then placed on top of this.
- The indifferent electrode should be placed about 25 cm proximal to the skin defect. For continuous direct current, an amplitude of 0.1 mA/cm^2 is set.

In order to (objectively) assess the results of the treatment(s), it is recommended to

- measure the wound surface area,
- determine the depth of the wound,
- if microorganisms are present in the wound, identify the type of these microorganisms,
- describe any other characteristic of the wound,
- photograph the wound together with a measuring tape (before starting electrostimulation and then once a week),
- record the results after each treatment.

TENS current types can also be used for wound healing. Lundeberg (1988) used an alternating rectangular pulse with a variable phase duration of 0.2–1.0 ms in the treatment of ulcers, postoperative wounds (skin flap surgery), and diabetic leg ulcers. For the initial treatment of diabetic, arterial, and venous ulcers, a phase duration of 1.0 ms and a frequency of 80 Hz are set. The amplitude should elicit a strong stabbing/tingling sensation (sensory – up to the motor stimulation threshold). If this is too painful for the patient or causes significant skin irritation, the phase duration can be reduced to 0.2 ms. Since a symmetrically alternating current is used, polarity does not matter in this case. The electrodes are placed as follows:

1. If sensation in the wound area is intact: place one electrode proximally and one electrode distally to the wound, as close to the wound edge as possible.
2. If sensation in the wound area is impaired, both electrodes are placed proximally to the wound, in areas where sensation is still intact.

The treatment duration is 20–30 (60) min and is performed twice daily at 6-h intervals. For the treatment of postoperative wounds, e.g., ischemic skin flaps, a phase duration of 0.4 ms and a frequency of 80 Hz are used. The treatment duration is 2 times 2 h daily.

According to Lundeberg's publications, healing is accelerated by this method and the recovery time can even be reduced by up to 110%. For the treatment of pressure ulcers, a phase duration of 1 ms is used, but a low frequency of 2 Hz is set. The amplitude is set higher; clearly perceptible contractions must occur in the wound area (motor stimulation threshold). The treatment duration is 20–30 min and is repeated twice daily at 6-h intervals.

Kaada uses his specific stimulation method to accelerate wound healing. He does not treat locally in the wound area, but stimulates at the acupuncture point Hegu dorsally in the thenar eminence, with stimulation parameters as in Low Frequency High Intensity TENS, up to 3 times daily for up to 40 min. For a detailed description, see "Nonsegmental Stimulation according to B. Kaada" above.

3.7 Further Options for Electrode Placement

3.7.1 Regional Electrode Placement

In this application, the electrodes are placed in the painful area. It is a simple application that is often effective in practice. As already mentioned, the cathode is usually placed proximally.

3.7.2 Paravertebral Electrode Placement

This placement is used in the treatment of spinal problems. In addition, the method is often used for segmental treatment when local treatment is not possible.

This form of therapy takes advantage of the fact that embryologically related tissue types, which originate from the same segment (dermatome, myotome, sclerotome, vasotome, viscerotome, etc.), remain connected to the spinal cord (neurotome) via the same nerve root and thus continue to be neurophysiologically linked. A disorder in one structure, for example in an organ, can therefore cause *symptoms* in another tissue, such as the skin, via the neural connection. A classic example: a myocardial infarction that can cause radiating pain toward the jaw and in the left arm. Note: It has never been proven that a *pathology* in one structure also leads to pathological changes in another, segmentally related structure.

Theoretically, any perceptible stimulus in a tissue anywhere in the body can trigger reflex reactions in another tissue, *as long as these tissues are segmentally related.* Because segmentation is well preserved at the dorsal ramus of the spinal nerve, paravertebral segmental placement is frequently used. The innervation areas of the dorsal rami must be carefully considered when placing the electrodes. It is important to realize that not only does the depiction of the segments vary from author to author, but segmental innervation can also vary from person to person. In addition, there is more or less significant overlap in all segments, with the maximum being around 50% in the arm. Therefore, there is no such thing as a 100% "correct" dermatome map. At this point, the interested reader is recommended the book by Dr. B. van Cranenburgh (2018).

Transitional Segments

Close to the spine, the innervation of the skin matches the exit segment well. However, ventrally on the trunk, so-called transitional segments must be considered, for example where the dermatome innervated by the ventral ramus of C4 borders the dermatome supplied by the ventral ramus of T1. This is because the ventral rami from C5 to C8 have grown into the arm. The dorsal rami, in the course of evolutionary development, have largely remained in their original position and therefore do not have such transitional segments. The relationship between the cause of pain and the symptomatic area can be demonstrated using the various cutaneous branches. This is illustrated below using the example of T12.

The skin directly paravertebral to T12 is innervated by the medial cutaneous branch, the skin dorsally-medially over the iliac crest by the lateral cutaneous branch, the skin in the groin by the ilioinguinal nerve (T12–L1), and the skin over the trochanter by the ventral ramus T12 and the iliohypogastric nerve (T12–L1). Thus, a T12 problem can trigger symptoms in quite distant and, if one is not familiar with the anatomy, sometimes unexpected locations.

With paravertebral placement, segmental therapy can be administered in a simple manner. Most often, the segments on the symptomatic side are treated. However, it is also possible to treat contralaterally or bilaterally.

3.7.3 Placement of Electrodes on Specific Stimulation Points

This is referred to as point treatment when an electrode is placed on a specific point in the painful area. However, points that are not located in the painful area are often stimulated. The condition, however, is that a strong afferent stimulus can be applied from such a point in the corresponding segment. Therefore, these are called "specific stimulation points." Of course, it is advantageous to know in which spinal cord segment the stimulus enters, so that targeted segmental treatment can be performed.

There are four categories of specific stimulation points:

- Nerve stimulation points, NP
- Motor points, MP
- Myofascial trigger points, MTrP
- Acupuncture points, AP

3.7.3.1 Nerve Stimulation Points

These are locations such as the "funny bone," where the ulnar nerve lies very superficially, or the area dorsal to the fibular head, where the common peroneal nerve is found. Since many neurons are relatively superficial and close together at these sites, these points are very well suited for treatment. Naturally, precise anatomical knowledge is also advantageous here, as well as knowledge of which spinal cord segments the individual nerves enter (see the relevant literature). Fortunately, most electrotherapy departments have more or less frequently noticed decorative wall charts for this purpose. A special nerve stimulation point is the stellate ganglion, a traditionally popular target for various electrotherapeutic applications. It has now been well documented that stimulation of this ganglion cannot induce sympathetic inhibition (Larsen et al. 1995). Nevertheless, stimulation in this area repeatedly achieves success in the treatment of diffuse painful conditions in the arm, including circulatory disorders (Barker et al. 2007; Liao et al. 2016). The underlying mechanism is unclear. However, if one looks at the neuroanatomical relationships in this area, it is not far-fetched to claim that strong afferent stimuli can be generated here, which can reflexively influence pain in the arm. However, it is definitely not a substitute for a proper chemical blockade.

3.7.3.2 Motor Points

Motor points are locations where innervated muscles can be optimally stimulated by electrical stimulation. It is the site where nerve branches and blood vessels penetrate the muscle, and afferent and efferent information is transmitted to and from muscle fibers, muscle spindles, free nerve endings, and capillaries. In this sense, motor points are also nerve points.

Motor points have a segmental relationship via the spinal nerve to other tissues belonging to the same segment. The points can sometimes be localized by measuring skin resistance, as skin resistance is sometimes lower here. Measurement probes are used for this purpose, as are used for locating acupuncture points, or electro-palpation (= galvanopalpation) is performed. Vance et al. (2015) studied the pressure pain sensitivity in healthy subjects after a High TENS application (100 Hz, 100 μs, 30 min, clearly perceptible but not painful) at sites with low skin resistance and with normal resistance. They found no difference in effect; the application led to an increase in pressure pain threshold in both groups.

3.7.3.3 Myofascial Trigger Points

A myofascial trigger point is generally understood to be a point that, when stimulated (mechanically, electrically), triggers not only local pain but also a characteristic referred pain.

Travell and Simons refer to "myofascial trigger points" (MTrP). The mechanism of their development will not be discussed here (see, for example, the books by Travell and Simons).

As already mentioned, trigger points can be very effectively targeted with a mobile stimulation electrode, while the indifferent second electrode is fixed at a conveniently accessible site. Both Low and High TENS can be used in treatment, with Low TENS having the anecdotal edge due to the muscle contractions it induces. For the hard-boiled, Intense TENS would be the method of choice here.

Dry needling is a valuable technique in trigger point therapy, but unfortunately is not yet accepted and permitted everywhere. For deep, intramuscular stimulation, needling can be very well combined with TENS; in fact, this is electroacupuncture, even if trigger point practitioners call it IMES: Intramuscular Electrical Stimulation. When the needle is correctly placed, the TENS stimulation is optimally localized. The cables are attached to the needles with small crocodile clips. Because the current spreads a few millimeters around the needle, the localization is not overly critical. With a modern electrotherapy device, it is usually possible to treat four MTrPs simultaneously with two channels. Good experience has been gained in EAP with Low TENS. The claim that the effect of dry needling can be explained by the gate control mechanism is incorrect. Activation of this system requires non-painful stimulation of Aβ fibers. Stimulation of Aδ fibers with needles, on the other hand, activates, in addition to central pain inhibition, the long-term depression mechanism and descending pain inhibition via monoaminergic raphe pathways. The author has had particularly good experience with this method for deep-seated trigger points, for example in the lumbar region. All superficial areas can be very well treated with normal electrodes.

Due to the risk of collapse, do not use EAP at Du20, H7, and P6. In TCM, P6 is stimulated in chemotherapy patients to suppress nausea, but only for a few minutes. Pregnancy: do not treat lumbar or abdominal areas. Do not use EAP in the first trimester. Caution with acupuncture points ST36, LI4, SJ4, GB34. But appropriately trained colleagues are aware of this.

3.7.3.4 Acupuncture Points

That AP points provide a good target for TENS has been demonstrated in many studies (see the reviews by Chen et al. 1998 and Cheing and Chan 2009). The use of these points for TENS appears to have gained popularity over the past 10 years, so the following will take a closer look at electroacupuncture (EAP). It is not absolutely necessary to use needles when treating via acupuncture points (AP points); these points can also be very well targeted with normal electrodes! Andersson et al. (1973) achieved better results with electrodes than with needles, possibly because stronger stimuli can be applied with electrodes.

Jean Baptiste Sarlandière, a French physician, described 1825 the treatment of pain with EAP, after Dr. Louis Berlioz (the father of the composer) had already experimented with it as early as 1810. He used needles made of gold and silver, connected to Leyden jars. One can only imagine these "impulses"... In China, EAP was not used until around 1934.

For electrical stimulation of AP points to be effective, the De-Qi sensation must occur. In electroacupuncture, the De-Qi sensation is elicited with fairly aggressive current forms: phase duration 100–400 μs, low frequencies of 1 to 5 Hz, and intensities of 3 to 6 T, clearly at the motor threshold. Sometimes, however, as with High TENS, frequencies between 50 and 200 Hz are used. The treatment duration for EAP is usually no more than 10–20 min. Typically, 1–3 pairs of points are treated, mostly on the same side of the body.

First, the needle is inserted and manually stimulated until the De-Qi sensation occurs, then the electrical stimulation device is connected. If the patient becomes accustomed to the current during treatment, the intensity is adjusted as with normal TENS.

The advantage of the method is that a constant, intensive stimulation can be administered over a longer period. In addition, as mentioned above, precise localization is not critical. It has been found that results with normal electrodes on the skin are sometimes better, probably because a larger area is stimulated and stronger muscle contractions can be elicited (Andersson et al. 1973). However, deeper points are better reached with EAP.

The single pulses used are quite unpleasant. The use of so-called bursts was found to be somewhat less effective but much more comfortable. In Burst TENS, a tetanizing pulse current, for example at 100 Hz, is interrupted several times, so that a certain number of short pulse series (bursts, salvos, volleys, pulse trains) are triggered per second. Since the effect is similar to that of EAP, this method is also called Acupuncture-like TENS (AL TENS). Some authors (Stux et al. 2003) still prefer treatment with single pulses.

Of the several hundred known acupuncture points, only about 50 are used for pain therapy, often in combination with other AP points. EAP has proven particularly valuable in the treatment of chronic pain and neurological diseases, including paralysis and spasticity.

There are repeated references to connections between acupuncture points, motor stimulation points, nerve points, and trigger points, which are then just as stubbornly denied by proponents of the various concepts. Melzack (1977) speaks of over 70% correspondence. A detailed overview can be found in Chang-Zern Hong (2000), who even assumes a 95% correspondence.

3.7.3.5 Trigger Points and Ah-Shi Points

In his publication, Hong points out, among other things, special features of localization and pain response. He assumes that all MTrPs are identical to so-called Ah-Shi points. These are sensitive, clinically relevant acupuncture points that are not related to a meridian. The sites are usually hardened and slightly thickened. Ah-Shi means in Mandarin: "Ouch!" or "Oh, yes!" and corresponds to what the patient says when such an Ah-Shi point is pressed. In other words: "Bingo! That's the point!"

In most active MTrPs, typical referred pain can be provoked with sufficient pressure. The same reaction can be triggered with acupuncture/dry needling if the needle is stimulated, for example by rotating it. The fact that the referred pain patterns when activating certain MTrPs are almost identical in different patients suggests anatomically determined connections to the spinal cord. This also applies to acupuncture points. Thus, the mechanism of pain relief by MTrP injection and dry needling could be the same as the mechanism of action of acupuncture (Bing et al. 1990; Le Bars 2002; Le Bars and Willer 2002).

Hong also observed that the De-Qi sensation elicited at the AP is similar to the local twitch response (LTR) in active MTrPs. The best results are also obtained when this phenomenon occurs during acupuncture, as with dry needling of MTrPs.

There are locations in the human body where several specific stimulation points are found close together, if they can be distinguished at all. For example, at the proximal third of the tibialis anterior muscle, one finds the AP point Stomach 36 (St36, Zusanli or Tsu-Sann-li, English St36), the trigger point for the tibialis anterior muscle, the motor point for the tibialis anterior muscle, and the termination of the lateral sural cutaneous nerve. Many other such sites can be identified.

For electrotherapy, these regions provide very good opportunities, because strong afferent stimuli can be generated here and it is possible to influence relatively large areas via these points, often "indirectly," i.e., without having to place the electrodes directly in the problematic area. It is therefore worthwhile to acquire a (simple) acupuncture book and compare the illustrations with tables from trigger point materials and muscle stimulation tables from electrotherapy books. A good book, which also deals in detail with EAP and pain inhibition, is *Basics of Acupuncture* by Stux et al. (2003).

> Don't forget! There are several well-conducted studies showing that stimulation of certain acupuncture points such as LI4 (Hegu) and GB34, either with High or Low TENS (with sufficiently high intensity!), also on the contralateral side, results in a significant increase in pain threshold (Chesterton et al. 2002, 2003; Wang et al. 1997).

3.7.4 Microcurrent Electrical Stimulation (MES), Study Results

There are not many publications on wound healing and MES. A PubMed search in September 2020 for "microcurrent, clinical trial" yielded 38 hits, with only one publication mentioning the treatment parameters. If the search is broadened, one finds publications with very different electrotherapeutic applications, equally varied parameters, and contradictory results. In general, it appears that MES, if applied with subsensory intensities, is ineffective in the treatment of poorly healing wounds (Houghton 2014).

Only when dosed at the motor threshold, as in high-voltage therapy, can an effect be expected. However, this is impossible with MES due to the low intensity.

- Ibrahim et al. (2019) compared wound healing in burn patients using MES and negative pressure (V.A.S. – Vacuum Assisted Closure) with a group of patients receiving standard wound care. MES parameters: 10 Hz, 300 μA, polarity change every second, 1 h per day, 3 times per week, 3 weeks, electrode placement unknown. In both the MES group and the V.A.S. group, wound areas decreased more rapidly than in the control group. The V.A.S. method showed less bacterial colonization than MES.

Studies on the effectiveness of MES in the treatment of pain are also contradictory and rare, with only 57 hits for "microcurrent AND pain" on PubMed (September 2020). Unfortunately, in this application as well, it is all too often only mentioned that MES was used, without specifying parameters.

- Weber et al. (1994) found no effect of MES in 40 healthy subjects in the treatment of DOMS (Delayed Onset Muscle Soreness). After a defined exercise sequence, one group of 10 subjects was massaged, a second group was treated with MES. Parameters: 0.3 Hz, 30 μA, alternating polarity every 2.5 s. The third group did a workout on a training device, a fourth group served as control. After 24 h, there was no difference between the groups in terms of performance and muscle pain.
- Lambert et al. (2002), on the other hand, found a reduction in muscle pain in 30 healthy young men after the application of an adhesive, MES-current-producing membrane that discharges over 48 h with a voltage of about 20 μA. The application was repeated after 48 h. The control group received an inactive membrane. The reduction in pain in the treatment group after 96 h (!) was small but significant.
- Allen et al. (1999) studied the effect of MES in 9 subjects with DOMS two, three, and four days after an intense training stimulus. MES parameters: 10 min 200 μA, 30 Hz, then 10 min 100 μA, (0.3 Hz). Another 9 received placebo MES. The groups did not differ.
- Using a painful cold stimulus, Johnson et al. 1997 found no difference in effect between real MES and placebo MES; both applications led to a significant increase in pain threshold. Parameters: MES biphasic, 600 μA, 100 Hz, 20 min.
- Rajpurohit et al. (2010) treated 30 patients with masticatory muscle pain due to bruxism with TENS (50 Hz, 500 μs, 20 min, once daily, 7 days, intensity "as tolerated") and another 30 with MES (0.5 Hz, 1000 μA, 20 min, 7 days, intensity "as tolerated"). Both groups showed pain relief, with the MES group making greater progress.
- Poltawski et al. (2012) conducted a pilot study using MES to treat patients with tennis elbow. In one experiment, they compared MES at 50 μA and 500 μA for 35 h (really…) and in a second experiment MES at 25 μA and different frequencies for 15 and 189 h, over 3 weeks. 93% of the 50 μA group considered themselves "cured" after 15 weeks, as did 47% of the 500 μA group. In the second experimental group, the success rate for both variations was about 75%.
- Ranker et al. (2020) found in a small study with patients with knee osteoarthritis that MES provided better pain relief than a placebo, although their parameters are unfortunately unclear. They used a preset program and intensities of 100 μA and 25 μA, 30 min, over 22 days.
- Vrouva et al. (2019) studied 42 patients with a partial rotator cuff tear. One group was treated with exercise therapy and TENS (100 Hz, 15 mA, 20 min, 4 electrodes around the shoulder, 15 sessions in 3 weeks), the second group with exercise therapy and MES (50 Hz, 100 μA, 24 min, 15 times in 3 weeks, electrode placement as in the TENS group). After 3 months, the groups did not differ significantly

in terms of ROM, SPADI, EuroQoL-5. However, the MES group had better results for pain, while the TENS group performed better in function and quality of life.

- Gossrau et al. (2011) treated 40 patients with diabetic neuropathy, 21 with MES, 19 with placebo MES. Parameters: 2 Hz bursts, 30–40 μA, 30 min, 3 times per week, for 4 weeks. In the placebo group, 10 patients showed improvement. In the treatment group, 6 did.

3.7.5 Summary of Electrode Placement

- For electrode placement, it is important to know whether a local or a referred problem is present. In the case of a local problem, treatment is usually also local, unless this is not possible for certain reasons, for example due to skin defects, marked local sensitivity, or a dressing.
- In the case of reflex, segmental irritation, one will first clarify whether there is primarily a paravertebral symptomatology or whether the symptomatology of specific stimulation points is predominant. In the case of paravertebral symptoms, segmental paravertebral treatment will be given accordingly; in the case of stimulation points, local treatment will be applied there.
- When using High TENS, it is important that the patient feels an electrical current sensation in the painful area. Here, if possible, treatment of nerve stimulation points will be chosen. It should be noted that treatment of MTrPs and acupuncture points can also lead to paresthesias in the painful area, so these may also be targeted.
- For muscular problems, it may be useful to induce muscle contractions. Here, targeting motor stimulation points and nerve points is optimal, sometimes also MTrPs. The same applies if one wishes to induce muscle contractions for more intensive Low TENS or AP-TENS treatment; then, local point stimulation will also be applied at motor and nerve points.
- With devices that allow 2-channel stimulation, the above-mentioned methods can be combined: one pair of electrodes can be used for segmental paravertebral or local transregional treatment, the second pair for point treatment at a corresponding segmentally appropriate site.

From the above discussion of acupuncture points, it is clear that these points provide a very good target for TENS.

3.8 High-Voltage Therapy

This form of electrotherapy is classified under TENS, as it involves transcutaneous nerve stimulation. Normally, for electrotherapy, the mains voltage (230 V) is reduced to about 24–50 V (low voltage). At this voltage and with a typical phase duration, relatively low current strengths are sufficient to trigger an action potential.

In high-voltage therapy, short, monophasic or asymmetrically compensated (double) pulses are used with a phase duration of 5–20 μs. In order for these short pulses to trigger an action potential at all, the applied voltage must be significantly higher than with conventional current forms. In fact, voltages between 150 and 500 V are used. This is where the name comes from: High Voltage Galvanic Current Stimulation (HVGC). The term High Voltage Pulsed Current Stimulation (HVPC) is also frequently seen, or simply high-voltage therapy in plain English. Strictly speaking, the term "high voltage" would be correct, but this designation is probably avoided because, for an electrical engineer, high voltage starts at 100,000 V. After all, you don't want to frighten this group of patients.

Due to the short pulse duration (as short as with High TENS), the treatment is significantly more comfortable than, for example, Low TENS. The usual frequencies of 1–200 Hz are used. The short pulses and the relatively very long pauses at these frequencies mean that hardly any chemical changes occur: 99% of the time, no current flows. At a frequency of 100 Hz and a phase duration of 10 μs, current flows for 1 s (= 1,000,000 μs) during 100 × 0.00001 s = 0.001 s. The risk of electrolysis or burns is also relatively low with non-compensated pulses, but not zero! Another reason for this is the fact that with HV stimulation, the device can be set to switch the polarity of the electrodes as an option. The rhythm, for example once per second or every 3–5 s, can usually be freely selected. Therefore, hyperemia normally does not occur, also because C fibers are only stimulated at phase durations of about 300–500 μs. However, if the C fibers are sensitized, as in the case of a local inflammatory reaction, redness may still occur under the electrodes. This is normal in such a case and is not related to an allergic reaction. Low frequencies (up to about 10 Hz, at motor threshold) are said, for reasons not further explained, to have a relaxing effect on tense muscles, medium frequencies (20–80 Hz) are said to be used for toning, and high frequencies (starting at 100 Hz) are said to have an analgesic effect. These are manufacturer claims; there is no clinical evidence, nor any physiological explanation for these different effects. On the topic of HVPC and pain, there is very little literature with comprehensible treatment parameters:

- Michlovitz et al. (1988) studied 30 patients after an inversion injury of the foot. One group received 30 min of ice, the second group received, in addition to ice, negatively polarized HVPC at 28 Hz, and the third group the same at 80 Hz. The three groups did not differ in the final outcome (28 Hz and 80 Hz, negatively polarized, clearly perceptible without muscle contractions, 30 min, once daily for 3 days).
- Stralka et al. (1998) used HVPC in the treatment of edema in patients with chronic hand problems (RSI). One group received a splint and daily 30 min HVPC, the control group received only a splint. The HVPC group showed less edema after 35 days than the control group. Parameters: 100 Hz, 30 min, 20 treatments over 35 days, (almost) imperceptible, polarity not mentioned.
- Sandoval et al. (2010) studied 28 patients with an inversion injury of the foot to assess the effect of either anodic, cathodic, or no HVPC, combined with a "standard" therapy for such injuries. The final outcome for the three groups was the same, but the cathodic HVPC group may have recovered somewhat faster. Parameters: 120 Hz, phase duration 75 μs, submotor threshold, 2 active electrodes locally (bimalleolar), one indifferent lumbar electrode.

The main area of application for HVPC is probably wound treatment. Reviews on this topic include some well-conducted clinical studies that demonstrate that HVPC can accelerate the healing of poorly healing wounds (Houghton et al. 2003). However, standard TENS parameters are used in treatments with HVPC. For example, Houghton used 100 Hz and pulses of 100 μs duration, unfortunately without precise information on intensity ("maximum 150 V"). The author is not aware of any studies in which the effects of HVPC and TENS were directly compared. Khouri et al. (2017) are the only ones who have established a kind of hierarchy showing that HVPC may have an edge in wound healing compared to other electrotherapies such as TENS and microcurrent. Polak et al. 2016 were able to show that HVPC and ultrasound (1 MHz, 0.5 W/cm^2, 20% pulse, 1–3 min per cm^2) led to the same result.

Since these devices are almost always CV types, the method is suitable for dynamic applications. If the active electrode is carefully placed or lifted, the resistance increases as the contact area increases or decreases. If the voltage (in volts) remains constant, the current, i.e., the intensity in mA, must decrease. The patient does not receive a shock.

3.8.1 High Voltage for Pain Relief and Wound Treatment

High voltage is about as effective as interferential current for pain relief, but not as effective as TENS. Electrode placement is similar to that of TENS; manufacturer recommendations regarding intensity vary from "pleasant, barely perceptible" and "pleasant, clearly perceptible" to "pleasant, motor." The mechanism of action is unclear; it is assumed that segmental inhibition is activated via stimulation of Aβ fibers. There is no in vitro evidence for this. High voltage does not have a significant effect on blood flow, except for a slight increase when dosed at the motor threshold, via the muscle pump. Heath and Gibbs (1992) found in a study that HVPC at frequencies of 2 Hz and 128 Hz improved blood flow in the calf of healthy subjects by about 30% (the 2 Hz group) and 13% (the 128 Hz group), respectively. An isometric contraction, performed as a control in the same study, improved blood flow by 330%. HVPC is effective in wound treatment. Compared to TENS, the effect is probably equally good. Please do not confuse a constant-voltage setting on the device with high voltage!

3.9 Microcurrent Electrical Stimulation, MES

Also known as microcurrent, Microcurrent Electrical Nerve Stimulation (MENS), microamperage stimulation, and low-intensity direct current. The term microelectrostimulation (MES) will be used below.

Frequencies of 0.5–150 Hz are used with current strengths in the μA range, i.e., one thousandth of the current strengths of TENS. Sometimes, during treatment, the polarity of the electrodes is switched in a certain rhythm. Either standard electrodes are used or probes for the treatment of acupuncture points. Clips are also used, which are attached to the earlobes for the treatment of headaches, sleep disorders, and stress (Taylor et al. 2013).

3.9.1 MES and Wound Healing

Between the surface of the skin and just below it, i.e., between the epithelium and endothelium, there is an electrical voltage difference, called the transepithelial potential difference, with the skin being negatively charged (Zhao et al. 2006). After an injury, the existing electrical balance is locally disturbed (Foulds and Barker 1983), resulting in a so-called current of injury of 10–60 mV 2–3 mm around the wound. The wound itself is negatively charged and the surrounding tissue is positive. This current of injury is important for wound healing, as it directs cells involved in wound healing toward the wound (Zhao 2009). Proponents of microcurrent now claim that MES stimulates this current of injury and thus supports healing. The application is also said to relieve pain, although it is unclear whether this occurs through activation of a pain inhibition system or whether the pain relief is secondary to wound healing. Since nothing is felt during the application, it can be assumed that microcurrent and TENS have different mechanisms of action.

3.9.2 Further Notes on MES

In pain treatment, regional application is often used; sometimes, for unclear reasons, two pairs of electrodes are crossed and applied around a painful area, possibly with a tetrapolar interferential analogy in mind. Acupuncture points are also often targeted. The mechanism of action of MES is unclear; the gate control mechanism is often cited, as the impulses are clearly too short to stimulate Aδ or even C fibers. Some authors mention the involvement of endorphins, without providing evidence.

3.10 Therapy with Medium-Frequency Currents

3.10.1 Definition

Medium-frequency therapy is the therapeutic application of alternating currents from the medium-frequency range. According to the classic classification by Edel, this is the range between 1000 and 300 kHz. The somewhat rough distinction is made due to the different physiological effects in the low-frequency, medium-frequency, and high-frequency ranges (Edel 1977).

With medium-frequency currents, nerves are stimulated through the skin. The impulses used are too short to directly trigger anything detectable in the muscle. Thus, these currents belong to the TENS applications.

Because MF currents, together with High and Low TENS, are among the most commonly used applications for the treatment of pain, the method will be discussed in detail below. See Table 3.7 for an MF-specific glossary.

3.10.2 Why This Distinction?

In the low-frequency range, the principle of period-synchronous stimulation (= cycle-synchronous stimulation) applies. This means that each impulse, provided phase duration and amplitude are sufficient, triggers an action potential. The action potentials are triggered at the same rhythm as the frequency of the current. A nerve fiber has a maximum depolarization frequency. This frequency is determined by the refractory period and is theoretically just over 300 Hz. In practice, frequencies above 200 Hz are rare (del Vecchio et al. 2019). Up to this threshold frequency range, each impulse will trigger an AP 1:1. If a nerve is stimulated with a frequency that exceeds the maximum depolarization frequency, the neural response changes. First, this leads after a few seconds to a conduction block, a so-called high frequency electrical conduction block (see following section). Second, several impulses are needed to trigger an action potential. Third, some of the impulses fall into the refractory period, so not every impulse can cause a depolarization. So, if a nerve is stimulated, for example, with 2000 impulses, not 2000 action potentials will come out at the other end, but only a few hundred, and these also irregularly. This phenomenon is called asynchronous depolarization or period-asynchronous stimulation. Therefore, the generously rounded distinction between low and medium frequency is made at 1000 Hz. In the *high-frequency* range, above 300 kHz, electromagnetic waves are used, which have a deep heating effect (diathermy) and do not trigger electrochemical and neuromuscular stimulation effects, except those related to heating.

3.10.3 High Frequency Electrical Conduction Block

The physiologist Wedensky described 1903 an interesting phenomenon, which he had already discovered in 1884. When stimulating Aα motoneurons, he noticed, among other things, that when using medium-frequency currents, the induced muscle contractions became very weak very quickly or even stopped altogether after a short time. When using lower frequencies, strong contractions could be triggered again immediately. There was no explanation for this phenomenon at the time; it was later called "Wedensky inhibition" (Bowman and McNeal 1986). Today, it is known that high frequencies have consequences for stimulation: Some of the impulses fall into the refractory period of the nerve. This makes repolarization of the membrane more difficult or even prevents it. This causes, after a few seconds, a rapidly reversible tonic depolarization of the membrane under the electrodes: the resting potential is no longer reached (Bhadra and Kilgore 2004; Kilgore and Bhadra 2004). As a result, no more action potentials can be conducted: a conduction block has been created.

This type of conduction inhibition is now referred to as high frequency electrical conduction block (Bowman and McNeal 1986). The phenomenon is clinically and therapeutically interesting for the inhibition of unwanted muscle activity, e.g., in spasticity, and perhaps in pain inhibition. In addition to this inhibition, continued stimulation leads to rapid depletion of neurotransmitter stores at the motor endplate. The depleted endplate is no longer able to transmit action potentials to depolarize the muscle fiber membrane. This phenomenon also manifests as inhibition and is an aspect of fatigue.

3.10.4 Why Therapy with MF Current?

Medium-frequency currents have thus been known for a long time, and as always, it is only a matter of time before people start thinking about their use. Usually, either the military or medicine takes the first step (ultrasound, infrasound, laser, microwaves, etc.), closely followed by industry.

With MF currents, it is possible to deliver stimuli in tissue, and Gildemeister found in his many experiments on humans that the current is not even that unpleasant and, despite high intensities, rarely leads to serious side effects (Gildemeister 1944). In addition, purely theoretically, the skin resistance should be lower due to the high frequency than with low frequency; more on this topic in Sect. 3.10.6. However, the problem was the aforementioned Wedensky inhibition. So what now? The current should be designed so that the nerve fibers have a chance to repolarize, so that the aforementioned inhibitory mechanisms do not occur. The basic idea: to create from a continuous MF alternating current a current that combines the impulse characteristics of an LF current with the advantages of an MF current. There are two solutions for this.

3.10.4.1 Solution 1

The simplest and, chronologically speaking, the second solution: It was devised in Russia at the end of the 1960s, some time after the Austrian engineer Nemec had developed his method. According to the Russian method, the medium-frequency current is interrupted in the device so that the nerve fibers have the opportunity to repolarize. Wedensky inhibition is thus prevented, as it only occurs after a few seconds of continuous stimulation. So-called MF impulses are generated, with the internal pulse frequency always corresponding to the frequency of the selected MF frequency; in Russia at that time, this was 5000 Hz. This means that if a stimulation frequency of, for example, 50 Hz is set, the MF current is interrupted 50 times per second. This type of current is called frequency-modulated medium-frequency current or MF impulse method; the pulse shape was sinusoidal (Fig. 3.7, variant c). Ward and Oliver (2007) now call it burst mode alternating current (BMAC), and the terms bursts or trains are used. Some readers may recognize the current as Russian stimulation avant la lettre, or—in a slightly modified form—as Aussie stimulation. More on this topic in the chapter on muscle stimulation (Sect. 4.7).

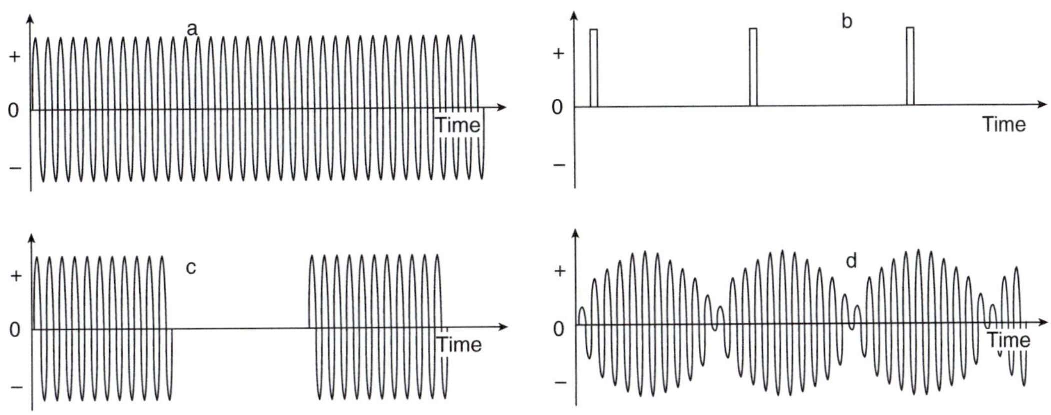

Fig. 3.7 (**a**) Continuous MF alternating current, (**b**) conventional monophasic impulse current, (**c**) rhythmically interrupted MF current (like Russian stimulation, frequency-modulated = BMAC), (**d**) amplitude-modulated MF current. From Ward 2009, with kind permission

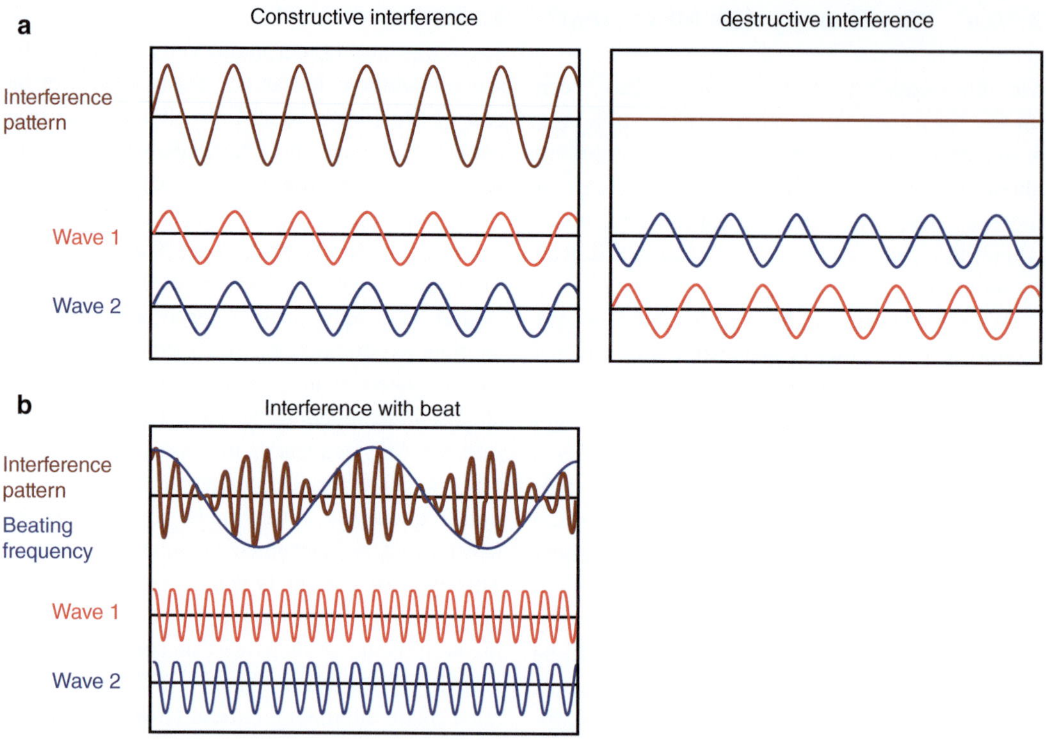

Fig. 3.8 (**a**) Interference. Left: The waves are congruent and reinforce each other. Right: The waves are shifted by half a phase and cancel each other out. © Jan Krieger, Wikimedia Commons, licensed under Creative Commons License by-sa-2.0-de, URL: http://creativecommons.org/licenses/by-sa/2.0/de/legalcode. (**b**) The waves are slightly offset from each other, creating a beat. © Jan Krieger, Wikimedia Commons, licensed under Creative Commons License by-sa-2.0-de, URL: http://creativecommons.org/licenses/by-sa/2.0/de/legalcode

3.10.4.2 Solution 2

The second solution is significantly more complicated, but probably gives the current a certain mystique (Johnson 1999). Although it can be demonstrably shown that the idea definitely does not work, it is in any case original (Treffene 1983; Beatti et al. 2011).

Starting point: When two waves meet, interference phenomena occur.

In Fig. 3.8, the superposition on the left leads to a doubling of the wave energy, on the right the waves cancel each other out: the net energetic result is zero. If the waves differ only slightly in frequency, they can never overlap exactly. This results in a so-called beat: the intensity then increases and decreases at a certain frequency; this is called the beat frequency. Guitar players among us use this principle when tuning their instrument with harmonics. The closer the tones, i.e., their frequencies, of two strings are, the lower the beat frequency; the further apart, the higher the beat frequency. If two tones are very close together, for example, the A string is nicely tuned to 440 Hz, the string to be tuned produces "almost" an A at 443 Hz, then a beat with a frequency of 3 Hz (443 minus 440) is produced as the difference tone. This becomes audible when tuning the guitar: it is still an A (almost), but the volume (the intensity) increases and decreases 3 times per second, you hear the beat of 3 Hz.

With so-called true interferential current (IF), it works as follows: An alternating current with a constant frequency of 4000 Hz (the so-called carrier frequency) is combined with an alternating current whose frequency can be set between 4000 and 4200 Hz. The difference between the two frequencies then results, as with sound waves, in the beat frequency. However, with IF, it is not called a beat, but the amplitude modulation frequency (AMF): the frequency remains constant, only the amplitude (the intensity) is modulated. Hence the official name: amplitude-modulated medium-frequency current.

Example: One circuit has a fixed frequency of 4000 Hz, the other circuit is set to 4050 Hz, the difference is 50 Hz. This is the AMF: the actual (supposed) stimulation frequency that is supposed to trigger something in the tissue and allegedly has the same properties as a low-frequency 50 Hz pulse current.

The low-frequency interruptions (the beats) actually prevent a conduction block with their gradual on-off phases: the continuous MF current is constantly interrupted. In this way, the cell membrane can repeatedly repolarize.

According to Nemec, two separate MF circuits are used in a technically quite complicated way with two pairs of electrodes, also called tetrapolar interference. The two circuits are supposed to be combined in the tissue to produce an LF stimulation character. This is called endogenous interference. If these two circuits are combined in the device, it is called exogenous interference, which is thus bipolar. In English, the terms "true interferential current" and "premodulated interferential current" are used.

At the interference location (in the so-called interference cross), in the theoretical ideal case, the amplitude (intensity) of the two intersecting circuits would almost double. As with ultrasound waves, there would be amplifications (increases in intensity) and attenuations (decreases in intensity) of the intensity set on the device in mA. The carrier frequency (in the example above, the tone A) remains the same.

3.10.5 Summation, Gildemeister Effect

At the beginning of the last century, the physiologist Gildemeister discovered that with MF, several impulses are necessary to trigger excitation (Gildemeister 1944). Each negative half-wave depolarizes the cell membrane a little more, until after a certain number of alternating current periods (Gildemeister calls this the effective time) the depolarization threshold is reached. An action potential is then triggered. The higher the amplitude, i.e., the set intensity, the shorter the effective time. Gildemeister recognized this phenomenon as summation. Bromm and Lullies (1966) further investigated the phenomenon and found that the cathodic half-waves of the sine wave cause the stepwise depolarization and that the immediately following anodic sine half-waves are not sufficient to counteract this depolarization. The effect occurs under both electrodes. Incidentally, exactly the same thing happens when symmetrically compensated rectangular pulses are used, only no summation occurs here (Bromm and Lullies 1966). This effect was later called the "Gildemeister effect." Knowledge of this phenomenon makes it more difficult to explain the effect of MF currents on tissue. We can never predict exactly at what frequency the target tissue will be stimulated. This will be explained in detail below.

3.10.6 Special Properties of Medium-Frequency Currents

Medium-frequency alternating current is a symmetrically compensated alternating current with a frequency between 1000 and 300,000 Hz. Typically, frequencies between 2500 and 10,000 Hz are used, most commonly—though for unclear reasons (Johnson 1999)—4000 Hz. Sinusoidal pulses are usually employed. Due to the symmetrical compensation, electrolytic effects generally do not occur.

However, MF is not harmless! In a study by Ward and Robertson (1998), after application in three healthy subjects, blisters appeared around the electrodes. Ford et al. in 2005 described a patient with third-degree burns after MF application to the knee following knee joint replacement surgery. Satter in 2008 described a patient with burns after MF treatment in an area containing osteosynthetic material.

The chemical changes that occur in the tissue during the short (125 μs at 4000 Hz), negative half-wave are counteracted by the subsequent positive half-wave, just as with compensated TENS pulses. Without chemical changes, there is no pH change in the tissue, and the risk of tissue damage is low. Due to the rapid polarity changes at the electrodes, the current is referred to as apolar. Wyss (1975) speaks of ambipolar stimulation, but since the processes under the electrodes do not occur exactly simultaneously, but rather with a half-phase shift, MF current also follows the laws of polar stimulation as usual (Bromm and Lullies 1966). But who wants to split hairs here. The short pulses (125 μs at 4000 Hz), like the equally short high TENS pulses, practically do not stimulate Aδ and C fibers, which is why the current is usually quite comfortable for the patient. Mind you: Depending on how high the intensity is set, MF current can also become unpleasant at high intensities (Ward and Robertson 1998; Palmer et al. 1999; Ward and Oliver 2007).

According to Nemec (1959, 1960, 1967, 1968), interferential current has three advantages:

1. Due to the high frequency, skin resistance is said to be lower, making it easier for the current to pass through the poorly conducting skin barrier. As a result, the sensory load for the patient would be lower, making the current more comfortable for the patient.
   - It's not that simple. First, because resistance depends not only on frequency but also on phase duration (Lykken and Venables 1971; Yamamoto and Yamamoto 1977), and at a frequency of 4000 Hz, the phase duration is 125 μs, in the same range as with TENS applications. The fact remains, however, that skin impedance is lower at medium frequency than at low frequency. The composition of the frequencies, however, depends crucially on the waveform. And it can happen that different waveforms produce the same impedance. Therefore, both applications can be about equally (un)pleasant, depending on intensity. Second, it actually doesn't matter that skin resistance is high. This high resistance is caused by the stratum corneum, where there are no sensors. The relevant sensors responsible for the sensory aspect of the current are located beneath this layer, where the electrical properties are the same as deeper in the tissue.
2. The two circuits would interfere with each other and form an area in the so-called interference cross where the target tissue is maximally stimulated (Fig. 3.9).
   - That is definitely not true. Interference phenomena occur almost everywhere between the four electrodes, but least of all in the center. First, as the distance from the electrode increases, the current density decreases, and thus it is lowest in the center between the electrodes. Stimulation is always strongest directly under the electrodes. Treffene showed in 1983 that interference phenomena in a plastic tank filled with water occur almost everywhere between the electrodes, but unfortunately weakest where they are supposed to—in the center; here they were minimal. Stimulation was greater between two adjacent electrodes than in the area where the circuits were supposed to cross.

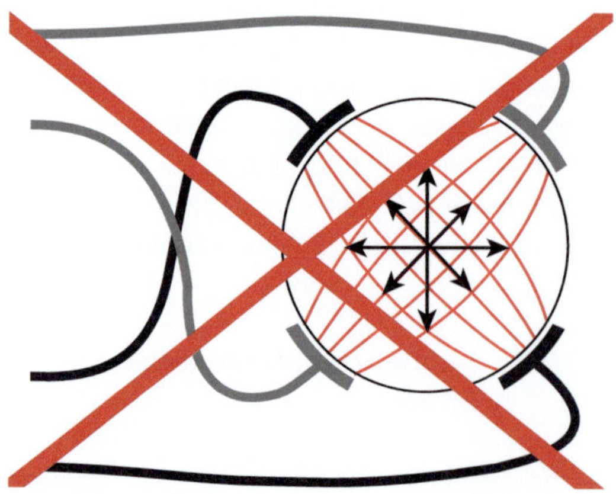

Fig. 3.9 Two circuits and a cross in the middle: This is definitely not how IF works. From Ward 2009, with kind permission

- Unlike the water tank mentioned above, the body is not homogeneous, so it is impossible for the voltage lines to run in such a way that they cross at the "correct" point for interference. Beattie et al. in 2011 performed measurements in humans on the medial quadriceps muscle to determine the voltage distribution during tetrapolar interferential current in the muscle. Measurement electrodes were inserted at various locations relative to the four stimulating electrodes. Result: The highest voltage was measured near a stimulating electrode, the lowest in the center at the supposed interference cross. A measurement electrode 5 cm outside the stimulation area of the four stimulating electrodes registered almost twice as high values as in the supposed interference cross. The authors also compared exogenous IF with endogenous IF and found that with exogenous IF, where the interference occurs in the device and not in the patient, the highest voltage, as expected, is measured superficially near the electrodes.

3. In the interference cross, an area would be formed with the actual stimulation frequency, the amplitude modulation frequency or AMF. The AMF, or beat frequency, is determined by the different frequencies of the two circuits and typically lies, depending on the setting, in the usual low-frequency range of 1 to 200 Hz. This AMF would not have the same properties as the LF frequencies, but rather "genuine MF stimulation effects due to the MF carrier frequency itself" (Edel 1977).
   - There are quite a few things wrong with that. First: see the point above. Second: The reason for the occurrence of "genuine MF stimulation effects" is physiologically at best vague. Third: It is nevertheless repeatedly claimed that tissue responds to this 50 Hz AMF in the same way as to a low-frequency current of the same frequency, and that effects such as pain relief and improved blood flow should occur with MF current just as with LF. More on that later. First, about the AMF: If low frequency is used to stimulate one end of a nerve fiber at 50 Hz, one can expect 50 action potentials at the other end. This works up to a certain physiological limit, and this limit, as already mentioned, is determined by the refractory period of the nerve. Let's take a closer look. The part of the pulse current intended to produce the stimulus consists of a short series of individual pulses (Fig. 3.7c, d), called a burst. The duration of such bursts is either fixed or variable depending on the device, as long as these 50 Hz "fit" into one second. If, for example, a burst lasts 10 ms, it consists (at 4000 Hz base frequency) of $10 \div 1000 \times 4000 = 40$ alternating current pulses. Now the refractory period comes into play. During the absolute refractory period, the fiber definitely cannot generate an action potential; this phase lasts about 1 ms. Afterwards, during the relative refractory period, the nerve fiber can generate an AP, but only if the stimulus is significantly stronger than normal. This phase lasts about 2 ms. For this reason, the refractory period only has an effect when firing rates occur with a frequency higher than about 300 Hz, something unusual in the human nervous system. These 300 Hz correspond to 1/13 of the 4000 Hz generated by the MF current. In other words: at most, every 13th MF pulse could trigger an action potential (Bowman and McNeal 1986). Each burst, with its 40 pulses, thus triggers at most about 3 action potentials in the nerve, and the 50 bursts per second trigger a total of 150 action potentials ($40 \div 13 \times 50$). The target tissue is therefore not stimulated at 50 Hz, but at 150 Hz. Perhaps. Because with the sinusoidal endogenous variant, some pulses remain subthreshold (Fig. 5.7 d); these probably do not trigger anything, but perhaps the Gildemeister effect plays a role here. However, we do not know how this effect plays into the process, since we do not know how many

individual MF pulses are needed to trigger an action potential by summation. Perhaps only 3 pulses per burst are needed. Or 8. Or it varies. But it will definitely not be exactly 50 Hz; rather, it will be a multiple of the set burst frequency. There is solid evidence for these claims (Bowman and McNeal 1986; Stefanovska and Vodovnik 1985; Laufer et al. 2001; Ward and Robertson 2000; Laufer and Elboim 2008). This tedious calculation is intended to make it clear that, despite the low AMF settings, the tissue is stimulated at quite high frequencies. Whether this is biologically meaningful is unclear and unresearched. Furthermore, the calculation is intended to make it clear that statements such as "The AMF determines the depolarization frequency" and "The AMF corresponds to the frequencies used in low frequency" (den Adel and Luykx 2005 in a therapy manual from a device manufacturer) are not correct. We definitely cannot apply the results of TENS research to MF current.

A bit more on the topic of skin load. In electrotherapy application, two well-conducting structures (sponge and subcutis) are separated by a very poorly conducting structure: the stratum corneum (R about 1000–500,000 Ohms). This corresponds to the structure of a capacitor. A capacitor presents no significant resistance to a high-frequency current. From the very simplified formula shown in Fig. 3.10, it can be seen that the capacitive resistance of a capacitor depends on the frequency of the applied current. At a higher frequency, the resistance would therefore decrease. Since the electrotherapy device in constant-current mode keeps the intensity (in mA) constant, a lower (skin) resistance results in a lower voltage at the electrodes (Ohm's law, U = I × R), so the current can pass through the skin relatively easily, which is supposed to be more comfortable for the patient. Allegedly, the current can therefore penetrate deeper, which, according to calculations by Lambert et al. (1989), unfortunately is not true. Because the current is distributed most diffusely between adjacent electrodes, little remains for depth (Table 3.5).

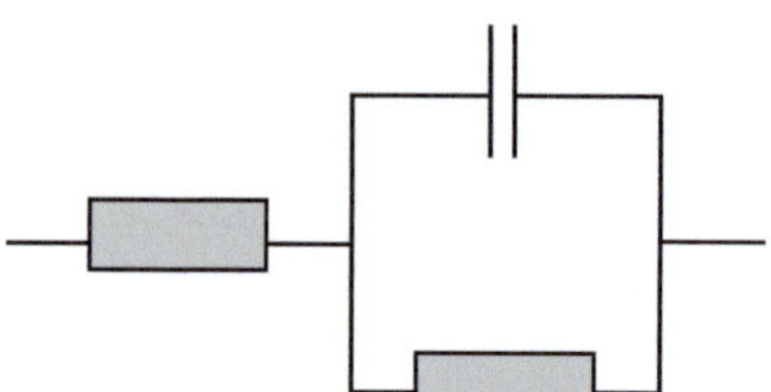

$$\text{RC (Ohm)} = \frac{1}{\text{C (farad)} \times 2\pi \text{f (Hz)}}$$

Fig. 3.10 Simplified representation of the equivalent circuit diagram of the skin

Table 3.5 Approximate skin resistance at different frequencies

50 Hz (DD)	3180 Ω
143 Hz (UR)	1110 Ω
2500 Hz (MF)	60 Ω
4000 Hz (MF)	40 Ω

3.10.7 Spectrum, Sweep, and Vector

To optimize the MF effect and avoid habituation, every clinical device offers various setting options, of which four are almost always present, though usually under different names. You can select the AMF, i.e., the "stimulation frequency." In addition, you can choose a so-called spectrum and the way the spectrum is "swept," as well as a vector. A spectrum, or "sweep" in English, is an AMF range that is automatically traversed stepwise. For example: you set a lower limit of 70 Hz and an upper limit of 120 Hz, and the device now changes the AMF from 70 to 120 Hz and back in a certain rhythm. Other devices require you to set, for example, 70 Hz and a spectrum of 50 Hz, and the device does the same as in the first example: 70 Hz → 120 Hz → 70 Hz. Sometimes you simply select program 42 because the device suggests it, and it does the rest. Here, it is worth studying the user manual. In addition, every device offers the option to select the sweep mode. These modes would make the sweep more aggressive or milder, depending on the acuteness of the problem. There are settings in which the aforementioned 70–120 Hz switch abruptly, for example, one second at 70 Hz and immediately after that one second at 120 Hz and back, or slowly increase from 70 to 120 Hz over 6 s and then slowly decrease again. This, of course, with any conceivable frequency combination.

Johnson and Tabasam (2003a, b) conducted two studies on healthy subjects using a painful cold stimulus (arm in ice-cold water) to investigate how these settings affect cold sensitivity. Settings in both studies: carrier frequency 4000 Hz, IF tetrapolar on the forearm, intensity very clearly perceptible but tolerable, duration 20 min. The subjects were "blinded." First study: 60 subjects, AMF frequencies 20, 60, 100, 140, 180, 220 Hz. In the second study, 40 subjects, AMF from 1 to 100 Hz, sweep 1–1 abrupt, 6–6 abrupt, 6–6 slow, and 100 Hz bursts (burst duration unclear). Result: IF increases the pain threshold for the cold stimulus, but neither the frequency nor the sweep mode has any effect on the outcome. Fuentes et al. (2010) found the same result with healthy subjects: IF increased the pressure pain threshold on the back equally with and without AMF sweep.

Then there is the vector. Whether it is an "isoplanar field," a "dipole vector," a "rotating vector," or whatever: the electronic trick is that either amplitude modulation takes place in the device or the intensity of the individual channels is continuously varied. Or both. This then feels as if the current is "wandering" around the treatment area. In reality, this means that electrode placement is less critical. Noble et al. (2000) found no added value for the outcome (a slight improvement in blood flow) when using a "rotating vector."

3.10.8 Use of Certain Electrotherapies, an Ethical Problem?

Herbert et al. (2011) define evidence-based physiotherapy as follows:

> *"Evidence-based physiotherapy is physiotherapy that is based on relevant, high-quality research. The practice of evidence-based physiotherapy should be shaped by relevant, high-quality clinical research, **the preferences of the patients** and the practical knowledge of the physiotherapist."* (Emphasis by the author)

Patient preferences include their expectations, views, and goals. Naturally, these are central.

Veras et al. (2016) found the definition insufficient because it does not take into account certain ethical aspects such as autonomy, appreciation, and justice. They wish to adapt the definition of the World Confederation for Physical Therapy (WCPT) and have made the following proposal:

> *"Evidence-based physiotherapy is a field of study, research, and practice in which clinical decisions are made based on the best available evidence, integrating professional practice and expertise with ethical principles."* (Transl. by the author)

Roman (2017) describes how manufacturers of medical devices and their users can find themselves in ethical conflicts when devices are manufactured, sold, and used for which there is either no or only little, sometimes contradictory, evidence. There are a multitude of devices on the market that any professional can easily recognize as dubious, for example, those that are claimed to be equally effective for psychological problems as well as rheumatic complaints. Note the wording "can be used".

But does this also apply to IF? With TENS, we have a well-researched application whose effectiveness has been confirmed. The application is almost free of side effects and, after appropriate instruction, can be performed by most patients at home at low cost. IF devices are expensive and large, and the patient must go to a clinic or practice for treatment, where the application requires the involvement of a professional. The evidence for effectiveness is thin, although proponents of the therapy repeatedly make claims about specific MF current properties that would distinguish the therapy from conventional electrotherapy. Properties for which no evidence has been provided.

Admittedly, there are special properties, but these are not necessarily specific to MF. TENS has such properties as well. However, to this day we cannot assess to what extent the results, for example from Dertinger (2000) and Phillipp et al. (2000), have clinical relevance or are applicable, except in psoriasis patients (1998, 2004). The investigators successfully used MF in a small study in psoriasis patients (Phillipp et al. 2000). There are no further, larger studies or long-term results; for various reasons, the therapy seems to have fallen out of use.

A brief digression: The researchers discovered that certain modulation frequencies of MF currents, under very specific conditions in cell cultures in the laboratory, stimulate the production of cAMP. There are frequencies that stimulate better than others, and some that inhibit. The investigators speak of a frequency window, roughly comparable to an absorption spectrum of light or laser. This cAMP (cyclic adenosine monophosphate) is a second messenger protein involved in a wide variety of biological processes, from spermatogenesis to regulation of the circadian rhythm, from metabolic and immune processes to pain memory (Silva et al. 1998; Serezani et al. 2008; Ould Amer and Hebert-Chatelain 2018). Incidentally, 50 Hz alternating current, TENS, and EAP also influence cAMP production, and not just in a petri dish, but in living rats (Ding et al. 2013) and mice (Kim et al. 2018). To attribute the supposedly specific effect of MF current to this would probably be somewhat simplistic or short-sighted, and as already mentioned: this knowledge has not yet had any clinical consequences.

Back to patient preferences. Does this also mean that the therapist must do what the patient wants?

An example: TENS and IF are among the most commonly used applications for pain relief, and their effects have been and continue to be studied worldwide both in the laboratory and clinically. The effect of TENS on a wide variety of pain types is considered established, of course only if the intensity is appropriate. IF does not fare badly in pain relief, although much remains unclear regarding the mechanisms of action. The most recent reviews (September 2020) generally attest that IF is more effective than placebo treatment in the management of various types of pain (Almeida et al. 2018; Ferreira et al. 2018, 2019; Resende et al. 2018; Galasso et al. 2020).

However: Shanahan et al. (2006) compared the effect of High TENS (100 Hz, 100 μs, 20 min) and IF (exogenous, AMF 100 Hz, 5000 Hz, phase duration 100 μs, 20 min) on raising the pain threshold for a painful cold stimulus. The intensity for both applications was adequate and the same: strong but comfortable. The result: TENS was significantly more effective, but the subjects preferred IF, *because this application was more pleasant*.

Such a result presents us with an ethical problem: Do I use a therapy whose effectiveness is proven, or do I do something that is less effective but the patient prefers? After all, money is also involved.

3.10.8.1 Over-, Under-, and Misprovision

The German Advisory Council for Concerted Action in Health Care defined a few terms in 2000 that are of interest in this context:

- Underprovision is
  - provision in the case of individual, professionally and scientifically recognized need, which is refused or not (reasonably) made available, even though services with sufficiently proven medical benefit and an acceptable benefit-cost ratio are in fact available.
- Overprovision refers to
  - services provided beyond individual needs and without or without sufficiently proven medical (additional) benefit (e.g., out of ignorance, courtesy, for marketing purposes, or for income interests).

- Misprovision is
  - any provision that causes avoidable harm or any provision of services whose harm or potential for harm clearly outweighs their (possible) benefit. The following subcases can be distinguished:
    Services that are in themselves appropriate to needs, i.e., neither over- nor underprovision and are efficient, but in the way they are applied do not meet recognized professional quality criteria (§§ 106 and 135–137 SGB V) and therefore imply avoidable risks or harm.

Omitted but indicated and in themselves appropriate services can also be interpreted as misprovision in terms of the outcome, since missed benefit means unnecessary harm; underprovision is, in this sense, also a form of misprovision. End of quote.

And what does this mean for us? When a therapist performs a treatment, they should be informed about which application is most likely to lead to success. Da Silva et al. (2015) investigated what physiotherapists think of EBM. These therapists have a positive opinion of EBM and believe that there is potential for optimization regarding their knowledge, skills, and behavior towards EBM. Obstacles in this context are

- too little time,
- insufficient knowledge of statistics,
- insufficient support from the employer,
- too few sources and tools,
- too little interest, and
- insufficient generalization of study results.

Other authors express the influences on EBP in physiotherapy more as facilitators than as barriers. For example, Bridges et al. (2007) identified several personal characteristics that can facilitate EBP:

- independent learning,
- postgraduate study (bachelor's, master's, continuing education courses),
- the conviction that research (especially in a "digested" format such as clinical guidelines) can be used in daily clinical decision-making without impairing productivity and efficient patient flow,
- nonconformity, i.e., not being afraid to deviate from traditional or usual practice when newer research demonstrates more effective methods.

The last point stands refreshingly in direct contrast to two excuses the author has often heard in electrotherapy courses when it comes to justifying a therapy choice. "Because we've always done it this way." And: "Because we've never done it that way."

3.10.8.2 Considerations for Therapy with Medium-Frequency Currents

There are a multitude of studies confirming the effectiveness of TENS. TENS is also easy to use, virtually free of side effects, the devices are handy and not expensive. The effectiveness of medium-frequency currents is confirmed; MF is better than placebo treatment, but not better than TENS (Table 3.6). The devices are expensive, the patient must travel to a clinic or practice for treatment, the explanations for the mechanisms of action are at best vague and sometimes completely untenable. The argument against IF that the devices cost more than TENS devices is no longer entirely valid; today there are Walkman-sized devices for home treatment in the same price range as very expensive TENS devices. Let's forget about the tetrapolar IF cross, which does not exist where you want it. If you use IF, you should choose the premodulated variant.

With a standard setting such as: carrier frequency 4000 Hz, AMF 80 Hz, spectrum 50 Hz, sweep 6/\6, intensity clearly perceptible but comfortable, you can go a long way with sensitive patients. By the way: the symbol "6/\6" on the device means "increasing slowly for 6 s, then decreasing for 6 s". The frequency setting (AMF) and the sweep program (swing pattern)

Table 3.6 Publications on the effectiveness of medium-frequency currents. Only publications with comprehensible treatment parameters were considered

Indication	Authors	Result
Muscle stimulation of innervated musculature, see NMES	1. Ward & Robertson (2000), Ward et al. (2004), Ward (2009) 2. Scott et al. (2015) 3. Vaz and Frasson (2018) 4. Lijima et al. (2018)	1. Good results with MF current, Russian Stim, Aussie-Stim. 2. LF better than MF 3. MF = LF 4. MF = LF
Pain in general (review, meta-analysis)	Fuentes et al. (2010)	Generally better than placebo
Temporomandibular joint pain	Taylor et al. (1987)	No effect
Shoulder impingement	1. Nazligul et al. (2018) 2. Gomes et al. (2018)	1. No effect 2. No effect
Shoulder pain after CVA	1. Eslamian et al. (2020) 2. Suriya-amarit et al. (2014)	1. EAP better than IF, no intensity data 2. Better than placebo
Low back pain	1. Facci et al. (2011) 2. Albornoz-Cabello et al. (2017) 3. Franco et al. (2018)	1. IF = TENS, better than control group 2. Short-term better than control group 3. IF combined with Pilates better than Pilates alone
Pain in knee OA review	Zeng et al. (2015)	Promising
Improvement of blood circulation	Noble et al. (2000)	Better skin blood flow in healthy subjects, comparable to low TENS
Wound healing (decubitus)	Shahrokhi et al. (2014)	Questionably better (no control group)
DOMS	Minder et al. (2002)	No effect

DOMS: Delayed Onset Muscle Soreness, LF: Low Frequency, MF: Medium Frequency, EAP: Electroacupuncture, NMES: Neuromuscular Electrical Stimulation

have no effect on the outcome (Johnson and Tabasam 2003a, b). You can therefore use the various settings on the device to make the application as comfortable as possible for the patient. The effect can most likely be explained by a gate control mechanism: fast-conducting nerve fibers are stimulated. However, there are no studies confirming this, as there are for TENS. The more the therapist tries to localize the interference cross at the right spot, the greater the placebo effect is likely to be.

Shanahan and Ward showed in 2006 that High TENS is objectively superior to IF in terms of pain relief. However, the subjects found the IF application more pleasant.

This is not unproblematic: Should we now follow the facts or the patients? In other words: It may not work as well, but it feels so nice?

Food for thought.

3.10.9 General Treatment Guidelines for MF Currents

If one decides to use MF currents, the interference should be applied exogenously, bipolarly, or as 2 + 2. The latter refers to an application with two separate circuits, for example, one circuit lumbar and one circuit simultaneously segmental in the area of radiation on the leg, or one circuit lumbar and one circuit on related trigger points. The endogenous application is problematic. It is not as if nothing happens with this application. The application can be made very comfortable and can be used as a good introduction to a more effective application. The same can be achieved with a carefully dosed High TENS application.

Low, abruptly changing frequencies would irritate the tissue more than higher, slowly changing ones. Because MF current is almost always perceived as very pleasant, this distinction is irrelevant. Johnson and Tabasam (2003a, b) could not find any difference in effect between different spectrum programs and various frequencies. It certainly makes sense to find the most comfortable setting for the patient, although this does not mean that it is also the most effective treatment. It should be emphasized again that to date, no different effects of the various settings have been found.

3.10.10 Indications for MF Currents

As discussed above, it is indeed possible to generate afferent stimuli with MF alternating currents. Although what is claimed does not happen exactly, there are nevertheless studies showing that MF current has a better analgesic effect than placebo treatment (Fuentes et al. 2010; Facci et al. 2011; Albornoz-Cabello et al. 2017). Unfortunately, there are also many studies that cannot demonstrate an effect, but this may also be due to IF being underdosed. Unfortunately, there are no comparative studies on this. IF is often applied only for a relatively short time; 15 min is not uncommon. This is because patients are said to show signs of fatigue during longer treatments. However, experiences with TENS in this regard contradict this concern. The 15 min may have become established rather because this corresponds to the usual treatment rhythm in a clinic.

MF currents are used for a variety of indications, and accordingly, there are many treatment guidelines and proposals. These proposals are based on the assumption that MF current, due to its high frequency, possesses special properties. Why this should be the case is unclear. This assumption has never been scientifically confirmed to date.

It should be noted that MF therapy has virtually no effect on blood circulation. Since there is no stimulation of Aδ and C fibers, activation of central pain-inhibiting systems is not to be expected. There are no studies in which, as with low TENS, it has been investigated whether an analgesic effect is prevented by administration of an opioid antagonist. A PubMed search with terms such as "interferential current, kilohertz current, naloxone, naltrindole, descending, central, inhibition" yielded no results (as of December 2021).

The common practice of transferring results from TENS studies to MF current is, in today's era of evidence-based practice—putting it mildly—problematic. This does not mean that MF current should not be used. However, a certain skepticism is warranted.

The alleged indications for MF are the same as for high and low TENS:

- Chronic and acute pain of various causes
- Diseases of the rheumatic spectrum
- Osteoarthritis, spondylosis, myalgia
- Pain points, trigger points
- Post-traumatic conditions, swelling
- Peripheral circulatory disorders

As with high and low TENS, a distinction is made between:

- Local treatment (pain point or trigger point treatment)
- Regional treatment, larger painful areas
- Neural and segmental treatment
- Muscular treatment (muscle stimulation is discussed in Chap. 4).

It is essential to note that only the analgesic effect of MF current has been confirmed; the mechanism remains unclear (Table 3.7).

Table 3.7 Glossary Medium Frequency

Amplitude	Intensity in mA
Phase duration/time, T (Time)	Pulse duration/time in ms or μs
Phase interval, R (Rest)	The time between 2 pulses in ms or μs, pulse pause
Frequency modulation	The regular interruption of the carrier frequency to prevent conduction block. English: Bursts, Trains
Spectrum or spectrum frequency	Running through a selected frequency range to avoid habituation. For example, from 100 to 150 Hz and back. English: Sweep
Amplitude modulation	The rhythmic increase and decrease of the amplitude to prevent conduction block
AMF, amplitude modulation frequency	The difference between the fixed carrier frequency and a variable frequency, supposedly the stimulation frequency. English: Beat
Sweep time, spectrum program	The time during which a current type changes its frequency. For example, 6/\6: in 6 s slowly up and in 6 s back down. English: Sweep Pattern
Carrier frequency	The fixed MF frequency, usually 2500 Hz or 4000 Hz
Vector	Enlargement of the effective stimulation area by automatically varying the intensity and/or frequency
Modulation depth	Extent of modulation in percent, indicates how much the intensity increases and decreases from one beat to the next

Some manufacturers use different terms for those mentioned here. See the user manual for details

3.11 Indications and Contraindications for TENS (including MF, MES, HVPC)

3.11.1 Indications

- Acute and chronic pain, including neurogenic pain
- Postoperative or post-traumatic pain
- Wound healing disorders

3.11.2 Contraindications

Contraindications are a tricky matter. If one consults various textbooks, unfortunately the authors do not always agree (Houghton et al. 2010). In particular, references are rarely mentioned. Not only because they do not exist, but also because in many cases common sense is sufficient. See the highly recommended review by Smith and Pell (2003) on the lack of studies on the use of parachutes. The subsequent RCT on their effectiveness is also worth reading (Yeh et al. 2008). Research can indeed be fun.

TENS should not be used

- in areas where it could cause malfunction of electronic devices, including pacemakers and implanted cardioverter-defibrillators (ICDs) (Vlay 1998; Holmgren et al. 2008). The recommended safety distance of at least 50 cm between electrodes and pacemaker is demonstrably insufficient (see below, 3.12.3). If necessary, consult with a cardiologist;
- in areas with implanted osteosynthesis material. The claim that IF/MF currents may be used with implanted osteosynthesis material is **definitely false**. Ford et al. (2005) and Satter (2008) have described serious burns in patients treated with interferential current in areas containing metal;
- on the lower back or abdomen of pregnant women in the first trimester,
- without specialized training on acupuncture points in pregnant women,
- in regions with known or suspected malignancy,
- on recently irradiated body areas,
- in persons with active deep vein thrombosis or thrombophlebitis (locally),
- in actively bleeding tissue or in persons with untreated hemorrhagic disorders,

- on infected tissue, in tuberculosis, or wounds with underlying osteomyelitis (locally),
- without specialized training on the thorax in persons with heart disease, cardiac arrhythmias, or heart failure,
- in the neck or head area of persons known to have epileptic seizures,
- transcranially without specialized training,
- without specialized training on areas near reproductive organs or genitals,
- on areas near or over the eyes,
- on the anterior neck or over the carotid artery,
- on damaged or compromised skin areas that would lead to uneven current conduction (except for open wounds where the specific intent is to use electrical stimulation for tissue healing),
- in areas with impaired sensation (Ward and Robertson 1998), relatively (monitor very closely! But see also Cuypers et al. 2010),
- in persons with cognitive or communication impairments that limit their ability to provide adequate feedback, relatively (monitor very closely!),
- in pain of unclear origin,
- in cases of general malaise, fever, relatively (monitor very closely!),
- in anxious individuals, general agitation, traumatized patients (torture victims).

3.12 Risks and Side Effects of TENS Applications (including MF)

3.12.1 Suction Electrodes

So-called suction electrodes are often used for MF current applications—flexible rubber cups with moist sponges inside. The devices used typically have a small container on the back to collect the water that is drawn out of the cups. In a personal study on risk management in physiotherapy, the author found in a hospital that this container, despite regular cleaning, was heavily colonized with Burkholderia cepacia (Fig. 3.11). The interior of the device was not examined.

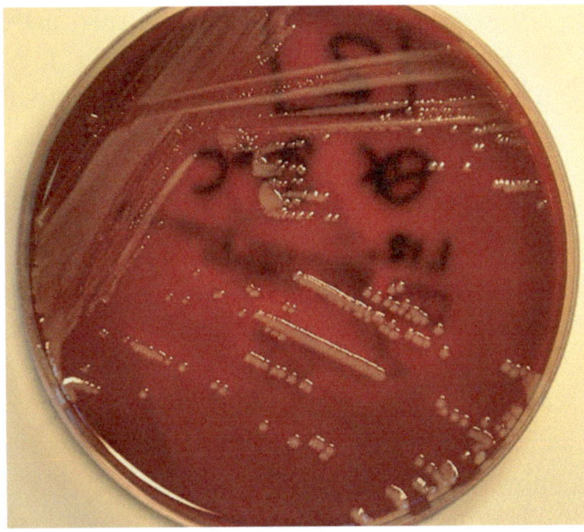

Fig. 3.11 Burkholderia cepacia

Burkholderia is a multi-resistant microorganism that causes onion rot and is found everywhere in groundwater and soil. We all have it on our shoes. For patients with cystic fibrosis in particular, infection with this organism can have very serious consequences. It is therefore strongly recommended to thoroughly clean and disinfect these water containers daily. Regular bacteriological testing certainly does no harm; at the same time, you can check the ultrasound heads and the gel.

3.12.2 Contact Dermatitis

- Dwyer et al. described 1994 a patient with contact dermatitis at the stimulation sites after repeated TENS application. Allergy tests showed that the patient reacted to propylene glycol in the contact gel. Reactions to this substance are common.
- Corazza et al. described 1999 a female patient with contact dermatitis a few minutes after a TENS treatment on the back. Allergy tests revealed a nickel allergy. Upon inquiry, the manufacturer stated that their electrodes contained no nickel, but gold-plated copper. An analysis of the electrodes detected nickel instead of gold.

- Castelain and Chabeau described 1986 three patients with contact dermatitis after lumbar TENS applications. The patients tested positive for allergy to propylene glycol. The electrode manufacturers were unwilling to provide information about the composition of the contact gel.
- Weber-Muller et al. described 2004 two patients with contact dermatitis due to an allergic reaction to several substances in the electrode gel. These included ethylene glycol dimethacrylate, ethyl acrylate, 2-hydroxyethyl acrylate, triethylene glycol diacrylate, 2-hydroxyethyl methacrylate, and 2-hydroxypropyl methacrylate.

This is the well-known tip of the iceberg. Since these are relatively harmless irritations and because there is not yet a proper reporting culture for so-called adverse events in physiotherapy, we have absolutely no idea how often these irritations occur. From personal experience and based on feedback from courses and continuing education, the author can confirm that it is "rather frequent." The treatment is simple: inform the patient, switch electrode manufacturers, treat the irritated area with an appropriate ointment or cream, and temporarily choose a different location for the electrodes. In the case of more severe irritations, which fortunately are truly rare, or if there is any uncertainty, a physician should definitely be consulted. Since almost everyone now has a camera with them, the affected area should be photographed.

3.12.3 Pacemakers

- Weitz et al. described 1997 how a postoperative parasternal TENS application in a 24-h ECG in a female patient simulated atrial fibrillation. The authors point out that this misinterpretation could have led to overdiagnosis and incorrect therapy.
- Vlay described a case in 1998 in which a patient with an implanted pacemaker and cardioverter-defibrillator (Implanted Cardioverter Defibrillator, ICD) received an electric shock during a TENS treatment. The electrodes were placed more than 50 cm from the pulse generator at the sacrum. Vlay points out that patients must be instructed to avoid these sources of electromagnetic interference.
- Crevenna et al. 2003 observed pacemaker disturbances in 3 out of 8 patients with so-called DDD-R pacemakers during muscle stimulation of the quadriceps with TENS-like parameters. Here too, the safety distance between electrodes and pacemaker was certainly more than 50 cm.
- Pyatt et al. described 2003 a patient with angina pectoris symptoms after bypass surgery and ICD implantation. Burst TENS was used for pain management. The electrodes were placed on the ventral thorax in the painful area. At a follow-up after 6 months, the patient reported that he had once received a shock during TENS application and that he became dizzy during every session. He also became bradycardic (hence the dizziness). As soon as he turned off the device, the symptoms disappeared. ICD testing showed that the TENS device was interfering with the ICD function. The application was discontinued. The authors point out that problems can develop even after initially uneventful use, and that patients must therefore be particularly well informed in this regard.
- Occhetta et al. 2006 investigated the incidence and clinical relevance of ICD disturbances due to external electromagnetic interference. In 13 out of 336 patients, unwanted shocks occurred between 1989 and 2005, in 2 patients due to an unspecified TENS treatment. Patients were advised to avoid this type of therapy, and no further disturbances occurred.
- Nägele and Azizi reported 2006 a case in which a patient was treated with TENS in the upper lumbar region (50 Hz, 40 mA). Practically immediately after the start of treatment, he experienced several shocks from his ICD; the treatment was immediately stopped and the patient was transferred to cardiology.

- Engelhardt et al. (2007) describe a case in which, after shoulder joint replacement, stimulation of the right brachial plexus with 1 ms, 1.4 mA led to complete temporary shutdown of the pacemaker (also on the right).
- Holmgren et al. investigated the influence of TENS on ICDs in 2008. In 30 patients with an ICD, TENS was applied under medical supervision at two different sites. The electrodes were first placed proximal to the nipples. In the second trial, the electrodes were placed over the anterior superior iliac spines (ASIS). Both low frequency TENS and high frequency TENS were used. Placement proximal to the nipples triggered interference with the ICD in 16 of 30 patients, placement over the ASIS in 7 of 30 (more than 50 cm!). The applications differed only minimally in terms of disturbances. The authors recommend not using TENS in patients with an ICD.
- Carlson et al. 2009 investigated the influence of TENS on implanted pacemakers. In 29 patients, TENS was applied under medical supervision at 2 Hz and 80 Hz. The electrodes were placed proximal to the nipples. In the first trial, both TENS applications were performed at normal pacemaker sensitivity. Then the pacemaker was set to maximum sensitivity. Only 5 of the 29 patients experienced no disturbances. At normal sensitivity, disturbances occurred at 80 Hz in 9 and at 2 Hz in 14 patients. At maximum sensitivity, disturbances occurred at 80 Hz in 17 and at 2 Hz in 22 patients. The authors advocate a controlled trial application before a TENS device is given to pacemaker patients, and subsequent monitoring of the treatment. They suggest setting the pacemaker to the lowest clinically acceptable sensitivity.
- Cenik et al. (2016) recommend clear precautions when using neuromuscular electrical stimulation (NMES) (with TENS-like parameters). Individual risks (dependence on the pacemaker, acute heart failure, unstable angina pectoris, ventricular arrhythmias in the last 3 months) must be excluded, NMES should only be used for the thigh and gluteal muscles, patient compliance, especially at home, must be ensured, and regular monitoring by the treating cardiologist is required.
- Badger et al. (2017) state in their review that the use of electrical stimulation on the lower extremity in pacemaker patients is probably safe. However, since there is too little reliable information, caution should still be exercised when using electrical stimulation in patients with a pacemaker or ICD.
- Egger et al. 2019 conducted measurements on a pyjama-like model consisting of several towels soaked in NaCl solution. They found that unilateral stimulation on the "thigh" and "upper arm" of the model did not cause disturbances in the respective pacemaker tested, but bilateral applications did. Their parameters are not specified, but were "typical for electrical stimulation" and were performed at the maximum possible intensity. Their conclusion: electrical stimulation can interfere with pacemakers, especially with bilateral applications. Unilateral applications appear to be safe.
- ... and there are many more such cases ...

Pacemakers and implanted cardioverter-defibrillators (ICDs) can demonstrably be disrupted by TENS and MF applications. For patients with ICDs, this means that they may receive one or more quite severe shocks while awake, even when the recommended safety distance of 50 cm between electrodes and ICD is observed.

The demand pacemaker measures and monitors heart activity via an electrode and only delivers impulses if the heart's own stimulation fails. Today, almost exclusively multiprogrammable demand pacemakers are implanted. Exogenous electrical stimuli (electrotherapy) and strong electromagnetic fields (high-frequency electrotherapy, e.g., shortwave and microwave) have been shown to disrupt the function of such devices. So-called "permanent pacemakers" are not affected by such external stimuli and therefore do not constitute a contraindication, only a relative one in the case of local application. These pacemakers deliver stimulation impulses continuously, but this type is now only used in exceptional cases.

Given this situation, pacemakers and implanted cardioverter-defibrillators must be considered absolute contraindications for any treatment with low-frequency electrical stimulation, TENS, and interferential current. This also applies to high-frequency applications, more on this in the relevant Chap. 7. The author himself has a "state of the art" ICD and can confirm that a low TENS application on the left elbow with a high-quality TENS device leads to rapid activation of the ICD. This is not the case on the right elbow. The ICD is located in the upper left thorax, about two fingerbreadths distal to the clavicle.

ICD Activation

What actually happens during such an interaction? Let's say the patient uses TENS and, by chance, becomes bradycardic at that very moment and the heart rate drops below the threshold set on the device. Normally, the demand pacemaker would intervene and deliver extra impulses to keep the pump working. However, the device can be misled by the TENS device and "think" that the patient's heart is already beating more or less regularly and does not need additional support. The patient becomes dizzy due to reduced cerebral perfusion and, if lucky, only loses consciousness. A well-informed patient knows this and turns off the TENS device at the first sign of dizziness. Nothing happened. With ICDs, it's different. ICDs are designed to deliver a series of impulses during arrhythmias to prompt the heart to return to sinus rhythm (the physician does not refer to these as shocks, but rather euphemistically as stimulations). These shocks become progressively stronger, depending on whether the disturbed rhythm is normalized or not. The initial stimulations feel like a series of quite forceful, dull blows to the thorax. If the ICD detects no change, the intensity of these stimulations increases. Normally, the patient is already unconscious and does not perceive the stimulations. Not so with TENS application—the patient remains awake. Ouch.

TENS is sometimes used for pain relief in patients with angina pectoris. The electrodes are placed ventrally on the thorax. Cardiologists recommend that this treatment be tried under close supervision before a device is given to the patient. Patients must, of course, be thoroughly informed about possible symptoms (bradycardia, dizziness) and monitored regularly.

3.12.4 TENS During Pregnancy

Pregnancy in the first trimester is considered an absolute contraindication for TENS treatment near the abdomen and lower back. Not that anyone has ever validated this statement, but sometimes you just don't need an RCT—see the parachute study mentioned above. There are, however, many women who experience lumbar or symphyseal discomfort during pregnancy, especially after the first trimester. In addition to the usual measures such as advice on activities of daily living, exercise therapy, and possibly some manual therapy, the use of TENS can certainly be considered. Literature on treatments in the last trimester shows that TENS can be used without risk to mother and child. Studies have been conducted with TENS in women with placental insufficiency, which even demonstrated that TENS was effective in this context (Kubista et al. 1987; Enzelsberger et al. 1991). A Cochrane review claims the opposite, but at least no adverse effects were reported (Gülmezoglu and Hofmeyr 2000). The parameters for the treatment of placental insufficiency by Kubista et al. can, taking into account more recent findings, also be used for back pain:

- 2 pairs of electrodes: 1 pair lumbar paravertebral between T10 and L1, 12 × 3 cm; 1 pair paravertebral sacral S2–S4, 8 × 3 cm.
- Intensity 20 to 40 mA, well tolerated. Today, one would say: as high as possible.
- Frequency 40 Hz. Today, for pain relief, 80–100 Hz would be recommended.
- Phase duration 250 μs, bipolar rectangular pulses. Shorter is also acceptable, around 100 μs.
- Treatment duration: 30 min twice daily.
- Treatment period: daily from the 29th to the 38th week of pregnancy.

TENS must, of course, never be used if there is even the slightest risk to mother or child, for example regarding the induction of labor. Dunn et al. (1989) attempted to induce labor in 20 women with overdue pregnancies using TENS over two suitable acupuncture points. Ten received TENS (30 Hz) at points Spleen 6 and Liver 3, a second group of ten women received a placebo treatment. During stimulation, the verum group experienced stronger and more frequent contractions. These stopped as soon as the stimulation ended.

There are acupuncture points that should be avoided during pregnancy. These points are LI4 (in the first dorsal interosseous muscle), SP6, BL60, BL67 (all three around the ankle), GB2 (middle area of the trapezius). Also mentioned are St36 and GB34 (at the fibular head). Therapists with appropriate training are, of course, aware of this. Therapists without such training should keep their hands off.

3.13 Patient Information TENS

Information Sheet for Patients

This chapter is intended as additional information for patients and does not replace the information in the TENS device user manual and/or the information provided by your therapist or physician.

It is only meant to supplement this information. The information sheet may be distributed to patients **free of charge** for non-commercial purposes without the author's permission, but please include the source. For commercial use, the author insists on being notified.

The author assumes that patients who receive this information sheet have been thoroughly informed and that the effectiveness of TENS treatment has been established for these patients.

It would be absolutely wrong and negligent to give a patient a device without first conducting a trial treatment of at least 6 TENS sessions in the practice or clinic.

The tips have been compiled to the best of the author's knowledge and belief. However, the author assumes absolutely no responsibility regarding the correctness of the indication when issuing a TENS device.

Dear Patient,

If you have purchased a TENS device from a department store or by mail order and are now experimenting with it, do not expect miracles from the treatment. The effectiveness of TENS depends on many factors. A specialist must determine which type of TENS is most effective for your specific problem and which settings need to be made on the device.

The information in the user manual is insufficient in this regard (and the salesperson in the department store is also not the right person to ask). It is better to contact a physiotherapist or doctor who is familiar with TENS treatment. It will be worth it.

You have a TENS device with which you can treat your pain at home yourself. In any case, always follow the instructions in your device's user manual and the directions given by your therapist or doctor.

If you are satisfied with the pain relief you achieve with your TENS device, you are certainly doing everything right. Do not change the settings on the device; continue as before. Let us assume that you are using new batteries, that the electrodes are still conducting well, and that your pain problem has not worsened. These are, in fact, the most common reasons why an initially successful TENS treatment may become less effective over time.

If you are not satisfied with the effect of TENS, you may be doing something incorrectly. With the following tips, you should have more success. Nevertheless, read the user manual carefully, as it often contains the technical information you need. Most TENS users experience almost immediate pain relief when they follow the user manual.

Are you following the prescribed treatment but still not having success? Then try the following tips, in any order you like:

1. High frequencies (the Hz value on the device) should feel like a very strong "tingling," "pins and needles," or "numbness," ideally in the area where you have your pain. However, the sensation must still be tolerable. Let us assume that you feel this tingling during TENS application. During the treatment (do not turn down the current!), change the pulse duration on the TENS device (the so-called pulse duration, pulse width, or phase duration). There is probably a μ symbol on the knob. This means "micro" and here stands for millionths of a second. You may not have a knob for this setting. In that case, there is often a small screw in the battery compartment that serves the same purpose. Now turn the knob (or screw) so that the pulse duration becomes longer. For example, if you started with 60 μs, slowly increase to 80–100 μs or even higher. If you now feel that the tingling sensation is spreading, i.e., the area where it tingles becomes larger, that is very good! It is also good if you feel that the current sensation goes deeper. Keep these settings and carry out the treatment. Make a note of the settings. If the tingling does not spread or the sensation does not go deeper, return the pulse duration to the initial setting (in this example, 60 μs). If the current sensation decreases during treatment, increase the intensity until the sensation is as strong as before.
2. You should clearly feel low frequencies as pulsing or twitching. Depending on the intensity, there will be more or less pronounced muscle twitching. This is generally desired! The treatment must last at least 25–30 min, but preferably 40–45 min, to stimulate the production of the body's own morphine-like substances (so-called endorphins). If you experience pain from the twitching during this long TENS treatment, the setting may be too high for you at that moment. Stop the treatment and wait until the pain subsides. This may be the same day or the next. For the next treatment, choose a shorter pulse duration so that the muscle twitches are less strong. If pain still occurs, trigger only very slight twitches in the next treatment by setting the intensity lower. If the reaction remains the same, then this form of TENS is probably too intense for you at the moment. If you wish, try once or twice more with the last, very gentle setting. Please keep in mind that with such intensive TENS treatments, a – usually mild – initial worsening is very common. Therefore, do not stop the treatment immediately and certainly do not lose heart! Talk to your therapist or doctor.
3. Make sure that the electrodes are always attached well and with even pressure. Instead of gel, try using a wet paper towel under the electrodes.
4. Try placing the electrodes in a different location. However, you should not do this for special treatments such as a stellate ganglion block or Kaada stimulation. In these cases, the placements are precisely specified and should not be changed.
5. If you are using TENS for back pain, place one electrode (for monophasic TENS, the cathode) directly on the painful spot and the second electrode on the opposite side of the spine, at the same distance from the spine as the first electrode. Or place the electrodes on both sides of the spine, about 2–3 cm apart, at the level of the pain.
6. Try different pulse frequencies during the treatment. For example, 10 min at a high frequency and then 10 min at a low frequency. Do not be afraid to experiment! Try each new setting for 2–4 days before possibly changing it again.
7. Gently move the painful body part during the TENS treatment.
8. Some patients have more success with the treatment if they cool the treated area for 10 min after TENS application. Take an ice cube and gently rub the painful area with it.

9. Keep in mind that it may take longer to respond to treatment if the pain has been present for a long time.
10. Heavy coffee or tea consumption can reduce the effectiveness of TENS. Halve your intake.
11. Sometimes it takes 2–3 treatments per day over several days before pain relief occurs, so do not stop the treatment after just a few attempts. Continue the therapy consistently for at least 2 weeks, unless the pain worsens! In that case, be sure to contact your therapist or doctor.
12. Be sure to continue taking your pain medication as usual. If you stop taking your medication during TENS treatment and the pain increases, you will not know whether the worsening is due to TENS or to taking less pain medication.

References

Aarskog R, Johnson MI, Demmink JH, Lofthus A, Iversen V, Lopes-Martins R, Joensen J, Bjordal JM (2007) Is mechanical pain threshold after Transcutaneous Electrical Nerve Stimulation (TENS) increased locally and unilaterally? A randomized placebo-controlled trial in healthy subjects. Physiother Res Int 12(4):251–263

den Adel RV, Luykx RHJ (2005) Nieder- und mittelfrequente Elektrotherapie. Therapie Handbuch, Enraf Nonius

Ainsworth L, Budelier K, Clinesmith M, Fiedler A, Landstrom R, Leeper BJ, Moeller LA, Mutch S, O'Dell K, Ross J, Radhakrishnan R, Sluka KA (2006) Transcutaneous electrical nerve stimulation (TENS) reduces chronic hyperalgesia induced by muscle inflammation. Pain 120:182–187

Albornoz-Cabello M, Maya-Martín J, Domínguez-Maldonado G, Espejo-Antúnez L, Heredia-Rizo AM (2017) Effect of interferential current therapy on pain perception and disability level in subjects with chronic low back pain: a randomized controlled trial. Clin Rehabil 31(2):242–249

Allen JD, Mattacola CG, Perrin DH (1999) Effect of microcurrent stimulation on delayed-onset muscle soreness: a double-blind comparison. J Athl Train 34(4):334–337

Almeida CC, Silva VZMD, Júnior GC, Liebano RE, Durigan JLQ (2018) Transcutaneous electrical nerve stimulation and interferential current demonstrate similar effects in relieving acute and chronic pain: a systematic review with meta-analysis. Braz J Phys Ther 22(5):347–354

Andersson SA, Ericson T, Holmgren E, Lindqvist G (1973) Electro-acupuncture. Effect on pain threshold measured with electrical stimulation of teeth. Brain Res 63:393–396

Antony AB, Mazzola AJ, Dhaliwal GS, Hunter CW (2019) Neurostimulation for the treatment of chronic head and facial pain: a literature review. Pain Pysician 22(5):447–477

Asadi MR, Torkaman G (2014) Bacterial inhibition by electrical stimulation. Adv Wound Care 3(2):91–97

Avendaño-Coy J, Bravo-Esteban E, Ferri-Morales A, Martínez-de la Cruz R, Gómez-Soriano J (2019) Does frequency modulation of transcutaneous electrical nerve stimulation affect habituation and mechanical hypoalgesia? A randomized, double-blind, sham-controlled crossover trial. Phys Ther 99(7):924–932

Back SK, Lee J, Hong SK, Na HS (2006) Loss of spinal μ-opioid-receptor is associated with mechanical allodynia in a rat modell of peripheral neuropathia. Pain 123:117–126

Badger J, Taylor P, Swain I (2017) The safety of electrical stimulation in patients with pacemakers and implantable cardioverter defibrillators: a systematic review. J Rehabil Assist Technol Eng 4. https://doi.org/10.1177/2055668317745498

Bai H, Forrester JV, Zhao M (2011) DC electric stimulation upregulates angiogenic factors in endothelial cells through activation of VEGF receptors. Cytokine 55(1):110–115

Barker R, Lang T, Hager H et al (2007) The influence of stellate ganglion transcutaneous electrical nerve stimulation on signal quality of pulse oximetry in prehospital trauma care. Anesth Analg 104(5):1150–1153

Beatti A, Rayner A, Chipchase L, Souvlis T (2011) Penetration and spread of interferential current in cutaneous, subcutaneous and muscle tissues. Physiotherapy 97(4):319–326

Beissner F, Brandau A, Henke C, Felden L, Baumgärtner U, Treede RD, Oertel BG, Lötsch J (2010) Quick discrimination of A(delta) and C fiber mediated pain based on three verbal descriptors. PLoS One 5(9):e12944

Bergeron-Vézina K, Corriveau H, Martel M, Harvey MP, Léonard G (2015) High- and low-frequency transcutaneous electrical nerve stimulation does not reduce experimental pain in elderly individuals. Pain 156(10):2093–2099

Bhadra N, Kilgore KL (2004) Direct current electrical conduction block of peripheral nerve. IEEE Trans Neural Syst Rehabil Eng 12(3):313–324

Bing Z, Villanueva L, Le Bars D (1990) Acupuncture and diffuse noxious inhibitory controls: naloxone-reversible depression of activities of trigeminal convergent neurons. Neuroscience 37(3):809–818

Bjordal JM, Johnson MI, Ljunggreen AE (2003) Transcutaneous electrical nerve stimulation (TENS)

can reduce postoperative analgesic consumption. A meta-analysis with assessment of optimal treatment parameters for postoperative pain. Eur J Pain 7(2):181–188

Bjordal JM, Johnson MI, Lopes-Martins RAB, Bogen B, Chow R, Ljunggren AE (2007) Short-term efficacy of physical interventions in osteoarthritic knee pain. A systematic review and meta-analysis of randomised placebo-controlled trials. BMC Musculoskelet Disord 22(8):51

Bouhassira D, Le Bars D, Villanueva L (1987) Heterotopic activation of A delta and C fibres triggers inhibition of trigeminal and spinal convergent neurones in the rat. J Physiol 389:301–317

Bowman BR, McNeal DR (1986) Response of single Alpha motoneurons to high frequency pulse trains: firing behaviour and conduction block phenomenon. Appl Neurophysiol 49(3):121–138

Bridges PH, Bierema LL, Valentine T (2007) The propensity to adopt evidence-based practice among physical therapists. BMC Health Serv Res 7:103

Bromm B, Lullies H (1966) Über den Mechanismus der Reizwirkung mittelfrequenter Wechselströme auf die Nervenmembran. Pflügers Arch. ges. Physiol 289:214–226

Buonocore M, Camuzzini N (2007) Increase of the heat pain threshold during and after high-frequency transcutaneous peripheral nerve stimulation in a group of normal subjects. Eura Medicophys 43(2):155–160

Buonocore M, Camuzzini N, Dall'Angelo A, Mandrini S, Dalla Toffola E (2015) Contralateral antalgic effect of high-frequency transcutaneous peripheral nerve stimulation. PM R 7(1):48–52

Burssens P, Forsyth R, Steyaert A, Van Ovost E, Praet M, Verdonk R (2003) Influence of burst TENS stimulation on the healing of Achilles tendon suture in man. Acta Orthop Belg 69(6):528–532

Calleja-Agius J, Brincat M, Borg M (2013) Skin connective tissue and ageing. Best Pract Res Clin Obstet Gynaecol 27(5):727–740

Carbonario F, Matsutani LA, Yuan SLK, Marques AP (2013) Effectiveness of high-frequency transcutaneous electrical nerve stimulation at tender points as adjuvant therapy for patients with fibromyalgia. Eur J Phys Rehabil Med 49(2):197–204

Carlson T, Andréll P, Ekre O et al (2009) Interference of transcutaneous electrical nerve stimulation with permanent ventricular stimulation: a new clinical problem? Europace 11(3):364–369

Castelain PY, Chabeau G (1986) Contact dermatitis after transcutaneous electric analgesia. Contact Dermatitis 15(1):32–35

Celik EC, Erhan B, Gunduz B, Lakse E (2013) The effect of low-frequency TENS in the treatment of neuropathic pain in patients with spinal cord injury. Spinal Cord 51(4):334–337

Cenik F, Schoberwalter D, Keilani M et al (2016) Neuromuscular electrical stimulation of the thighs in cardiac patients with implantable cardioverter defibrillators. Wien Klin Wochenschr 128(21–22):802–808

Cheing GLY, Chan WWY (2009) Influence of choice of electrical stimulation site on peripheral neurophysiological and hypoalgesic effects. J Rehabil Med 41(6):412–417

Chen CC, Johnson MI (2009) An investigation into the effects of frequency-modulated transcutaneous electrical nerve stimulation (TENS) on experimentally-induced pressure pain in healthy human participants. J Pain 10(10):1029–1037

Chen CC, Johnson MI (2010) A comparison of transcutaneous electrical nerve stimulation (TENS) at 3 and 80 pulses per second on cold-pressor pain in healthy human participants. Clin Physiol Funct Imaging 30(4):260–268

Chen L, Tang J, White PF, Sloninsky A, Wender RH, Naruse R, Kariger R (1998) The effect of location of transcutaneous electrical nerve stimulation on postoperative opioid analgesic requirement: acupoint versus nonacupoint stimulation. Anesth Analg 87(5):1129–1134

Chesterton LS, Barlas P, Foster NE, Lundeberg T, Wright CC, Baxter GD (2002) Sensory stimulation (TENS): effects of parameter manipulation on mechanical pain thresholds in healthy human subjects. Pain 99(1–2):253–262

Chesterton LS, Foster NE, Wright CC, Baxter GD, Barlas P (2003) Effects of TENS frequency, intensity and stimulation site parameter manipulation on pressure pain thresholds in healthy human subjects. Pain 106(1–2):73–80

Chiang C (1974) A physical theory of acupuncture anesthesia. Physiol Chem Phys 6(1):85–86

Claydon LS, Chesterton LS, Barlas P, Sim J (2008) Effects of simultaneous dual-site TENS stimulation on experimental pain. Eur J Pain 12(6):696–704

Claydon LS, Chesterton LS, Barlas P, Sim J (2011) Dose-specific effects of transcutaneous electrical nerve stimulation (TENS) on experimental pain: a systematic review. Clin J Pain 27(7):635–647

Corazza M, Maranini C, Bacilieri S, Virgili A (1999) Accelerated allergic contact dermatitis to a transcutaneous electrical nerve stimulation device. Dermatology 199(3):281

Cosmo P, Svensson H, Bornmyr S, Wikström SO (2000) Effects of transcutaneous nerve stimulation on the microcirculation in chronic leg ulcers. Scand J Plast Reconstr Surg Hand Surg 34(1):61–64

Cramp AF, Gilsenan C, Lowe AS, Walsh DM (2000) The effect of high- and low-frequency transcutaneous electrical nerve stimulation upon cutaneous blood flow and skin temperature in healthy subjects. Clin Physiol 20(2):150–157

van Cranenburgh B (2018) Segmentale Phänomene. Ein Beitrag zu Diagnostik und Therapie, überarb. u. erw. Aufl. KIENER, München, ISBN-13: 978-3943324334

Crevenna R, Mayr W, Keilani M, Pleiner J, Nuhr M, Quittan M, Pacher R, Fialka-Moser V, Wolzt M (2003) Safety of a combined stretch and endurance training using NMES of thigh muscles in patients with heart failure and bipolar sensing cardiac pacemakers. Wien Klin Wo 115(19–20):710–714

Cuypers K, Levin O, Thijs H, Swinnen SP, Meesen RL (2010) Long-term TENS treatment improves tactile sensitivity in MS patients. Neurorehabil Neural Repair 24(5):420–427

Daguet I, Bergeron-Vézina K, Harvey MP, Martel M, Léonard G (2018) Transcutaneous electrical nerve stimulation and placebo analgesia: is the effect the same for young and older individuals? Clin Interv Aging 13:335–342

Dailey DL, Rakel BA, Vance CGT, Liebano RE, Amrit AS, Bush HM, Lee KS, Lee JE, Sluka KA (2013) Transcutaneous electrical nerve stimulation reduces pain, fatigue and hyperalgesia while restoring central inhibition in primary fibromyalgia. Pain 154(11):2554–2562

Defrin R, Ariel E, Peretz C (2005) Segmental noxious versus innocuous electrical stimulation for chronic pain relief and the effect of fading sensation during treatment. Pain 115(1–2):152–160

Del Vecchio A, Negro F, Holobar A, Casolo A, Folland JP, Felici F, Farina D (2019) You are as fast as your motor neurons: speed of recruitment and maximal discharge of motor neurons determine the maximal rate of force development in humans. J Physiol 597(9):2445–2456

Dertinger H (2000) Interferenzstrom: Wirkungsmechanismen und klinische Anwendung. Nachrichten Forschungszentrum Karlsruhe 32:1–2

Desantana JM, Santana-Filho VJ, Sluka KA (2008) Modulation between high- and low-frequency transcutaneous electric nerve stimulation delays the development of analgesic tolerance in arthritic rats. Arch Phys Med Rehabil 89(4):754–760

DeSantana JM, Da Silva LF, De Resende MA, Sluka KA (2009) Transcutaneous electrical nerve stimulation at both high and low frequencies activates ventrolateral periaqueductal grey to decrease mechanical hyperalgesia in arthritic rats. Neuroscience 163(4):1233–1241

Ding L, Song T, Yi C et al (2013) Transcutaneous electrical nerve stimulation (TENS) improves the diabetic cytopathy (DCP) via up-regulation of CGRP and cAMP. PLoS One 8(2):e57477

Dorsher PT (2008) Can classical acupuncture points and trigger points be compared in the treatment of pain disorders? Birch's analysis revisited. J Altern Complement Med 14(4):353–359

Dunn PA, Rogers D, Halford K (1989) Transcutaneous electrical nerve stimulation at acupuncture points in the induction of uterine contractions. Obstet Gynecol 73(2):286–290

Dwyer CM, Chapman RS, Forsyth A (1994) Allergic contact dermatitis from TENS gel. Contact Dermatitis 30(5):305

Edel H (1977) Fibel der Elektrodiagnostik und Elektrotherapie, 4. Aufl. Verlag Theodor Steinkopff, Dresden

Egger F, Hofer C, Hammerle FP et al (2019) Influence of electrical stimulation therapy on permanent pacemaker function. Wien Klin Wochenschr 131(13–14):313–320

Elboim-Gabyzon M, Najjar SA, Shtarker H (2019) Effects of transcutaneous electrical nerve stimulation (TENS) on acute postoperative pain intensity and mobility after hip fracture: a double-blinded, randomized trial. Clin Interv Aging 14:1841–1850

Engelhardt L, Grosse J, Birnbaum J, Volk T (2007) Inhibition of a pacemaker during nerve stimulation for regional anaesthesia. Anaesthesia 62(10):1071–1074

Enzelsberger H, Skodler WD, Kubista E (1991) Zur Verbesserung der Doppler-Sonographiebefunde nach transkutaner Elektrostimulation bei Frauen mit Plazentainsuffizienz [Improvement of Doppler ultrasonography findings following transcutaneous electrostimulation in women with placental insufficiency]. Z Geburtshilfe Perinatol 195(4):172–175

Eriksson M, Sjölund B (1976) Acupuncture-like electroanalgesia in TNS resistant chronic pain. In: Zotterman Y (Hrsg) Sensory functions of the skin. Pergamon Press, Oxford/New York, S 575–581

Eslamian F, Farhoudi M, Jahanjoo F, Sadeghi-Hokmabadi E, Darabi P (2020) Electrical interferential current stimulation versus electrical acupuncture in management of hemiplegic shoulder pain and disability following ischemic stroke-a randomized clinical trial. Arch Physiother 10(10):2

Facci LM, Nowotny JP, Tormem F, Trevisani VF (2011) Interferential currents (IFC) in patients with nonspecific chronic low back pain: randomized clinical trial. Sao Paulo Med J 129(4):206–216

Ferreira RM, Duarte JA, Gonçalves RS (2018) Non-pharmacological and non-surgical interventions to manage patients with knee osteoarthritis: an umbrella review. Acta Reumatol Port 43(3):182–200

Ferreira RM, Torres RT, Duarte JA, Gonçalves RS (2019) Non-pharmacological and non-surgical interventions for knee osteoarthritis: a systematic review and meta-analysis. Acta Reumatol Port 44(3):173–217

Ford KS, Shrader MW, Smith J, McLean TJ, Dahm DL (2005) Full-thickness burn formation after the use of electrical stimulation for rehabilitation of unicompartmental knee arthroplasty. J Arthroplast 20(7):950–953

Foulds IS, Barker A (1983) Human skin battery potentials and their possible role in wound healing. Br J Dermatol 109(5):515–522

Francis RP, Marchant P, Johnson MI (2011a) Conventional versus acupuncture-like transcutaneous electrical nerve stimulation on cold-induced pain in healthy human participants: effects during stimulation. Clin Physiol Funct Imaging 31(5):363–370

Francis RP, Marchant PR, Johnson MI (2011b) Comparison of post-treatment effects of conventional and acupuncture-like transcutaneous electrical nerve stimulation (TENS): a randomised placebo-controlled study using cold-induced pain and healthy human participants. Physiother Theor Pract 27(8):578–585

Franco YR, Franco KF, Silva LA, Silva MO, Rodrigues MN, Liebano RE, Cabral CM (2018) Does the use of interferential current prior to pilates exercises accelerate improvement of chronic nonspecific low back pain? Pain Manag 8(6):465–474

Fuentes CJ, Armijo-Olivo S, Magee DJ, Gross D (2010) Does amplitude-modulated frequency have a role in the hypoalgesic response of interferential current on pressure pain sensitivity in healthy subjects? A randomised crossover study. Physiotherapy 96(1):22–29

Galasso A, Urits I, An D et al (2020) A comprehensive review of the treatment and management of myofascial pain syndrome. Curr Pain Headache Rep 24(8):43

Gardner SE, Blodgett NP, Hillis SL, Borhart E, Malloy L, Abbott L, Pezzella P, Jensen M, Sommer T, Sluka KA, Rakel BA (2014) HI-TENS reduces moderate-to-severe pain associated with most wound care procedures: a pilot study. Biol Res Nurs 16(3):310–319

Gemmell H, Hilland A (2011) Immediate effect of electric point stimulation (TENS) in treating latent upper trapezius trigger points: a double blind randomised placebo-controlled trial. J Bodyw Mov Ther 15(3):348–354

George SZ, Dannecker EA, Robinson ME (2006) Fear of pain, not pain catastrophizing, predicts acute pain intensity, but neither factor predicts tolerance or blood pressure reactivity: an experimental investigation in pain-free individuals. Eur J Pain 10(5):457–465

Gildemeister M (1944) Untersuchungen über die Wirkung der Mittelfrequenzströme auf den Menschen. Pflugers Arch 247:366–404

Giuffrida O, Simpson L, Halligan PW (2010) Contralateral stimulation, using TENS, of phantom limb pain: two confirmatory cases. Pain Med 11(1):133–141

Gomes CAFP, Dibai-Filho AV, Moreira WA, Rivas SQ, Silva EDS, Garrido ACB (2018) Effect of adding interferential current in an exercise and manual therapy program for patients with unilateral shoulder impingement syndrome: a randomized clinical trial. J Manipulative Physiol Ther 41(3):218–226

Gossrau G, Wähner M, Kuschke M et al (2011) Microcurrent transcutaneous electric nerve stimulation in painful diabetic neuropathy: a randomized placebo-controlled study. Pain Med 12(6):953–960

Gülmezoglu AM, Hofmeyr GJ (2000) Transcutaneous electrostimulation for suspected placental insufficiency (diagnosed by Doppler studies). Cochrane Database Syst Rev 1996(2):CD000079

Hamza MA, White PF, Ahmed HE, Ghoname EA (1999) Effect of the frequency of transcutaneous electrical nerve stimulation on the postoperative opioid analgesic requirement and recovery profile. Anesthesiology 91(5):1232–1238

Han JS (2003) Acupuncture: neuropeptide release produced by electrical stimulation of different frequencies. Trends Neurosci 26(1):17–22

Han JS, Chen XH, Sun SL, Xu XJ, Yuan Y, Yan SC, Hao JX, Terenius L (1991) Effect of low- and high-frequency TENS on Met-enkephalin-Arg-Phe and dynorphin A immunoreactivity in human lumbar CSF. Pain 47(3):295–298

Heath ME, Gibbs SB (1992) High-voltage pulsed galvanic stimulation: effects of frequency of current on blood flow in the human calf muscle. Clin Sci (Lond) 82(6):607–613

Herbert R, Jamtvedt G, Hagen KB, Mead J (2011) Practical evidence-based physiotherapy, 2. Aufl. Churchill Livingstone, London, ISBN: 9780702054501

Hettrick HH, O'Brien K, Laznick H et al (2004) Effect of transcutaneous electrical nerve stimulation for the management of burn pruritus: a pilot study. J Burn Care Rehabil 25(3):236–240

Hingne PM, Sluka KA (2007) Differences in waveform characteristics have no effect on the anti-hyperalgesia produced by Transcutaneous Electrical Nerve Stimulation (TENS) in rats with joint inflammation. J Pain 8(3):251–255

Hoare JI, Rajnicek AM, McCaig CD, Barker RN, Wilson HM (2016) Electric fields are novel determinants of human macrophage functions. J Leukoc Biol 99(6):1141–1151

Hofmann SG (2008) Cognitive processes during fear acquisition and extinction in animals and humans: implications for exposure therapy of anxiety disorders. Clin Psychol Rev 28(2):199–210

Holmgren C, Carlsson T, Mannheimer C, Edvardsson N (2008) Risk of interference from transcutaneous electrical nerve stimulation on the sensing function of implantable defibrillators. Pacing Clin Electrophysiol 31(2):151–158

Hong CZ (2000) Myofascial trigger points. Pathophysiology and correlation with acupuncture points. Acupunct Med 18:41–47

Houghton PE (2014) Clinical trials involving biphasic pulsed current, MicroCurrent, and/or low-intensity direct current. Adv Wound Care (New Rochelle) 3(2):166–183

Houghton PE (2017) Electrical stimulation therapy to promote healing of chronic wounds: a review of reviews. Chronic Wound Care Manag Res 4:25–44

Houghton PE, Kincaid CB, Lovell M, Campbell KE, Keast DH, Woodbury MG, Harris KA (2003) Effect of electrical stimulation on chronic leg ulcer size and appearance. Phys Ther 83(1):17–28

Houghton PE, Nussbaum EL, Hoens AM (2010) Electrophysical agents. Contraindications and precautions: an evidence-based approach to clinical decision making in physical therapy. Physiotherapy 62(5). Special Issue ISSN-0300-0508 E-ISSN-1708-8313

Hughes GS Jr, Lichstein PR, Whitlock D, Harker C (1984) Response of plasma beta-endorphins to transcutaneous electrical nerve stimulation in healthy subjects. Phys Ther 64(7):1062–1066

Hugosdottir R, Mørch CD, Andersen OK, Helgason T, Arendt-Nielsen L (2019) Preferential activation of small cutaneous fibers through small pin electrode also depends on the shape of a long duration electrical current. BMC Neurosci 20:48

Hui KKS, Nixon EE, Vangel MG, Liu J, Marina O, Napadow V, Hodge SM, Rosen BR, Makris N, Kennedy DN (2007) Characterization of the "deqi" response in acupuncture. BMC Complement Altern Med 7:33

Hunckler J, de Mel A (2017) A current affair: electrotherapy in wound healing. J Multidiscip Healthc 10:179–194

Ibrahim ZM, Waked IS, Ibrahim O (2019) Negative pressure wound therapy versus microcurrent electrical stimulation in wound healing in burns. J Wound Care 28(4):214–219

Ignelzi RJ, Nyquist JK (1976) Direct effect of electrical stimulation on peripheral nerve evoked activity: implications in pain relief. J Neurosurg 45(2):159–165

Ignelzi RJ, Nyquist JK (1979) Excitability changes in peripheral nerve fibres after repetitive electrical stimulation. Implications in pain modulation. J Neurosurg 51:824–833

Iijima H, Takahashi M, Tashiro Y, Aoyama T (2018) Comparison of the effects of kilohertz- and low-frequency electric stimulations: A systematic review with meta-analysis. PLoS One 13(4):e0195236

Janko M, Trontelj JV (1980) Transcutaneous electrical nerve stimulation: a microneurographic and perceptual study. Pain 9(2):219–230

Jin DM, Xu Y, Geng DF, Yan TB (2010) Effect of transcutaneous electrical nerve stimulation on symptomatic diabetic peripheral neuropathy: a meta-analysis of randomized controlled trials. Diabetes Res Clin Pract 89(1):10–15

Johnson MI (1999) The mystique of interferential currents when used to manage pain. Physiotherapy 85(6):294–297

Johnson MI (2014) Transcutaneous Electrical Nerve Stimulation (TENS). Research to support clinical practice. Oxford University Press, Oxford, ISBN-13: 978-0199673278

Johnson MI (2017) Transcutaneous electrical nerve stimulation (TENS) as an adjunct for pain management in perioperative settings: a critical review. Expert Rev Neurother 17(10):1013–1027

Johnson MI, Tabasam G (2003a) A single-blind investigation into the hypoalgesic effects of different swing patterns of interferential currents on cold-induced pain in healthy volunteers. Arch Phys Med Rehabil 84(3):350–357

Johnson MI, Tabasam G (2003b) An investigation into the analgesic effects of different frequencies of the amplitude-modulated wave of interferential current therapy on cold-induced pain in normal subjects. Arch Phys Med Rehabil 84(9):1387–1394

Johnson MI, Ashton CH, Thompson JW (1991) An in-depth study of long-term users of transcutaneous electrical nerve stimulation (TENS). Implications for clinical use of TENS. Pain 44:221–229

Johnson MI, Penny P, Sajawal MA (1997) An examination of the analgesic effects of microcurrent electrical stimulation (MES) on cold-induced pain in healthy subjects. Physiother Theor Pract 13:293–301

Julka IS, Alvaro M, Kumar D (1998) Beneficial effects of electrical stimulation on neuropathic symptoms in diabetes patients. J Foot Ankle Surg 37(3):191–194

Kaada B (1982) Vasodilation induced by transcutaneous stimulation in peripheral ischemia (Raynaud's phenomenon and diabetic polyneuropathy). Eur Heart J 3(4):303–314

Kaada B, Eielsen O (1983) In search of mediators of skin vasodilation induced by transcutaneous nerve stimulation: II. Serotonin implicated. Gen Pharmacol 14(6):635–641

Kaada B, Melesse W (1988) Promoted healing of leprous ulcers by transcutaneous nerve stimulation. Acup Elec-Ther Res 13(4):165–176

Kaada B, Hognestad S, Havstad J (1989) Transcutaneous nerve stimulation (TNS) in tinnitus. Scand Audiol 18(4):211–217

Kalra A, Urban MO, Sluka KA (2001) Blockade of opioid receptors in rostral ventral medulla prevents antihyperalgesia produced by transcutaneous electrical nerve stimulation (TENS). J Pharmacol Exp Ther 298:257–263

Katz J, Melzack R (1990) Pain 'memories' in phantom limbs: review and clinical observations. Pain 43(3):319–336

Katz J, France C, Melzack R (1989) An association between phantom limb sensations and stump skin conductance during transcutaneous electrical nerve stimulation (TENS) applied to the contralateral leg: a case study. Pain 36(3):367–377

Kawamura H, Ito K, Yamamoto M, Yamamoto H, Ishida K, Kawakami T, Tani T, Kaho K, Masaki Y (1997) The transcutaneous electrical nerve stimulation applied to contralateral limbs for the phantom limb pain. J Phys Ther Sci 9(2):71–76

Kayman-Kose S, Arioz DT, Toktas H, Koken G, Kanat-Pektas M, Kose M, Yilmazer M (2014) Transcutaneous electrical nerve stimulation (TENS) for pain control after vaginal delivery and cesarean section. J Matern Fetal Neonatal Med 27(15):1572–1575

Khadilkar A, Odebiyi DO, Brosseau L, Wells GA (2008) Transcutaneous electrical nerve stimulation (TENS) versus placebo for chronic low-back pain. Cochrane Database Syst Rev 2008(4):CD003008

Khouri C, Kotzki S, Roustit M, Blaise S, Gueyffier F, Cracowski JL (2017) Hierarchical evaluation of electrical stimulation protocols for chronic wound healing: an effect size meta-analysis. Wound Repair Regen 25(5):883–891

Kilgore KL, Bhadra N (2004) Nerve conduction block utilising high-frequency alternating current. Med Biol Eng Comput 42(3):394–406

Kim YR, Ahn SM, Pak ME et al (2018) Potential benefits of mesenchymal stem cells and electroacupuncture on the trophic factors associated with neurogenesis in mice with ischemic stroke. Sci Rep 8(1):2044

King EW, Audette K, Athman GA, Nguyen HO, Sluka KA, Fairbanks CA (2005) Transcutaneous electrical nerve stimulation activates peripherally located alpha-2A adrenergic receptors. Pain 115(3):364–373

Kordestani SS (2019) Atlas of wound healing. A tissue regeneration approach, 1. Aufl. Elsevier, Philadelphia, ISBN: 9780323679688

Kowarschik J (1957) Physikalische Therapie. 2. Aufl. Springer, Wien

Kubista E, Skodler W, Pateisky N, Heytmanek G (1987) Sonographischer Nachweis der Durchblutungssteigerung bei Plazentainsuffizienz nach TNS-Therapie mit Hilfe des gepulsten Doppler-Ultraschalls [Sonographic detection of increased perfusion in placental insufficiency following TNS therapy using pulsed Doppler ultrasound]. Geburtshilfe Frauenheilkd 47(9):594–596

Kumar D, Marshall HJ (1997) Diabetic peripheral neuropathy: amelioration of pain with transcutaneous electrostimulation. Diabetes Care 20(11):1702–1705

Lambert H, De Bisschop F, De Mey G, De Cuyper H, Demurie S, Vanderstraeten G, Blondé W (1989) Electric current distribution in tissues upon electrotherapy. Acta Belg Med Phys 12(2):31–40

Lambert MI, Marcus P, Burgess T, Noakes TD (2002) Electro-membrane microcurrent therapy reduces signs and symptoms of muscle damage. Med Sci Sports Exerc 34:602–607

Lang PM, Stoer J, Schober GM, Audette JF, Irnich D (2010) Bilateral acupuncture analgesia observed by quantitative sensory testing in healthy volunteers. Anesth Analg 110(5):1448–1456

Larsen B, Macher F, Bolte M, Larsen R (1995) Blockade des Ganglion stellatum mit transkutaner elektrischer Nervenstimulation (TENS): Eine Doppelblindstudie an gesunden Probanden [Stellate ganglion block with transcutaneous electric nerve stimulation (TENS): a double-blind study with healthy probands]. Anasthesiol Intensivmed Notfallmed Schmerzther 30(3):155–162

Laufer Y, Elboim M (2008) Effect of burst frequency and duration of kilohertz-frequency alternating currents and of low-frequency pulsed currents on strength of contraction, muscle fatigue, and perceived discomfort. Phys Ther 88(10):1167–1176

Laufer Y, Ries JD, Leininger PM, Alon G (2001) Quadriceps femoris muscle torques and fatigue generated by neuromuscular electrical stimulation with three different waveforms. Phys Ther 81(7):1307–1316

Lauretti GR, Chubaci EF, Mattos AL (2013) Efficacy of the use of two simultaneously TENS devices for fibromyalgia pain. Rheumatol Int 33(8):2117–2122

Lazarou L, Kitsios A, Lazarou I, Sikaras E, Trampas A (2009) Effects of intensity of Transcutaneous Electrical Nerve Stimulation (TENS) on pressure pain threshold and blood pressure in healthy humans: a randomized, double-blind, placebo-controlled trial. Clin J Pain 25(9):773–780

Le Bars D (2002) The whole body receptive field of dorsal horn multireceptive neurones. Brain Res Brain Res Rev 40(1–3):29–44

Le Bars D, Willer JC (2002) Pain modulation triggered by high-intensity stimulation: implication for acupuncture analgesia? Int Congr Ser 1238:11–29. https://doi.org/10.1016/S0531-5131(02)00412-0

Lee JE, Watson D, Frey-Law LA (2013) Psychological factors predict local and referred experimental muscle pain: a cluster analysis in healthy adults. Eur J Pain 17(6):903–915

Lee KH, Chung JM, Willis WD Jr (1985) Inhibition of primate spinothalamic tract cells by TENS. J Neurosurg 62(2):276–287

Léonard G, Goffaux P, Marchand S (2010) Deciphering the role of endogenous opioids in high-frequency TENS using low and high doses of Naloxone. Pain 151(1):215–219

Léonard G, Cloutier C, Marchand S (2011) Reduced analgesic effect of acupuncture-like TENS but not conventional TENS in opioid-treated patients. J Pain 12(2):213–221

Li CL, Bak A (1976) Excitability characteristics of the A- and C-fibers in a peripheral nerve. Experimental Neurology 50(1):67–79

Li L, Gu W, Du J et al (2012) Electric fields guide migration of epidermal stem cells and promote skin wound healing. Wound Repair Regen 20(6):840–851

Liao CD, Tsauo JY, Liou TH, Chen HC, Rau CL (2016) Efficacy of noninvasive stellate ganglion blockade performed using physical agent modalities in patients with sympathetic hyperactivity-associated disorders: a systematic review and meta-analysis. PLoS One 11(12):e0167476

Liebano RE, Abla LE, Ferreira LM (2008) Effect of low-frequency transcutaneous electrical nerve stimulation (TENS) on the viability of ischemic skin flaps in the rat: an amplitude study. Wound Repair Regen 16(1):65–69

Liebano RE, Rakel B, Vance CGT, Walsh DM, Sluka KA (2011) An investigation of the development of analgesic tolerance to TENS in humans. Pain 152(2):335–342

Lullies H, Trincker D (1974) Taschenbuch der Physiologie, Bd 3/1. Gustav Fischer, Stuttgart, ISBN: 3437001213/3-437-00121-3

Lundeberg T, Kjartansson J, Samuelsson U (1988) Effect of electrical nerve stimulation on healing of ischemic skin flaps. Lancet 2:712–714

Lundeberg TC, Eriksson SV, Malm M (1992) Electrical nerve stimulation improves healing of diabetic ulcers. Ann Plast Surg 29(4):328–331

Lykken DT, Venables PH (1971) Direct measurement of skin conductance: a proposal for standardization. Psychophysiology 8(5):656–672

Mackenzie RA, Burke D, Skuse NF, Lethlean AK (1975) Fibre function and perception during cutaneous nerve block. J Neurol Neurosurg Psychiatry 38(9):865–873

Maeda Y, Lisi TL, Vance CG, Sluka KA (2007) Release of GABA and activation of GABA(A) in the spinal cord mediates the effects of TENS in rats. Brain Res 1136(1):43–50

Mahure SA, Rokito AS, Kwon YW (2017) Transcutaneous electrical nerve stimulation for post-operative pain relief after arthroscopic rotator cuff repair: a prospective double-blinded randomized trial. J Shoulder Elb Surg 26(9):1508–1513

Marchand S, Charest J, Li J, Chenard JR, Lavignolle B, Laurencelle L (1993) Is TENS purely a placebo effect? A controlled study on chronic low back pain. Pain 54(1):99–106

Marchand S, Li J, Charest J (1995) Effects of caffeine on analgesia from transcutaneous electrical nerve stimulation. N Engl J Med 333(5):325–326

Martínez-Rodríguez A, Bello O, Fraiz M, Martinez-Bustelo S (2013) The effect of alternating and biphasic currents on humans' wound healing: a literature review. Int J Dermatol 52(9):1053–1062

Melzack R (1975) Prolonged relief of pain by brief intense transcutaneous somatic stimulation. Pain 1:357–373

Melzack R (1981) Myofascial triggerpoints. Relation to acupuncture and mechanism of pain. Arch Phys Med Rehabil 62:114–117

Melzack R, Stillwell D, Fox EJ (1977) Triggerpoints and acupuncturepoints for pain. Correlations and implications. Pain 3:3–23

Michlovitz SL, Smith W, Watkins M (1988) Ice and high voltage pulsed stimulation in treatment of acute lateral ankle sprains. J Orthop Sports Phys Ther 9(9):301–304

Minder PM, Noble JG, Alves-Guerreiro J, Hill ID, Lowe AS, Walsh DM, Baxter GD (2002) Interferential therapy: lack of effect upon experimentally induced delayed onset muscle soreness. Clin Physiol Funct Imaging 22(5):339–347

Moran F, Leonard T, Hawthorne S, Hughes CM, McCrum-Gardner E, Johnson MI, Rakel BA, Sluka KA, Walsh DM (2011) Hypoalgesia in response to Transcutaneous Electrical Nerve Stimulation (TENS) depends on stimulation intensity. J Pain 12(8):929–935

Nägele H, Azizi M (2006) Inappropriate ICD discharge induced by electrical interference from a physio-therapeutic muscle stimulation device. Herzschrittmacherther Elektrophysiol 17(3):137–139

Namer B, Barta B, Ørstavik K, Schmidt R, Carr R, Schmelz M, Handwerker HO (2009) Microneurographic assessment of C-fibre function in aged healthy subjects. J Physiol 587(2):419–428

Nardone A, Schieppati M (1989) Influences of transcutaneous electrical stimulation of cutaneous and mixed nerves on subcortical and cortical somatosensory evoked potentials. Electroencephalogr Clin Neurophysiol 74(1):24–35

Nazligul T, Akpinar P, Aktas I, Unlu Ozkan F, Cagliyan Hartevioglu H (2018) The effect of interferential current therapy on patients with subacromial impingement syndrome: a randomized, double-blind, sham-controlled study. Eur J Phys Rehabil Med 54(3):351–357

Nemec H (1959) Interferential therapy: a new approach in physical medicine. Br J Physiother 12:9–12

Nemec H (1960) Reizstromtherapie mit Interferenzströmen. Dtsch Badebetrieb 12:320–322

Nemec H (1967) Endogene Elektrostimulierung durch mittelfrequente und Interferenzströme. Rehabilitation (Bonn) 20:1–11

Nemec H (1968) Elektrostimulierung in endogener Anwendung: Aktionsmechanismus der Interferenztherapie. Physikalische Medizin und Rehabilitation 9:73–75

Noble JG, Henderson G, Cramp AF, Walsh DM, Lowe AS (2000) The effect of interferential therapy upon cutaneous blood flow in humans. Clin Physiol 20(1):2–7

Occhetta E, Bortnik M, Magnani A, Francalacci G, Marino P (2006) Inappropriate implantable cardioverter-defibrillator discharges unrelated to supraventricular tachyarrhythmias. Europace 8(10):863–869

Ould Amer Y, Hebert-Chatelain E (2018) Mitochondrial cAMP-PKA signaling: what do we really know? Biochim Biophys Acta Bioenerg 1859 9:868–877

Palmer ST, Martin DJ, Steedman WM, Ravey J (1999) Alteration of interferential current and transcutaneous electrical nerve stimulation frequency: effects on nerve excitation. Arch Phys Med Rehabil 80(9):1065–1071

Pantaleão MA, Laurino MF, Gallego NLG, Cabral CMN, Rakel B, Vance C, Sluka KA, Walsh DM, Liebano RE (2011) Adjusting pulse amplitude during Transcutaneous Electrical Nerve Stimulation (TENS) application produces greater hypoalgesia. J Pain 12(5):581–590

Phillipp A, Wolf GK, Rzany B, Dertinger H, Jung EG (2000) Interferential current is effective in palmar psoriasis:an open prospective trial. Eur J Dermatol 10:195–198

Polak A, Taradaj J, Nawrat-Szoltysik A et al (2016) Reduction of pressure ulcer size with high-voltage pulsed current and high-frequency ultrasound: a randomised trial. J Wound Care 25(12):742–754

Poltawski L, Johnson M, Watson T (2012) Microcurrent therapy in the management of chronic tennis elbow: pilot studies to optimize parameters. Physiother Res Int 17(3):157–166. https://doi.org/10.1002/pri.526

Pyatt JR, Trenbath D, Chester M, Connelly DT (2003) The simultaneous use of a biventricular implantable cardioverter defibrillator (ICD) and transcutaneous electrical nerve stimulation (TENS) unit: implications for device interaction. Europace 5(1):91–93

Radhakrishnan R, Sluka KA (2003) Spinal muscarinic receptors are activated during low or high frequency TENS-induced antihyperalgesia in rats. Neuropharmacology 45(8):1111–1119

Radhakrishnan R, Sluka KA (2005) Deep tissue afferents, but not cutaneous afferents, mediate transcutaneous electrical nerve stimulation-Induced antihyperalgesia. J Pain 6(10):673–680

Rajpurohit B, Khatri SM, Metgud D, Bagewadi A (2010) Effectiveness of transcutaneous electrical nerve stimulation and microcurrent electrical nerve stimulation in bruxism associated with masticatory muscle pain – a comparative study. Indian J Dent Res 21(1):104–106

Rakel B, Frantz R (2003) Effectiveness of transcutaneous electrical nerve stimulation on postoperative pain with movement. J Pain 4(8):455–464

Rakel BA, Zimmerman MB, Geasland K, Embree J, Clark CR, Noiseux NO, Callaghan JJ, Herr K, Walsh D, Sluka KA (2014) Transcutaneous electrical nerve stimulation for the control of pain during rehabilitation after total knee arthroplasty: a randomized, blinded, placebo-controlled trial. Pain 155(12):2599–2611

Ranker A, Husemeyer O, Cabeza-Boeddinghaus N, Mayer-Wagner S, Crispin A, Weigl MB (2020) Microcurrent therapy in the treatment of knee osteoarthritis. Could it be more than a placebo-effect? A randomized controlled trial. Eur J Phys Rehabil Med. https://doi.org/10.23736/S1973-9087.20.05921-3

Resende L, Merriwether E, Rampazo ÉP et al (2018) Meta-analysis of transcutaneous electrical nerve stimulation for relief of spinal pain. Eur J Pain 22(4):663–678

Rodríguez-Fernández AL, Garrido-Santofimia V, Güeita-Rodríguez J, Fernández-de-Las-Peñas C (2011) Effects of burst-type transcutaneous electrical nerve stimulation on cervical range of motion and latent myofascial trigger point pain sensitivity. Arch Phys Med Rehabil 92(9):1353–1358

Roman N (2017) Physiotherapy devices able to generate ethical dilemma. MATEC Web Conf 112:08001. https://doi.org/10.1051/matecconf/201711208001

Rouabhia M, Park HJ, Zhang Z (2016) Electrically activated primary human fibroblasts improve in vitro and in vivo skin regeneration. J Cell Physiol 231(8):1814–1821

Sabino GS, Santos CM, Francischi JN, de Resende MA (2008) Release of endogenous opioids following transcutaneous electric nerve stimulation in an experimental model of acute inflammatory pain. J Pain 9(2):157–163

Sachverständigenrat für die Konzertierte Aktion im Gesundheitswesen (2000) http://dipbt.bundestag.de/doc/btd/14/068/1406871.pdf. Zugriff Mai 2021

Salar G, Job I, Mingrino S, Bosio A, Trabucchi M (1981) Effect of transcutaneous electrotherapy on CSF β-endorphin content in patients without pain problems. Pain 10:169–172

Salter MW, Henry JL (1987) Evidence that adenosine mediates the depression of spinal dorsal horn neurons induced by peripheral vibration in the cat. Neuroscience 22(2):631–650

Salter MW, De Koninck Y, Henry JL (1993) Physiological roles for adenosine and ATP in synaptic transmission in the spinal dorsal horn. Prog Neurobiol 41(2):125–156

Sandoval MC, Ramirez C, Camargo DM, Salvini TF (2010) Effect of high-voltage pulsed current plus conventional treatment on acute ankle sprain. Rev Bras Fis 14(3):193–199

Sarlandière JB (1825) Memoires sur l'electro-puncture, consideré comme moyen nouveau de traiter efficacement la goute, les rhumatismes et les affections nerveuses. (Paris). https://gallica.bnf.fr/ark:/12148/bpt6k5832681w/f4.image.texteImage. Zugriff Juli 2021

Satter EK (2008) Third-degree burns incurred as a result of interferential current therapy. Am J Dermatopathol 30(3):281–283

Scott W, Adams C, Cyr S, Hanscom B, Hill K, Lawson J, Ziegenbein C (2015) Electrically elicited muscle torque: comparison between 2500-Hz burst-modulated alternating current and monophasic pulsed current. J Orthop Sports Phys Ther 45(12):1035–1041

Serezani CH, Ballinger MN, Aronoff DM, Peters-Golden M (2008) Cyclic AMP: master regulator of innate immune cell function. Am J Respir Cell Mol Biol 39(2):127–132

Shahrokhi A, Ghorbani A, Aminianfar A (2014) Impact of interferential current on recovery of pressure ulcers grade 1 and 2. Iran J Nurs Midwifery Res 19(7 Suppl 1):S91–S96

Shanahan C, Ward AR, Robertson VJ (2006) Comparison of the analgetic efficacy of interferential therapy and transcutaneous electrical nerve stimulation. Physiotherapy 92:247–253

Shimizu T, Koja T, Fujisaki T, Fukuda T (1981) Effects of methysergide and naloxone on analgesia induced by the peripheral electric stimulation in mice. Brain Res 208(2):463–467

Silva AJ, Kogan JH, Frankland PW, Kida S (1998) CREB and memory. Annu Rev Neurosci 21:127–148

da Silva TM, Costa Lda C, Garcia AN, Costa LO (2015) What do physical therapists think about evidence-based practice? A systematic review. Man Ther 20(3):388–401

Simon CB, Riley JL 3rd, Fillingim RB, Bishop MD, George SZ (2015) Age group comparisons of TENS response among individuals with chronic axial low back pain. J Pain 16(12):1268–1279

Sivaramakrishnan A, Solomon JM, Manikandan N (2018) Comparison of transcutaneous electrical nerve stimulation (TENS) and functional electrical stimulation (FES) for spasticity in spinal cord injury – a pilot randomized cross-over trial. J Spinal Cord Med 41(4):397–406

Sjölund BH (1985) Peripheral nerve stimulation suppression of C-fiber-evoked flexion reflex in rats. Part 1: parameters of continuous stimulation. J Neurosurg 63(4):612–616

Sjölund BH (1988) Peripheral nerve stimulation suppression of C-fiber-evoked flexion reflex in rats. Part 2: parameters of low-rate train stimulation of skin and muscle afferent nerves. J Neurosurg 68(2):279–283

Sjölund BH, Eriksson MB (1979) The influence of Naloxone on analgesia by peripheral conditioning stimulation. Brain Res 173:295–301

Sjölund BH, Terenius L, Eriksson M (1977) Increased cerebrospinal fluid levels of endorphines after elektro-acupuncture. Acta Physiol Scand 100:382–384

Sluka KA (1999) Spinal blockade of opioid receptors prevents the analgesia produced by TENS in arthritic rats. J Pharm Exper Ther 289:840–846

Sluka KA, Walsh D (2003) Transcutaneous electrical nerve stimulation: basic science mechanisms and clinical effectiveness. J Pain 4(3):109–121

Sluka KA, Deacon M, Stibal A, Strissel S, Terpstra A (1999) Spinal blockade of opioid receptors prevents the analgesia produced by TENS in arthritic rats. J Pharmacol Exp Ther 289(2):840–846

Sluka KA, Judge MA, McColley MM, Reveiz PM, Taylor BM (2000) Low frequency TENS is less effective than high frequency TENS at reducing inflammation-induced hyperalgesia in morphine-tolerant rats. Eur J Pain 4:185–194

Sluka KA, Bjordal JM, Marchand S, Rakel BA (2013) What makes transcutaneous electrical nerve stimulation work? Making sense of the mixed results in the clinical literature. Phys Ther 93(10):1397–1402

Smith GC, Pell JP (2003) Parachute use to prevent death and major trauma related to gravitational challenge: systematic review of randomised controlled trials. BMJ 327(7429):1459–1461

Somers DL, Clemente FR (2006) Transcutaneous electrical nerve stimulation for the management of neuropathic pain: the effects of frequency and electrode position on prevention of allodynia in a rat model of complex regional pain syndrome type II. Phys Ther 86(5):698–709

Somers DL, Clemente FR (2009) Contralateral high or a combination of high- and low-frequency transcutaneous electrical nerve stimulation reduces mechanical allodynia and alters dorsal horn neurotransmitter content in neuropathic rats. J Pain 10(2):221–229

Stefanovska A, Vodovnik L (1985) Change in muscle force following electrical stimulation. Dependence on stimulation waveform and frequency. Scand J Rehabil Med 17(3):141–146

Stralka SW, Jackson JA, Lewis AR (1998) Treatment of hand and wrist pain. A randomized clinical trial of high voltage pulsed, direct current built into a wrist splint. AAOHN J 46(5):233–236

Stux G, Berman B, Pomeranz B (2003) Basics of acupuncture, 5th rev. ed. Springer, Berlin/Heidelberg, ISBN 3-540-44273

Sun S, Xu Q, Guo C, Guan Y, Liu Q, Dong X (2017) Leaky gate model: intensity-dependent coding of pain and itch in the spinal cord. Neuron 93(4):840–853.e5

Suriya-amarit D, Gaogasigam C, Siriphorn A, Boonyong S (2014) Effect of interferential current stimulation in management of hemiplegic shoulder pain. Arch Phys Med Rehabil 95(8):1441–1446

Taylor AG, Anderson JG, Riedel SL, Lewis JE, Kinser PA, Bourguignon C (2013) Cranial electrical stimulation improves symptoms and functional status in individuals with fibromyalgia. Pain Manag Nurs 14(4):327–335

Taylor K, Newton RA, Personius WJ, Bush FM (1987) Effects of interferential current stimulation for treatment of subjects with recurrent jaw pain. Phys Ther 67(3):346–350

Tong KC, Lo SK, Cheing GL (2007) Alternating frequencies of transcutaneous electric nerve stimulation: does it produce greater analgesic effects on mechanical and thermal pain thresholds? Arch Phys Med Rehabil 88(10):1344–1349

Toroski M, Nikfar S, Mojahedian MM, Ayati MH (2018) Comparison of the cost-utility analysis of electroacupuncture and nonsteroidal antiinflammatory drugs in the treatment of chronic low back pain. J Acupunct Meridian Stud 11(2):62–66

Travell J, Simons D (1992a) Myofascial pain and dysfunction. The trigger point manual, Bd 1. Williams and Wilkins, Baltimore, ISBN 0-683-08366-X

Travell J, Simons D (1992b) Myofascial pain and dysfunction. The trigger point manual, Bd 2. Williams and Wilkins, Baltimore, ISBN 0-683-08367-8

Treffene RJ (1983) Interferential fields in a fluid medium. Aust J Physiother. 29(6):209–216

Vance CG, Rakel BA, Blodgett NP, DeSantana JM, Amendola A, Zimmerman MB, Walsh DM, Sluka KA (2012) Effects of transcutaneous electrical nerve stimulation on pain, pain sensitivity, and function in people with knee osteoarthritis: a randomized controlled trial. Phys Ther 92(7):898–910

Vance CG, Rakel BA, Dailey DL, Sluka KA (2015) Skin impedance is not a factor in transcutaneous electrical nerve stimulation effectiveness. J Pain Res 8:571–580

Vance CG, Chimenti RL, Dailey DL, Hadlandsmyth K, Zimmerman MB, Geasland KM, Williams JM, Merriwether EN, Munters LA, Rakel BA, Crofford LJ, Sluka KA (2018) Development of a method to maximize the transcutaneous electrical nerve stimulation intensity in women with fibromyalgia. J Pain Res 11:2269–2278

Vaz MA, Frasson VB (2018) Low-frequency pulsed current versus kilohertz-frequency alternating current: a scoping literature review. Arch Phys Med Rehabil 99(4):792–805

Veras M, Kairy D, Paquet N (2016) What is evidence-based physiotherapy? Physiother Can 68(2):95–98

Vlaeyen JW, Linton SJ (2012) Fear-avoidance model of chronic musculoskeletal pain: 12 years on. Pain 153(6):1144–1147

Vlay SC (1998) Electromagnetic interference and ICD discharge related to chiropractic treatment. Pacing Clin Electrophysiol 21(10):2009

Vrouva S, Batistaki C, Paraskevaidou E et al (2019) Comparative study of pain relief in two non-pharmacological treatments in patients with partial rotator cuff tears: a randomized trial. Anesth Pain Med 9(2):e88327

Walsh DM, Lowe AS, McCormack K, Willer JC, Baxter GD, Allen JM (1998) Transcutaneous electrical nerve stimulation: effect on peripheral nerve conduction, mechanical pain threshold, and tactile threshold in humans. Arch Phys Med Rehabil 79(9):1051–1058

Wang B, Tang J, White PF, Naruse R, Sloninsky A, Kariger R, Gold J, Wender RH (1997) Effect of the intensity of transcutaneous acupoint electrical stimulation on the postoperative analgesic requirement. Anesth Analg. 85(2):406–413

Wang Y, Zhang Y, Wang W, Cao Y, Han JS (2005) Effects of synchronous or asynchronous electroacupuncture stimulation with low versus high frequency on spinal opioid release and tail flick nociception. Exp Neurol 192(1):156–162

Ward AR (2009) Electrical stimulation using kilohertz-frequency alternating current. Phys Ther 89(2):181–190

Ward AR, Oliver WG (2007) Comparison of the hypoalgesic efficacy of low-frequency and burst-modulated kilohertz frequency currents. Phys Ther 87(8):1056–1063

Ward AR, Robertson VJ (1998) Sensory, motor, and pain thresholds for stimulation with medium frequency alternating current. Arch Phys Med Rehabil 79(3):273–278

Ward AR, Robertson VJ (2000) The variation in fatigue rate with frequency using kHz frequency alternating current. Med Eng Phys 22(9):637–646

Ward AR, Robertson VJ, Makowski RJ (2002) Optimal frequencies for electric stimulation using medium-frequency alternating current. Arch Phys Med Rehabil 83(7):1024–1027

Ward AR, Robertson VJ, Ioannou H (2004) The effect of duty cycle and frequency on muscle torque production using kilohertz frequency range alternating current. Med Eng Phys 26(7):569–579

Weber MI, Servedio FJ, Woodall WR (1994) The effects of three modalities on delayed onset muscle soreness. J Orthop Phys Ther 20:236–242

Weber-Muller F, Reichert-Penetrat S, Schmutz JL, Barbaud A (2004) Eczéma de contact aux polyacrylates du gel conducteur des électrodes de neurostimulation [Contact dermatitis from polyacrylate in TENS electrode]. Ann Dermatol Venereol. 131(5):478–480. French

Wedensky NE (1903) Die Erregung, Hemmung und Narkose. Pflugers Arch 100:1–144

Weitz SH, Tunick PA, McElhinney L, Mitchell T, Kronzon I (1997) Pseudoatrial flutter: artifact simulating atrial flutter caused by a transcutaneous electrical nerve stimulator (TENS). Pacing Clin Electrophysiol 20(12 Pt 1):3010–3011

Whitaker C (2001) The use of TENS for pruritus relief in the burns patient: an individual case report. J Burn Care Rehabil 22(4):274–276

Wikström SO, Svedman P, Svensson H, Tanweer AS (1999) Effect of transcutaneous nerve stimulation on microcirculation in intact skin and blister wounds in healthy volunteers. Scand J Plast Reconstr Surg Hand Surg 33(2):195–201

Woolf CJ, Mitchell D, Barrett GD (1980) Antinociceptive effect of peripheral segmental electrical stimulation in the rat. Pain 8(2):237–252

Wyss OAM (1975) Prinzipien der elektrischen Reizung. Kommissionsverlag Leemann AG, Zürich

Yamamoto T, Yamamoto Y (1977) Analysis for the change of skin impedance. Med Biol Eng Comput 15(3):219–227

Yeh RW, Valsdottir LR, Yeh MW, Shen C, Kramer DB, Strom JB, Secemsky EA, Healy JL, Domeier RM, Kazi DS, Nallamothu BK, Investigators PARACHUTE (2008) Parachute use to prevent death and major trauma when jumping from aircraft: randomized controlled trial. BMJ 13(363):k5094

Zeng C, Li H, Yang T, Deng ZH, Yang Y, Zhang Y, Lei GH (2015) Electrical stimulation for pain relief in knee osteoarthritis: systematic review and network meta-analysis. Osteoarthritis Cartilage 23(2):189–202

Zhao M (2009) Electrical fields in wound healing – an overriding signal that directs cell migration. Semin Cell Dev Biol 20(6):674–682

Zhao M, Song B, Pu J et al (2006) Electrical signals control wound healing through phosphatidylinositol-3-OH kinase-gamma and PTEN. Nature 442(7101):457–460

Zhu Y, Feng Y, Peng L (2017) Effect of transcutaneous electrical nerve stimulation for pain control after total knee arthroplasty: a systematic review and meta-analysis. J Rehabil Med 49(9):700–704

4 Neuromuscular Electrical Stimulation (NMES)

Neuromuscular electrical muscle stimulation (NMES) and electromyostimulation (EMS) refer to the induction of contractions in muscle groups or individual muscles using an electrical stimulus. The terminology does not distinguish whether the muscle is innervated or denervated. In this application, it is not only the muscle that is stimulated. Over the past 20 years, evidence has accumulated that cortical, subcortical, and segmental neural networks are also activated in a manner similar to active training sequences (Smith et al. 2003; Blickenstorfer et al. 2009; Francis et al. 2009; Chipchase et al. 2011). The criticism that NMES is merely "dumb muscle training" because the CNS is bypassed is completely unfounded. Therefore, the term "neuromuscular electrical stimulation" is actually quite appropriate, even though in innervated muscles it is not the muscle itself that is directly stimulated, but always the innervating nerve. The sometimes-used terms "therapeutic electrical stimulation" or "transcutaneous electrical stimulation" (TES) are not particularly meaningful and should not be used, not least because the term TES is also used in place of TENS.

When the induced contractions are coordinated in such a way that a function such as standing, walking, or grasping is supported or taken over, this is referred to as functional electrical stimulation (FES). This term was coined as early as 1962 by Moe and Post. In fact, this is a type of neuroprosthesis (Popović 2014; Prochazka 2019). Unfortunately, this term is repeatedly used when NMES is actually meant, and this is fundamentally incorrect. NMES uses clearly different parameters than FES, which leads to confusion.

NMES is used in research and clinically as a rehabilitation/training method and is then mostly referred to as "retraining."

The method is used to maintain and restore muscle mass and function during prolonged periods of disuse or immobilization, as well as to improve muscle function in healthy individuals, for example in older adults, recreational and elite athletes. When the method is used preoperatively, it is sometimes referred to as prehabilitation. Areas of application include cardiovascular medicine, for example in patients with heart failure and COPD patients, in orthopedics after knee surgery or fractures, in neurology after a CVI or in CP patients, in general medicine for terminal patients, for incontinence, in geriatrics and sports medicine—and not to forget in space travel. Interestingly, despite the enormous variety of possibilities, the focus has mainly (in 60% of cases) been on the quadriceps femoris muscle (Filipovic et al. 2011).

P. van Kerkhof, *Evidence-Based Electrotherapy*, https://doi.org/10.1007/978-3-662-73019-5_4

4.1 Muscle Fiber Types

The distribution of muscle fibers varies enormously between individuals. Muscle biopsies from the vastus lateralis muscle of several subjects showed the following distribution (Staron et al. 2000):

- 15–85% type I fibers
- 18–50% type IIA fibers
- 12–34% type IID fibers

The basis for distinguishing muscle fiber types is the so-called isoforms of myosins (Schiaffino and Reggiani 2011; Zoladz 2018). An isoform is a molecule of identical composition but different structure compared to a second molecule. Isoforms perform similar but not identical functions. There are two different schemes for classifying muscle fibers. Both are based on specific chemical stains. The classic distinction between "fast" (fast-twitch) and "slow" (slow-twitch) fibers is based on the detection of myofibrillar adenosine triphosphatase (mATPase: an enzyme that catalyzes the splitting of ATP and thus triggers the myosin-actin cross-bridge). This analysis distinguishes three metabolically different muscle fiber types: FG (fast glycolytic), FOG (fast oxidative-glycolytic), and SO (slow oxidative). These three fiber types differ molecularly in the composition of their myofibrillar apparatus, metabolically in their enzymatic equipment, and functionally in their contraction properties. However, the distinction is somewhat crude for the fast fibers, as the boundary between glycolytic and oxidative is not sharply defined. The second method provides a more precise separation. This method examines the mATPase activity of the myosin heavy chain (MHC) and its isoforms. Using this method, a third fast fiber type was identified in rodents in addition to type IIA and IIB: type IID (= IIX). These three types (A, B, and D) contain different isoforms of the MHC. IIB fibers contain MHCIIb, IID fibers contain MHCIId, and IIA fibers contain MHCIIa. Now, type IID is histochemically quite similar to type IIB, which is why it was recognized relatively late, and even today, the two types are often not distinguished. However: the muscle fiber type referred to as type IIB in humans actually corresponds to type IID in rodents. The "true" type IIB is found only in small mammals. The larger the animal, the lower the proportion of IIB fibers. Dogs, pigs, sheep, llamas, and horses do not possess this isoform, and in humans it is practically absent. Therefore, it is preferable to refer to type IID rather than type IIB in humans.

It is confusing when the FG-FOG-SO classification is mixed up with the type I-IIA-IIB/D classification, as both are based on different criteria. Type I probably corresponds to the SO type, but for the fast fibers, the correspondence is no longer 100%.

In addition to the "pure" types, there are so-called hybrid fibers that simultaneously express two or more MHC isoforms. About 10 different types are known. The hybrid fibers occur in varying degrees depending on the type of load, especially in situations involving fiber type transformation.

The following sections introduce the individual muscle fiber types.

4.1.1 Type I Fiber

Also called slow twitch (ST), slow oxidative (SO), or tonic. These fibers have the smallest cross-sectional area. They contract slowly (twitch duration up to 100–200 ms) with little force development. In a physiological situation, these fibers always contract first. They fatigue only slowly and recover quickly. The fibers are well supplied with blood. Due to the large number of mitochondria and the cytochromes they contain, as well as the myoglobin stored in the fibers, the muscles are distinctly dark red in color. In the quadriceps femoris, they are located more deeply (Henriksson-Larsén et al. 1985) and therefore, depending on muscle size, contract only at very high stimulation intensities, if at all.

4.1.2 Type IIA Fiber

Also called fast twitch, oxidative (FO), fast twitch oxidative-glycolytic (FOG), phasic, or fast contracting, fatigue resistant (FR). These fibers have both oxidative (aerobic) and glycolytic metabolism. They fatigue less quickly and recover faster than FG fibers. They are relatively well supplied with blood. They contain more mitochondria and myoglobin than type IID fibers and are whitish-red in color. Their contractions are less rapid (50–100 ms) and less forceful than those of IID fibers. In laboratory electrical stimulation, type II fibers always contract first together with IID fibers. Inactivity leads to atrophy of this fiber type, together with IID fibers.

4.1.3 Type IID (IIX) Fiber

Also called fast twitch, glycolytic (G), fast twitch glycolytic (FG), phasic or fast contracting similar to type IIA, fatigueing (FF). According to current views (Pette and Staron 2000), the designation IIB is not correct, as this type occurs only in small mammals. In German literature, the term "IID" is now used, while Americans (among others) use the designation "IIX" for this fiber type (Smerdu et al. 1994). These fibers have predominantly glycolytic (anaerobic) metabolism and only little oxidative (aerobic) metabolism. In response to stimulation, the fibers produce a short (7.5–50 ms), strong twitch. The power output, especially at high speeds and force development, is greater in type IID than in type IIA. Type IID fibers have the highest ATP consumption (tension cost). Their speed thus comes at the expense of high ATP consumption, whereas the slow type I fibers work more economically. The fibers fatigue quickly and recover slowly. In a normal mixed muscle such as the quadriceps femoris, these fibers are found more superficially, which explains why they are easily accessible with NMES (Vanderthommen and Duchateau 2007). The fiber cross-section is relatively large, so the fibers can develop a lot of force. They are rather poorly supplied with blood. Due to the small number of mitochondria and the cytochromes they contain, and the lower amount of myoglobin, the muscles appear whitish. In laboratory electrical stimulation, the fibers contract first together with type IIA fibers. Inactivity also leads to atrophy of this fiber type. Today, the expression of the IID gene is considered a kind of default setting. People who sit a lot have a higher content of myosin IID in their muscles than physically active people. The number of these fibers decreases with increasing activity in favor of myosin IIA. If the activity level is reduced again, the process is reversed.

4.1.4 Type IIB Fiber

The designation IIB should no longer be used in humans in cases where type IID is actually meant, such as in the quadriceps femoris. Type IIB is found in humans only in the larynx (specifically the arytaenoidus transversus muscle), in the eye muscles, and sometimes in the masseter muscle (Andersen et al. 2002). In small mammals, type IIB is metabolically and in terms of performance superior to type IID. In rodents, there are hybrid muscle fibers that express two MHC isoforms: type IIX and IIB.

4.2 Innervation

Each muscle fiber is innervated by a motor nerve fiber, an Aα-motoneuron, and each nerve fiber in turn innervates a certain number of muscle fibers depending on the muscle. A group of muscle fibers innervated by the same nerve fiber is called a motor unit. The smaller the motor units, the finer and more coordinated the movements performed. All muscle fibers in a motor unit always contract simultaneously when activated. Eye muscles have very small motor units, about 1700 with about 13 muscle fibers each (innervation ratio 1:13). The biceps brachii consists of about 780 motor units with about 750 muscle fibers each (innervation ratio 1:750), the gastrocnemius has an innervation ratio of 1:1600. All muscle fibers in a motor unit are of the same type, which is why the terms "phasic" and "tonic" motor units are sometimes used. The terms "phasic" or "tonic" muscle are outdated and incorrect.

Muscle fibers with the largest cross-sectional area are innervated by very fast-conducting, thickly myelinated Aα-motoneurons, while the thinner muscle fibers are innervated by somewhat thinner and slightly slower-conducting nerve fibers of the same type. In a physiological contraction, type I fibers are activated first; if more force is required, type IIA fibers are recruited, and finally, in very forceful contractions, type IID fibers are involved. In activities requiring little force, such as "maintaining posture," mainly type I fibers are involved. The contraction speed of muscle fibers is influenced by the different rates at which ATP is split and consumed at the myosin heavy chain. "Fast" myosin from type II fibers splits ATP faster than "slow" myosin from type I fibers. This is one of the reasons for the faster contraction speed of type II fibers.

4.3 Activation Sequence

If one compares the SD curve of a motor nerve with that of a denervated muscle fiber, it becomes clear that direct stimulation of a muscle fiber requires much higher intensity and longer impulses than stimulation of a nerve fiber. This means that with electrical stimulation of an intact muscle-nerve complex, it is always the innervating nerve that is activated first. This transmits the stimulus to the muscle, which ultimately leads to contraction. In everyday life, innervation follows Henneman's size principle (Henneman et al. 1965). This principle describes that the physiological recruitment sequence within a muscle proceeds from the small to the large motor units. Type I (SO) fibers contract first, as they have the smallest motor units. If more force is required, IIA fibers (FR) with their somewhat larger motor units are recruited. Finally, in very forceful contractions, IID fibers (IIX, FF) with the largest motor units and the highest stimulation thresholds are involved. The nerve fibers that respond first in vitro during NMES are the fast-conducting Aα fibers, as these have the lowest stimulation threshold; consequently, during NMES, type II muscle fibers should always contract first: in principle, an unphysiological situation. That this is different in practice has already been demonstrated by several researchers (Mesin et al. 2010; Bergquist et al. 2011; Rodriguez-Falces and Place 2013; Watanabe et al. 2015). Due to local anatomical conditions (muscle size, fat layer, location of nerve fibers), stimulation parameters, and electrode placement, the various muscle fiber types are stimulated in a rather arbitrary manner (Gregory and Bickel 2005; Jubeau et al. 2007; Bickel et al. 2011). Placing the electrodes directly on the innervating nerve appears to result in a more physiological contraction sequence and is therefore better suited for NMES (Gobbo et al. 2011). Bergquist et al. (2012) see this type of stimulation more as a supplement, as more motor units are probably recruited and the contraction is likely more physiological, but less force is developed.

However, it is precisely this unphysiological sequence that makes NMES so interesting for patients who have atrophy of their fast muscle fibers. It is possible to stimulate these type II fibers with relatively low training doses when the patient cannot or is not allowed to do so themselves. It even appears that more severely affected patients respond better to NMES (Morrissey 1988; Roig and Reid 2009).

What actually happens?

When a muscle fiber is stimulated with an electrical impulse, it responds with a so called twitch. When a series of impulses is applied, the resulting contraction becomes increasingly smooth as the stimulation frequency increases. This leads to summation of contractions, which, as the frequency increases, manifests as a smooth tetanic contraction.

As frequency increases, contraction force also increases, with maximum force development being reached at about 50–60 Hz.

- 1–10 Hz: single twitches
- 10–20 Hz: fibrillations
- 20–80 Hz: tetanic contractions
- over 90 Hz: muscle waves (myokymia)

There are literally thousands of studies demonstrating that NMES leads to morphological and functional adaptations in the stimulated muscle.

- The phenotype of the stimulated muscle fibers changes, sooner or later, depending on the imposed stimulation frequency, from fast-to-slow or from slow-to-fast, and
- depending on the stimulation parameters, the stimulated muscle becomes stronger or more enduring in vitro.

Interestingly, during the first 3–4 weeks of an NMES treatment, little to nothing happens in the muscle itself. Strength increases significantly and the muscle becomes more resistant to fatigue, yet no morphological changes are observed (Hortobágyi et al. 2000; Maffiuletti 2010), similar to normal active strength training (del Vecchio et al. 2019). These adaptations are neural effects such as improved recruitment of motor units and processes that probably occur cortically, subcortically, and segmentally and are not yet fully understood (Hortobágyi et al. 2000).

The only problem with morphological adaptations is that studies are very often conducted on rather small rodents. However, the triceps surae of a rat is not comparable to the human quadriceps femoris, and the latter is used in 60% of studies involving Homo sapiens. It is easy to stimulate all muscle fibers in a rat calf for days with NMES. In the human quadriceps, however, things are quite different. At best, about 40% of the muscle fibers are stimulated, and depending on topographical conditions and the pain tolerance of the subjects, different muscle fiber types are targeted. If the electrodes remain in the same place during a session, the same motor units are always activated. This is one reason why unexpected study results sometimes occur (Gondin et al. 2011). Another reason is the fact that many studies use a wide variety of treatment parameters, making comparison of results impossible.

Some authors claim that certain muscle fibers should be stimulated with specific frequencies to target training for strength or endurance. The frequency is said to determine the training outcome. Appell (1992), for example, claims that fast-twitch fibers (type II) do not contract with stimulation frequencies below 35 Hz. Bossert et al. (2006) claim that these fibers should be maximally stimulated with frequencies of around 50–60 Hz. Other authors (Caiozzo et al. 1997; Veldman et al. 2016; Maffiuletti et al. 2018) believe that it is not the frequency but the work performed during NMES that determines the training effect. Most authors favor the second theory.

Let us take a closer look at this, as it is not that simple.

The way NMES is used depends on the treatment goal. For example, do you want to increase walking distance in a weakened COPD patient by stimulating the quadriceps femoris? Or improve jump strength in a well-trained elite athlete? Interestingly, according to several sources, the treatment parameters are practically the same for both individuals (Filipovic et al. 2011, 2012; Veldman et al. 2016; Maffiuletti et al. 2018). In the thousands of publications on NMES (October 2024: 9,065 hits for "neuromuscular electrical stimulation" on PubMed), very different parameters are often used. Nevertheless, successful applications almost always use the following settings for strength and hypertrophy training and for endurance training:

- Biphasic impulses, rectangular
- Phase duration 100–500 µs
- Frequency 50–100 Hz
- Gradually increasing impulse series, "ramp-up" 1–3 s

- Duty cycle 20–25% (= 100/total ON time PLUS_SPI OFF time), ON time 3–10 s, OFF time 15–50 s.
- Session duration: 10–30 min
- Once daily, 3 to 5 times per week
- Intensity: tolerance limit, pain threshold, "supramaximal"
- Always combined with active training

Very different training protocols are used. For example, there is the protocol of Russian Stimulation (more on this below). This 10–50–10 protocol requires a very strong contraction for 10 s, followed by 50 s of rest. This is repeated 10 times. There is also a 10–20–30 scheme: In the first 10 s, the amplitude is greatly increased up to the tolerance limit to trigger a very strong contraction. (Some authors leave the increase to the subject and are later surprised by varying results.) This contraction is held for 20 s. If muscle tension decreases during these 20 s, the current must be readjusted. At the end, there is a pause of at least 30 s to replenish ATP stores. After a maximal effort lasting 6–10 s, all immediately available energy sources are depleted (cf. 100 m sprint). These energy sources are the small amount of ATP freely available in the muscle, which is sufficient for 2–3 maximal contractions, and the ATP obtained from the creatine phosphate system. The time required to replenish about half of these energy sources after maximal effort is about 20 s. It therefore makes sense to allow a sufficiently long pause between individual maximal contractions. Whether the 20 s contraction is actually useful because of the HFF is questionable. In the two patients mentioned above, only the training intensities will differ greatly. It is common to specify training intensity as a percentage of the maximum voluntary contraction (MVC) of the muscle to be trained. The athlete will only benefit from NMES treatment if at least 50% of the MVC of the target muscle is achieved. In the COPD patient, we can only estimate the value, as the patient is often not adequately loadable. It may be about 5–10% of their MVC. The tolerance limit for impulse intensity will probably also be lower in our COPD patient than in the athlete, yet our patient will respond very well to stimulation (Roig and Reid 2009). The other parameters are still the same for both patients. Maffiuletti (2010) and Filipovic et al. (2011, 2012) recommend applying NMES with the parameters mentioned above, but always in combination with appropriately targeted conventional training (explosive strength, coordination, etc.).

Now to frequency specificity. For improving endurance, NMES with a frequency of 10–20 Hz is better suited than NMES with a higher frequency, simply because it is more comfortable (Thériault et al. 1996; Nuhr et al. 2003; Miyamoto et al. 2016). High-frequency NMES, if dosed for strengthening, is very demanding and leads to rapid fatigue, long before the physiological processes for improving endurance are activated. Nevertheless, this type of stimulation also interestingly leads to improved endurance. However, low-frequency stimulation is much more comfortable and is therefore well tolerated for longer periods—up to 4 h at a time! The author is unfortunately not aware of any studies in humans in which high-frequency NMES was simply applied at a lower intensity.

Aα-motoneurons vary in thickness (8–20 μm), conduction velocity (70 to 120 m/s), and excitability. The faster a nerve fiber conducts, the lower its stimulation threshold. Some authors use the designation Aα-1 for the faster and Aα-2 for the somewhat slower Aα-motoneurons. A sufficiently long and strong impulse triggers an action potential in the more sensitive and therefore faster-responding Aα1 nerve fiber, independent of frequency. This action potential is transmitted to the type IIA and IID muscle fibers. Whether these impulses stimulate the nerve at a frequency of 20 or 100 Hz does not matter: the faster, more sensitive Aα1 nerve fiber is always depolarized first. Only at higher stimulation intensities are the thinner and less sensitive Aα2 motoneurons depolarized, and as a result, the type I muscle fibers contract. At the same time, of course, the type II fibers are also stimulated. As already mentioned, this is irrelevant in vivo.

The somewhat slower-conducting Aα2 fibers cannot transmit such high stimulation frequencies as the faster-conducting Aα1 fibers due to their longer refractory period. However, this does not mean that type I muscle fibers do not contract at all at higher frequencies. At low and high stimulation frequencies, all muscle fiber types are always stimulated at sufficiently high stimulation intensity. This is subject to the aforementioned caveat that activation occurs in a rather disordered manner (Gregory and Bickel 2005; Jubeau et al. 2007; Bickel et al. 2011).

The so-called optimal stimulation frequency indicates the discharge frequency at which the respective muscle fibers exhibit a tetanic contraction; in other words, the discharge frequency at which the innervating nerve brings "its" muscle fiber type to a tetanic contraction and thus to maximum force development. Because type I fibers contract slowly, the second impulse can arrive a little later while the tetanic contraction is maintained: only a low stimulation frequency is required, around 20–30 Hz. Type II fibers contract only very briefly and rapidly: to maintain a tetanic contraction, the impulses must therefore arrive at a higher frequency, around 60 Hz.

When stimulation is applied at a low frequency (20–30 Hz), all motor units located in the stimulation area are activated, with type I muscle fibers tending to contract tetanically and develop their force optimally. The simultaneously stimulated type II fibers do not develop a smooth tetanic contraction, so their overall force development is less optimal. Due to the greater excitability of the Aα1 motoneuron, contractions can still be quite strong depending on the stimulation intensity. At higher frequencies, type II muscle fibers develop their maximum force due to the now occurring tetanic contraction. Type I fibers will also contract at sufficiently high stimulation intensity, perhaps not optimally, but they will contract nonetheless. The use of different frequencies in NMES therefore does not lead to specific stimulation of the different fiber types. What matters is the work performed (Hudlická et al. 1980; Nix and Vrbova 1986; Chan Kwan Kit-lan 1991; Caiozzo et al. 1997; Maffiuletti et al. 2018).

4.4 Fatigue

Fatigue occurs as a result of changes at multiple levels and manifests as a decrease in performance. Certain changes lead to an increase in performance, while others are merely disruptive (Carriker 2017; Burnley and Jones 2018).

Normally, during muscle activity, the central nervous system initiates efferent signal transmission via Aα-motoneurons. These signals are transmitted at the neuromuscular junction through the release of acetylcholine onto the muscle fiber membrane and are then propagated across the entire membrane. The excitation is conducted into the interior of the muscle fiber via the T-tubule system, leading to the release of calcium from the endoplasmic reticulum. These calcium ions bind to troponin molecules, and this binding activates the actin-myosin cross-bridge, which ultimately forms the basis for muscle contraction.

Fatigue can occur at any of the aforementioned levels. Central fatigue refers to performance-reducing changes that occur before the neuromuscular junction. Peripheral or local fatigue occurs at or after the neuromuscular junction.

Electrical stimulation with frequencies above 50–100 Hz leads to strong contractions but also to very rapid fatigue. As a result, contraction strength decreases sharply after just a few seconds. This type of fatigue is based on mechanisms such as a lack of neurotransmitters and changes in K^+ and Na^+ concentrations in the T-tubule system (Jones et al. 1979). It does not occur during voluntary contractions. This type of fatigue is called high frequency fatigue (HFF). The affected muscle fibers are unable to perform adequately due to HFF and, as a result, are not trained. HFF therefore does not contribute to performance improvement. Training requires physiological local fatigue: this must be caused by metabolic changes within the muscle fibers themselves. HFF must therefore be avoided. This means that it makes no sense to trigger strong, long contractions lasting up to 20 s with frequencies above about 60 Hz (Jones et al. 1979). Short, strong contractions lasting only a few seconds are not a problem.

In functional electrical stimulation (FES), it makes sense to vary the parameters, as this can prevent rapid onset of fatigue (Thrasher et al. 2005; Graham et al. 2006; Vromans and Faghri 2018). Here, the goal is not performance improvement, but rather the restoration of a function. If the musculature were to fatigue rapidly during this stimulation, the patient would, for example, only be able to stand for a short period. A program with varied stimulation parameters is more effective for this purpose than a monotonous program (Binder-Macleod and Russ 1999; Vromans and Faghri 2018). When stimulating with a fixed frequency, the same motor units in the immediate vicinity of the electrodes are repeatedly activated according to the all-or-nothing principle. This leads to very rapid exhaustion of the affected muscle fibers. To prevent such exhaustion, it is indeed sensible to modulate stimulation parameters such as frequency, phase duration, intensity, and electrode placement so that different motor units are activated each time—"just like in real life." However, such modulation should not be implemented only after 10–20 min, but ideally during a contraction, for example with special devices with multiple electrodes that are activated sequentially. Only in this way can previously loaded muscle fibers recover. This would also more closely resemble a physiological process.

The purpose of frequency modulation in NMES is therefore not a frequency-specific effect on different muscle fibers in the direction of strength or endurance training, but rather the prevention of rapid exhaustion. How training can nevertheless be directed in a specific direction is described in Sect. 4.6.

4.5 Muscle Fiber Transformation

The muscle fiber type is determined by the innervating nerve, and this is genetically predetermined. This also applies to the distribution of muscle fibers within individual muscles. A healthy average adult has about as many slow as fast fibers, depending on the muscle in a 4:5 or 5:4 ratio. However, there are large individual differences in the structure of muscles of the same type. It is likely that "gifted" marathon runners or sprinters are born with an exceptional muscle composition. Future long-distance runners, for example, would already stand out in early physical education classes due to a relatively high density of type I fibers. Naturally, the sport in which one excels with relative ease is more enjoyable, and one is more motivated to continue. This would explain why successful athletes sometimes have an extremely unbalanced muscle fiber distribution: it is not the training or the sport that determines the distribution, but rather the fiber type that determines the preferred sport. A basketball player does not grow taller just because he plays basketball.

Muscle fibers are extraordinarily plastic. Studies in athletes have shown that the type of training (aerobic or anaerobic) can cause a reversible shift in muscle composition, from "fast" to "slow" and vice versa (Steinacker et al. 2002). The basis for this transformation is altered gene expression: the "slow" myosin chains of one type are replaced by the "fast" ones of the same type. In addition, there are changes in certain membrane properties (for example, the Na/K pump) and specific metabolic enzyme reactions. When the stimulating factors are removed (cessation of training), the genes that produce the "slow" proteins are reactivated. Animal studies have shown that after replacing the innervating nerve (cross-innervation), the muscle fiber type changes: depending on the muscle and nerve, from fast to slow or slow to fast.

In humans, both high-frequency and low-frequency NMES lead to a fast-to-slow transformation (Thériault et al. 1996; Nuhr et al. 2003; Gondin et al. 2011). Minetto et al. (2013) found in their 14 healthy subjects a significant increase in strength and muscle girth after 24 high-frequency NMES sessions. They also found the complete spectrum of possible transformations: a fast-to-slow transition (4 subjects), bidirectional transformation of MHC-1 and MHC-2X isoforms to the MHC-2A isoform (7 subjects), shift to MHC-2X (2 subjects), no change in MHC distribution (1 subject). Their parameters: a warm-up phase: 200 μs, 5 Hz, 5 min, submaximal intensity. The actual training: 40 contractions/session, biphasic rectangular pulses, 8 weeks. Stimulation: 75 Hz, 400 μs, duty cycle 24%, 6.25 s ON, of which 1.5 s ramp-up and 0.75 s ramp-down, 20 s OFF, intensity at tolerance threshold. The investigators were able to demonstrate that NMES, despite very different individual adaptations in the muscle, can lead to the same result in all subjects (increase in strength and girth). The reason for this unexpected result: probably the intramuscular variations in muscle fiber distribution, perhaps also the different individual tolerance thresholds, as the subjects could determine themselves how high to turn up the intensity. Porcelli et al. (2012) studied 7 healthy subjects to determine whether the changes found in vitro after an NMES series, namely the improved oxidative properties that should accompany a fast-to-slow transition, are actually objectively measurable. Surprisingly, this was not the case. The investigators suspect that hypertrophy impedes peripheral O_2 diffusion. In any case, the improved muscle strength did not impair oxidative metabolism. Their parameters: warm-up 5 min, 5 Hz, 200 μs. Training: 400 μs, 75 Hz, 1.5 s ramp-up, 4 s hold, 0.75 s ramp-down, 20 s rest, 40 contractions, 25 sessions, 18 min, 8 weeks, 3/ week, intensity at tolerance threshold.

A slow-to-fast transformation has been observed under non-physiological conditions such as weightlessness in space (Caiozzo et al. 1994) and during immobilization (Andersen et al. 1999). The transformation probably occurs here for economic reasons: fast fibers require less oxygen for their metabolic processes. In addition, a slow-to-fast transformation has been observed in diseases such as hyperthyroidism and diabetes. Hypothyroidism has the opposite effect (Pette and Staron 2000).

However, in various studies, the transformation was not only dependent on the *stimulation frequency* but also on the *stimulation intensity*, i.e., the type of work performed. Stimulation with a frequency of 100 Hz or 25 Hz and very strong contractions led to the same result after 4 weeks (16 sessions, 40 contractions each) in a rat calf: the IIB-MHC protein isoform decreased by about 50%, the type IIX-MHC isoform increased independently of frequency (Caiozzo et al. 1994). Ausoni et al. (1990) found that high-dose stimulation of the rat calf with 150 Hz (15 s rest each) led to a decrease in the IIX isoform, while low-dose stimulation (15 min rest each) with the same frequency led to an increase. Again, the work performed was decisive.

Most authors believe that the purpose of sequential training with different frequencies is not to stimulate different fiber types, but that the use of different stimulation parameters such as phase duration, phase interval, and pulse shape can help avoid overly rapid exhaustion and activate as many muscle fibers as possible. The stimulation frequency is also not decisive, but rather the total work performed: if this work is more tonic, the training leads to different adaptations than if the training is more strength-oriented. The frequency used does not matter (Hudlická et al. 1980; Nix and Vrbova 1986).

4.6 Application

In physiotherapy, artificially induced muscle contractions are used for various purposes:

- To maintain neuromuscular functions during a period of immobilization, for example after an accident, surgery, or illness. See, for example, Dirks et al. (2014, 2015) and Kamel and Yousif (2017).
- To restore neuromuscular functions after an accident, surgery, or illness. See, for example, Vieira et al. (2014), Maddocks et al. (2016(, Spector et al. (2016), Qi et al. (2018) and Mäkelä et al. (2019).
- To improve neuromuscular functions in healthy individuals, for example in

recreational athletes, elite athletes, or older adults. See, for example, Seyri and Maffiuletti (2011) and Sanjuán Vásquez et al. (2019).
- To take over or support impaired functions in the sense of a neuroprosthesis using functional electrical stimulation (FES). See, for example, Thrasher and Popovic (2008), Popović (2014) and Prochazka (2019).

The targeted goals are diverse and the results influence each other. NMES leads to strengthening and improved endurance as well as improved circulation, which results in prophylaxis against atrophy and fibrosis and can even be used for muscle building (Kern et al. 2004, 2005; Carraro et al. 2015). Depending on the problem being treated, normalization of muscle tone in the sense of detoning and toning can be observed (Morrissey 1989), and the involvement of neural networks leads to improvement or maintenance of kinesthetics (Ridding et al. 2000; Chipchase et al. 2011; Meesen et al. 2011). Muscle stimulation is also used diagnostically in the creation of a so-called SD curve.

4.6.1 Improvement of Neuromuscular Function

It is well documented that muscle function can be improved with NMES. The method is used successfully in both patients and athletes, and the parameters are essentially the same. Apart from the intended goals, only the stimulation intensities used differ. The parameters for muscle strengthening have already been discussed above. With these parameters, changes occur in the musculature that not only strengthen the muscle but also make it more resistant to fatigue (Veldman et al. 2016). Erickson et al. (2017) studied in spinal cord injury patients how low-frequency NMES affects the oxidative properties of the musculature. Unfortunately, their description does not make it clear whether the investigators used bursts (which would be high-frequency NMES) or single pulses (which would actually be low-frequency NMES). They mention 2–7 Hz, 200 μs pulse duration with a 50 μs interval (literally "pulse duration/interval = 200/50 μs"). This would suggest pulse trains with an internal burst frequency of 40 Hz. And that is not low-frequency NMES. However, the authors refer to "twitch contractions," and the contractions were strong ("vigorous"). Treatment duration: 10–75 min, 3 to 5 times per week. They started with 10 min, 2 Hz; if this training was tolerated for 30 min, the frequency was increased weekly by 1 Hz up to 7 Hz. After that, the treatment duration was gradually extended to up to 75 min. The oxidative (aerobic) capacity improved by an average of about 120%. Muscle composition and blood values showed no change.

4.6.2 Muscle Stimulation for Detoning and Toning

To claim that NMES has a toning effect would imply that the application acts directly on the musculature, and this cannot be demonstrated. If the musculature becomes flaccid due to pain (reflex inhibition, pain inhibition) and it is possible to reduce the pain with NMES, secondary toning in the sense of normalization can occur. Whether this is a local or central mechanism is unclear. Local mechanisms discussed at the knee, for example, include the flexion reflex and the γ-spindle loop, but central neurological mechanisms must also be considered (Rice and McNair 2010).

Example: An active extension deficit at the knee due to reflex inhibition of the quadriceps muscle can improve dramatically if the pain is successfully eliminated. In 1984, Spencer et al. described how swelling of the knee joint leads to reflex inhibition of the quadriceps femoris. They injected certain amounts of a 0.9% NaCl solution into the knees of healthy subjects and found that at 20–30 ml, the Hoffmann reflex of the vastus medialis decreased by about 50%, and at 50–60 ml, there was an additional inhibition of about 40% of the rectus and vastus lateralis. If the knees were anesthetized with lidocaine beforehand, this inhibition did not occur. The investigators do not mention whether the subjects experienced pain during the first examination. Fahrer et al. 1988 used an isokinetic dynamometer to determine that knee patients with a "mild" chronic effusion performed significantly less on the affected side (about 300 Nsec versus about 480 Nsec). After aspiration of the effusion (about 50 ml), performance improved by a good 13%, and additional anesthesia of the joint brought another 8% improvement. In addition, after aspiration, EMG activity was increased, which according to the authors indicates a neurogenic mechanism. Harkey et al. (2014) analyzed in their review which applications can resolve this reflex inhibition and concluded that TENS and NMES are most effective, better than, for example, cryotherapy. Hopkins et al. (2002) compared TENS and cryotherapy in this context, and both applications were able to suppress the inhibition, as measured by the Hoffmann reflex. Their parameters: 60 ml physiological saline, injected intra-articularly. The cryo group: 2 plastic bags with 1.5 L of crushed ice each, applied for 30 min ventrally and dorsally to the knee. The TENS group: 100 μs, 120 Hz, 30 min, 4 electrodes around the knee, no visible contractions. Effective, despite underdosing. Incidentally, the soleus was not inhibited by an effusion in the knee (Hopkins et al. 2001).

Many knee patients who undergo postoperative muscle stimulation observe a reduction in their pain and improved mobility after stimulation. Such stimulation of the quadriceps muscle can even result in the immediate resolution of an active extension deficit. The cause? Central processes are triggered during NMES that we do not yet fully understand (Rice and McNair 2010). We know that NMES acts not only locally but also activates cortical and subcortical networks, similar to voluntary movements. For example, NMES applied to the right quadriceps immediately improves, regardless of dose, the force development of a simultaneous quadriceps contraction on the left side (Cattagni et al. 2018). We also know that the use of long pulses (1 ms, 100 Hz, so-called wide pulse NMES, Collins et al. 2001, 2002; Collins 2007) leads to processes that trigger increased recruitment of spinal motoneurons. This affects the excitability of the musculature in the periphery (Bergquist et al. 2011; Klakowicz et al. 2006). Whether these processes influence hyper- or hypotonia is not known. Perhaps there is a centrally controlled normalization of muscle tone due to a TENS-like effect. The strong contractions triggered by NMES (Aδ stimulation), the impulses used (200–400 μs: Aδ and C fiber stimulation), and the treatment duration (30 min and longer: β-endorphin production) fulfill almost all the requirements of a low-TENS treatment, except for the frequency (not 2–3 Hz). That NMES has an influence on reflex processes was demonstrated by Morrissey (1988).

What has been demonstrated at the knee joint can, of course, also occur at other joints.

Spasticity

NMES is used successfully in the treatment of spastic paresis, for example in hemiplegic patients (Stein et al. 2015; Lee et al. 2017; Hong et al. 2018; Alamer et al. 2020) and CP patients (Karabay et al. 2016; Qi et al. 2018) in three ways:

1. Stimulation of the antagonists of a spastic muscle group
2. Stimulation of the spastic muscle group itself
3. Alternating stimulation of the spastic agonists and their antagonists

Ad 1. Stimulation of the antagonists results in antagonist-agonist inhibition. For example, the wrist and finger extensors of a spastic hand can be stimulated, and during the subsequent "therapy window," the improved hand function can be actively practiced.

Ad 2. Stimulation of the spastic musculature leads to signal conduction toward the anterior horn, which can result in activation of Renshaw cells. The activated Renshaw cells inhibit both the agonist and antagonist motoneurons (recurrent inhibition). In other words: the neuron that controls the agonist inhibits its own activation and, via the same interneuron (the Renshaw cell), also reduces the inhibition of the antagonist. In addition, stimulation of the spastic musculature leads to its fatigue, which could allow the antagonists to be better activated.

Ad 3. By combining stimulation of the agonists and antagonists, all mechanisms can be activated.

Of course, such stimulation should be performed by the treating "neuro" therapist and not in the electrotherapy department half an hour before the patient goes to neurotherapy.

4.6.3 Muscle Stimulation to Improve Circulation

It has long been known that electrical stimulation can be used to improve blood flow with the help of the so-called muscle pump. Schnizer et al. investigated this plethysmographically in 1980 and found that blood flow in the lower leg of healthy subjects was slightly improved after 6 min of surge current application (500 μs phase duration, 10 Hz, 2 s ON 2 s OFF, motorically dosed) (from just over 1 ml per 100 ml tissue per minute to over 10 ml per 100 ml tissue per minute). CP (Bernard, motorically dosed) achieved a near doubling after 6 min, comparable to ultrastimulation (2–5, Träbert's current) and medium frequency (4000 Hz, AMF 1 s 50 Hz, 1 s 100 Hz, motorically). However, it could not be determined in which tissue this improvement in blood flow occurred. Miller et al. (2000) compared NMES application with medium-frequency current to active contractions to investigate improvement in calf blood flow. Their parameters: 2500 Hz, 20 Hz bursts, one electrode (20 cm^2) on the tibial nerve, the second (20 cm^2) on the medial gastrocnemius belly, 4 s ON, 4 s OFF, strong contractions. When the force development (measured with a pressure sensor under the foot) was the same, the improvement in blood flow was also the same in both groups. Initial values: 4.5 ml/100 ml/min, after stimulation and active contractions 10–11 ml/100 ml/min, practically the same as in Schnizer et al. (1980). The improvement lasted for 15 s after stimulation. For comparison and perspective: active isometric contractions with 50% of maximum force increase quadriceps blood flow from 4.5 ml/min/100 ml tissue to 257 ml/min/100 ml, almost 60 times as much (Walløe and Wesche 1988). The effect of surge current is therefore rather modest.

Pérez et al. (2002) demonstrated in healthy subjects that after a 6-week NMES application, not only did a fast-to-slow adaptation occur in the vastus lateralis muscle, but there was also increased capillarization in the type II fibers. Their parameters: 45–60 Hz, 12 s ON, 8 s OFF, 30 min/day, 3 times/week. In rodents, this is a well-known phenomenon and is explained by increased release of angiotensin II and VEGF (vascular endothelial growth factor) (Amaral et al. 2001).

Pseudoatrophy?

Incidentally: If for any reason a muscle group is not used, the girth of that muscle often decreases dramatically in a very short time. Especially knee patients repeatedly manage to shock their doctors and therapists postoperatively after 1–2 days with their—supposedly—atrophied vastus medialis. The subsequent therapy successes are just as impressive: just a few stimulations and the muscle is back!

The following should be noted: tissue that is not used is immediately less well perfused. This saves energy and is therefore sensible. There is, of course, great joy when, after just a few NMES treatments, the "atrophied" muscle, especially the notorious vastus medialis, has "gained mass" again and the quadriceps girth, conscientiously measured 10–15 cm proximal to the patella, is almost the same on both sides.

What have we observed here? Acute atrophy? And then a lightning-fast hypertrophy? Probably not. Reduced blood flow can cause a decrease in girth of up to several centimeters within minutes. The reverse is also true: after intensive muscle stimulation, there is an immediate improvement in blood flow due to the work performed. With 10 ml of blood per 100 ml of tissue instead of 1 ml/100 ml muscle mass, a few centimeters are quickly added.

4.6.4 Preservation and Improvement of Kinesthesia (Sense of Movement)

The term kinesthesia means sense of movement and refers to the ability to perceive spatial, force, speed, and tension relationships of one's own movement. The terms proprioception or deep sensation are also frequently used (Brandes et al. 2019). The literature contains a multitude of definitions for these two terms, and they are often used interchangeably. In sports physiology, "sense of movement" is defined as "a complex disposition for the differentiated, purposeful reception and processing of sensorimotor information during the execution of one's own movement actions." In this context, the term "body schema" is also used: the mental representation of one's own body regarding its spatial extension and position in space. In English, the term "kinesthetic awareness" is used, which refers to a kinesthetic consciousness of body parts and the relationship of these parts to each other and to objects in the environment. Afferent signals from kinesthetic receptors in and around joints, in muscles, tendons, and in the skin project to areas of the somatosensory cortex and trigger sensations of recognition and localization. This is related to the body model, which provides information about the size and shape of body parts. Kinesthesia, together with vision and touch, is associated with the sense of body ownership (Proske and Gandevia 2018).

So, the topic is quite complex. What is certain is that this sensation is a very complex process involving peripheral and central neural systems, and it is not just about the correct movement sequence, but also about the emotions associated with it. This is called the joy of movement, and here not only the sensorimotor cortex is involved, but also the limbic system.

In the 1930s, Penfield and colleagues conducted extensive intraoperative electrical stimulations on the brains of patients with epilepsy or tumors. The motor and sensory responses to these stimulations (the patients had local anesthesia) were meticulously recorded in sessions lasting hours, enabling the investigators to roughly represent the human body as a topographical projection on the somatosensory cortex. The medical illustrator Hortense Cantlie used a bit of artistic license to create the famous homunculus from this (Fig. 4.1) (Penfield and Boldrey 1937; Pogliano 2012; Gandhoke et al. 2019). In later publications, Penfield and his coauthors repeatedly emphasized that this homunculus should be used as a teaching tool and mnemonic, but is by no means anatomically correct. Not that the localizations are incorrect, but with modern methods it has since been confirmed that it is impossible to construct a representation with even approximately humanoid features from the measurement data (Gandhoke et al. 2019). Penfield himself never had a problem with the media spreading the idea, and the somewhat grotesque little man was well received by the general public. What is certain is that there are more or less well-defined cortical areas that are afferently and efferently connected to the periphery. And these areas are highly plastic.

From the many studies on brain plasticity, we know that reorganization of the projection area belonging to the denervated region takes place on the somatosensory cortex just a few minutes after denervation (Lundborg 2000; Björkman et al. 2004; Lundborg 2005; Rosén et al. 2012). The "orphaned" area is literally taken over by its neighbors. In other words: the receptive fields of the neighboring segments enlarge, and this already has functional consequences after 24 h (Kolasinski et al. 2016). Specialized hand therapists use various methods after hand, finger, or arm replantation and after nerve reconstructions to reverse this state; this is called reinnervation training. Not only are various methods of sensory stimulation used, such as TENS, but also mirrors (Wand et al. 2014), artificial hands (Lee et al. 2015), and acoustic stimuli (Lundborg 2003) to trick the CNS (Lundborg and Rosén 2007; Ehrsson et al. 2008; Kaas et al. 2013;

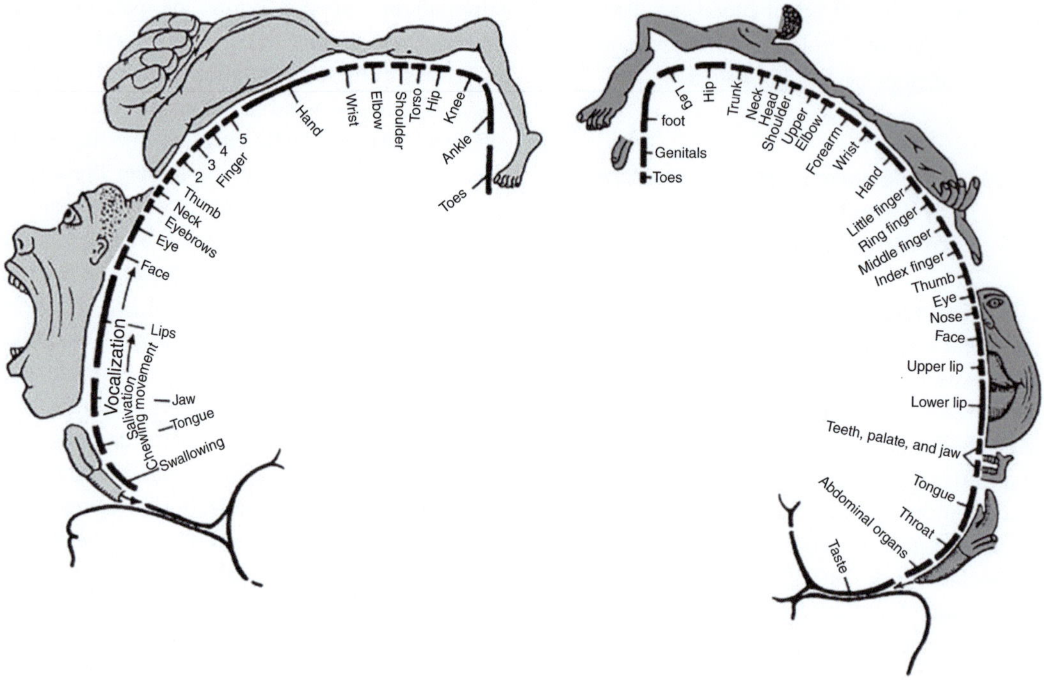

Fig. 4.1 Penfield's homunculus. Left motor, right sensory. Image with permission, © Lexikon der Neurowissenschaft by Hartwig Hanser, Springer Nature

Dempsey-Jones et al. 2019). We know that electrical stimulation in the periphery, via a nerve or a motor point, increases the activity of the motor cortex in the corresponding projection area (Ridding et al. 2000; Charlton et al. 2003), especially if the stimulation triggers contractions (Chipchase et al. 2011). The response of the sensorimotor cortex is dose-dependent: the more intense the NMES, the stronger the response measured by functional Magnetic Resonance Imaging (fMRI) (Smith et al. 2003). When NMES is combined with active movement, fMRI shows a stronger cortical activation than with NMES alone or activity alone (Joa et al. 2012). Prolonged stimulation with TENS leads to an enlargement of the cortical area corresponding to the stimulated muscle (Meesen et al. 2011)—an effect that can also be demonstrated with fMRI during acupuncture (Jiang et al. 2013).

These explanations are intended to make it clear that muscle stimulation does not just "do something to the muscle," but has far-reaching consequences for cognitive properties correlated with movement.

Moreover, this is perhaps the most important reason to perform stimulation of denervated muscles in patients after a peripheral nerve lesion. If reinnervation occurs after many months, the reinnervated muscle should ideally have a functioning, communicative brain area.

Otherwise, unfortunately, it will be: "No connection at this number."

4.6.5 Incontinence

It would go beyond the scope of this book to discuss all aspects of incontinence in detail; there are good specialized books for that. Therefore, only some general aspects will be addressed below. Urinary incontinence refers to the inability to retain urine, fecal incontinence is the inability to retain stool. Both have a number of subtypes. The most common types of urinary incontinence are stress incontinence, urge incontinence (to urge = to press), or a combination of both. Stress incontinence is characterized by urine loss as a result of an increase in intra-abdominal pressure during physical exertion, leading to an increase in intravesical pressure that in this case exceeds the maximum urethral closure pressure. This occurs, for example, when coughing, sneezing, laughing, climbing stairs, or jumping. In urge incontinence, there is a strong so-called imperative urge to urinate, which does not correlate with the degree of bladder filling; the patient constantly feels the need "to go." The mild form is also called overactive bladder or (nervous) irritable bladder. In the mixed form, the symptoms occur together.

In addition to pharmacological and surgical measures with implanted stimulators, there is the possibility of treating incontinence with NMES/TENS (Allon 2019; Mazur-Bialy et al. 2020). The method is successful in many cases, although the latest Cochrane review, of course, lists the usual shortcomings of the studies assessed: groups too small, no control groups, no blinding, different treatment parameters, etc. Nevertheless, in 2017 the authors concluded that the method is a valuable addition to standard therapies and that such treatment should definitely be combined with targeted active therapy (Stewart et al. 2017). NMES is performed either with standard (adhesive) electrodes, which can be placed in various locations, for example, sacral for stimulation of the sacral nerves, on the medial lower leg for stimulation of the posterior tibial nerve, or on the sensory branch of the pudendal nerve: in women on the clitoral nerve, in men on the dorsal nerve of the penis (Fig. 4.2). For asymmetrically compensated pulses, the cathode is placed on the site to be stimulated. For symmetrically compensated pulses, it does not matter. Special probes can also be used, which are inserted vaginally or rectally to get close to the pudendal nerve in the pelvis (Fig. 4.3). The use of such a probe is effective but can lead to infections (Dmochowski et al. 2019). Such probes sometimes have pressure sensors that can be used to assess the performance of the pelvic floor muscles. Therapeutic success often occurs after just

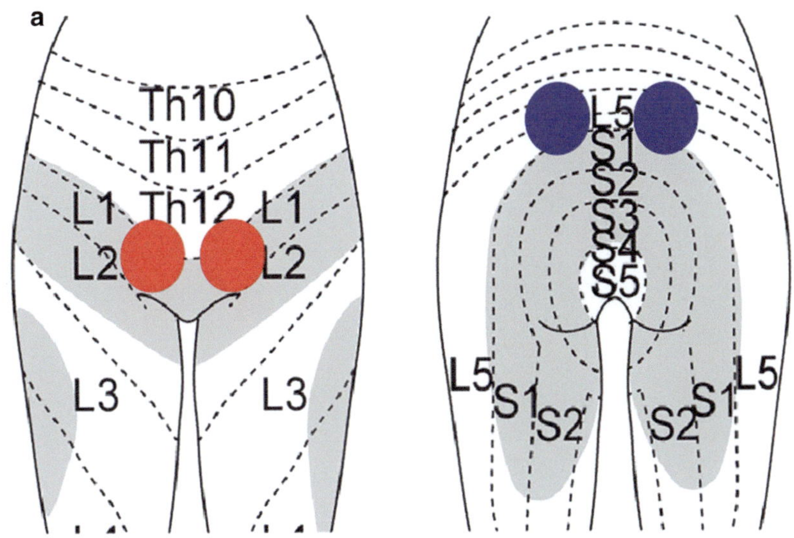

Fig. 4.2 (**a**) The position of the cathode and anode must be determined. Cathode blue. Positioning of the anode either at the perineum or sacral. © Schwa-Medico AG, Ehringshausen, with kind permission. (**b**) The position of the cathode and anode must also be determined here. Positioning of the anode either at the perineum or sacral. © Schwa-Medico AG, Ehringshausen, with kind permission. (**c**) Device for stimulation in incontinence. © Schwa-Medico AG, Ehringshausen, with kind permission

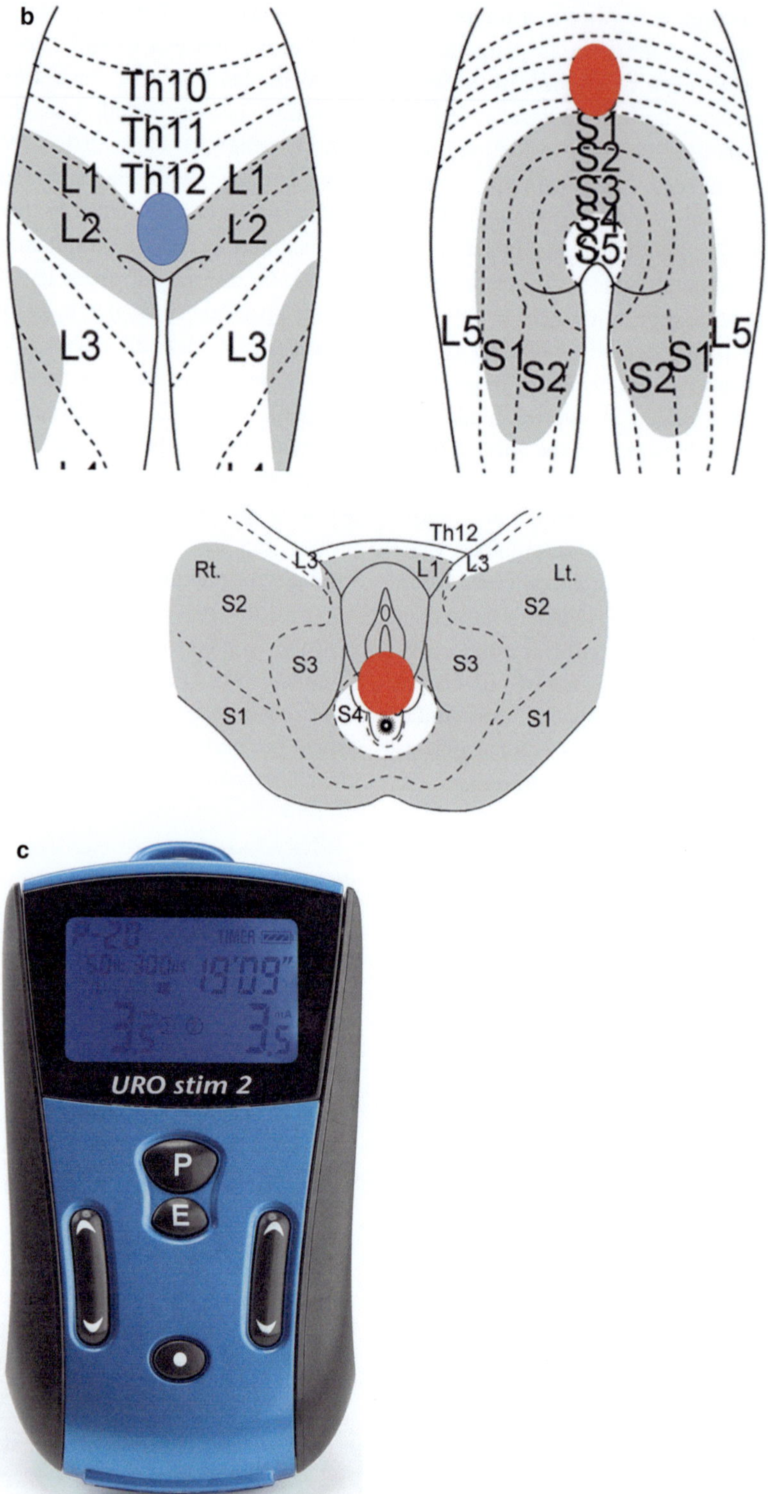

Fig. 4.2 (continued)

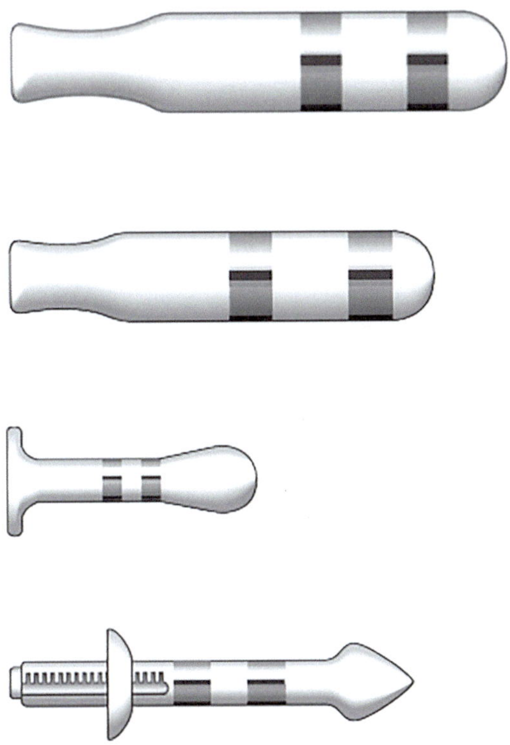

Fig. 4.3 Special electrodes. © Schwa-Medico AG, Ehringshausen, with kind permission

a few treatments, and it is reasonable to attribute at least part of this to the central neurological mechanisms discussed above.

The parameters used are very heterogeneous (Berghmans et al. 2000). Various current forms are used. Most often, TENS-like, low-frequency currents are used, but medium-frequency currents are also employed, either premodulated (endogenous interference, i.e., in the device) or tetrapolar, exogenous, classically according to Nemec, a method we know does not work, but which can still have a local sensory effect. As described under TENS (for example, in Sect. 3.10.8), patients often find MF application more pleasant than TENS—a benefit that can be exploited in applications in this sensitive area. The stimulation parameters differ in terms of frequencies, phase duration, and stimulation intensity, and to date, no optimal uniform combination of parameters has been found. La Rosa et al. (2019a, b) recommend, based on various reviews, stimulation at 50 Hz for the treatment of stress incontinence and at 10–20 Hz for the treatment of urge incontinence; this with the subjectively highest possible pulse intensity. The treatment, lasting 15–30 min, should be performed daily for 4–12 weeks. The parameters may indicate that, apart from neurologically caused incontinence and surgical applications, improvement of kinesthesia via sensory input is involved in the effect of this application, as they do not differ significantly from NMES for the quadriceps femoris muscle.

4.6.5.1 P-PTNS

A very interesting approach is percutaneous stimulation of the posterior tibial nerve (Percutaneous Posterior Tibial Nerve Stimulation, P-PTNS) (de Wall and Heesakkers 2017). In this application, the aim is to stimulate the sacral plexus via cross-communication through the posterior tibial nerve and to achieve neuromodulation (Fig. 4.4). Neuromodulation is defined here as the effect of "crosstalk" between sympathetic and parasympathetic postganglionic nerve endings and synapses, which is intended to cause a change in the nerve signals involved in the voiding reflex (de Groat et al. 2015; Janssen et al. 2017). For this, either a needle is placed as close as possible to the nerve and electrically stimulated, or conventional adhesive electrodes are used (Ramírez-García et al. 2019). The method has its roots in Traditional Chinese Medicine. Acupuncturists have apparently been using, among other things, the acupuncture point SP6 (Spleen 6) for centuries to treat incontinence (Janssen et al. 2017), and the location of this point corresponds to where the mentioned nerve is stimulated. SP6 is a so-called master point for all obstetric-gynecological indications. P-PTNS is usually applied for 12 weeks, 2 to 3 times per week, each session lasting 30 min. Stimulation parameters: 20 Hz, 200 μs, up to 10 mA. The intensity is increased until the sole of the foot begins to tingle and the big toe flexes or the toes spread. After these 12 weeks, monthly maintenance sessions are recommended. The method was initially met with great skepticism, but after Finazzi-Agrò et al.

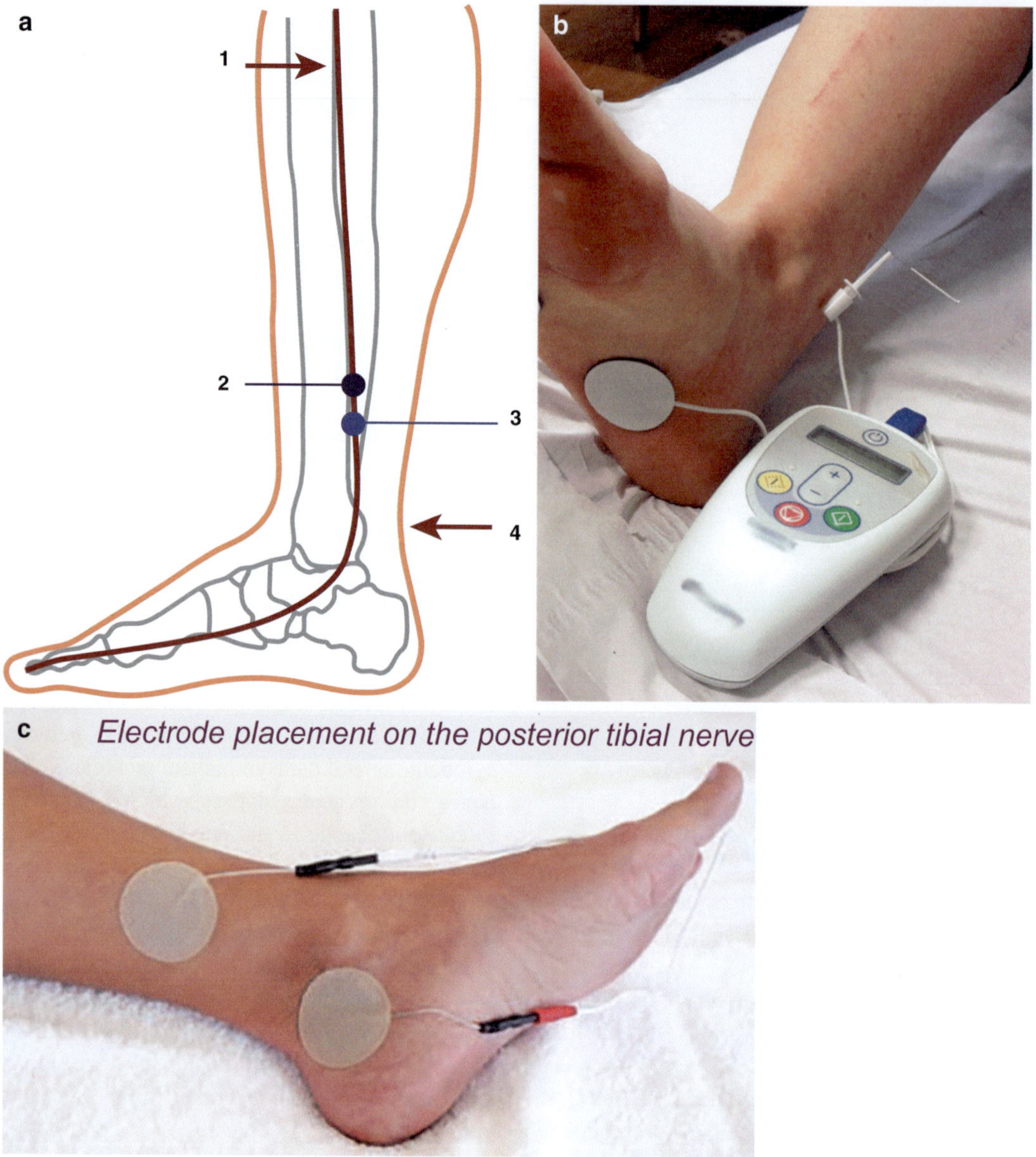

Fig. 4.4 (**a**) P-PTNS. 1 = posterior tibial nerve, 2 = SP6 (Sanyinjiao), 3 = insertion point for needle, 4 = medial malleolus. From de Wall and Heesakkers 2017, with kind permission. (**b**) P-PTNS. Needle 3 fingerbreadths proximal to the upper edge of the medial malleolus. From Knowles et al. 2015, with kind permission. (**c**) Stimulation of the posterior tibial nerve with adhesive electrodes. Cathode on SP6. © Schwa-Medico AG, Ehringshausen, with kind permission

(2010) and Peters et al. (2010) confirmed the effectiveness of the treatment with well-conducted RCTs, even the greatest skeptics were convinced, and the method is now included in the treatment guidelines of several international bodies (International Continence Society, American Urological Association, European Association of Urology) (Janssen et al. 2017). In the case of fecal incontinence, the application appears to have no effect (Knowles et al. 2015).

4.6.5.2 Studies on the Topic

Certain standard measurements are performed to monitor the effectiveness of this application. In addition to various quality-of-life questionnaires, the number of incontinence episodes is recorded and urine loss is assessed over a certain period using pads.

- Ramírez-García et al. (2019) compared the effect of percutaneous PTNS (P-PTNS) with transcutaneous PTNS (T-PTNS) in patients with overactive bladder. To recap: in the percutaneous version, a needle is placed near the posterior tibial nerve, the second electrode is a standard adhesive electrode placed nearby, often on the sole of the foot. In T-PTNS, two standard adhesive electrodes are used, one directly over the nerve (5 cm cranial to the medial malleolus), the second a few centimeters further cranial or under the sole of the foot. Parameters for both groups: 20 Hz, 30 min, 12 times, 1/week. Intensity: tingling in the sole of the foot and flexion of the big toe. After the treatment series, both groups showed the same improvement compared to the control group. Due to the lower burden, without a needle, the transcutaneous version is preferable. This method is also easy to perform at home.
- Jacomo et al. (2020) compared the effect of T-PTNS (10 Hz, 200 µs, submotor, 30 min) with transcutaneous sacral stimulation (adhesive electrodes distal to the PSIS paravertebrally over S2–S4, 10 Hz, 700 µs, 30 min, intensity "as tolerated") and found both applications effective in treating overactive bladder in older individuals. T-PTNS had the greater effect.
- Scaldazza et al. (2017) compared the effect of P-PTNS (standard parameters) as a solo treatment with electrical stimulation using an intravaginal (IV) electrode (30 min, 30 s 20 Hz, 30 s 5 Hz), combined with pelvic floor training. Both groups showed significant improvements, with P-PTNS (without PF training) being more effective.
- Correia et al. (2014) compared treatment with an IV electrode to standard adhesive electrodes (1 pair suprapubic, 1 pair on the ischial tuberosities) in women with stress incontinence. Parameters for both groups: 50 Hz, 20 min, 4 s ON, 8 s OFF, 2 s ramp up, 2 s ramp down, tolerance limit. Both groups showed significant improvements after 12 sessions (2/week), with the IV group showing the greater increase in pelvic floor muscle strength.
- Guo and Kang (2018) applied TENS in stroke patients with urinary incontinence. Parameters: 1 pair of electrodes on S2 paravertebral, 1 pair bilaterally halfway between PSIS and ischial tuberosity, 50 Hz, 250 µs, 10 s ON, 30 s OFF, 30 min, intensity up to tolerance limit. This was done daily for 10 weeks. The treatment group was significantly better than the control group.
- Elmelund et al. (2018) compared the effect of pelvic floor training alone and PF training combined with electrical stimulation using an IV electrode in women with incomplete spinal cord injury and incontinence and found no differences in the final outcome. Stimulation parameters (two different programs were used in succession): first 40 Hz, 250 µs, up to 10 min, 30 contractions of about 10 s with 10 s pause, during which the women were to contract as well. Then 10 Hz, 250 µs, 10–20 min continuously, during which the women were to relax. Intensity in each case up to tolerance limit.
- Tan et al. (2019) were able to show after analyzing controlled studies on the treatment of fecal incontinence and constipation that significant improvements also occurred in the control groups. This indicates a not insignificant placebo effect and should be taken into account when using this method for these diagnoses.

4.6.6 Improving the Sense of Movement

To improve kinesthesia, NMES can be used as follows; here is an example on the forearm:

- Of course, the patient should be informed about the purpose of the treatment. The usual contraindications must be observed (general measures before treatment).

- The device should be set to constant voltage (CV) so that the electrode can be moved easily and the patient does not get a shock if the stimulating electrode slips.
- All frequencies above 20 Hz are tetanizing. A frequency should be set that is comfortable for the patient, usually around 50 Hz.
- The longer the phase duration, the stronger the contraction at the same intensity. 150–200 μs is usually sufficient for beginners, but of course, it should be adjusted to the patient.
- Biphasic symmetrical rectangular pulses are best suited for eliciting muscle contractions and do not cause skin irritation as with uncompensated pulses.
- A large (about 7 × 12 cm) indifferent electrode (if asymmetrically compensated pulses are not used: the anode) is attached to the upper arm. If compensated pulses are used, an adhesive electrode can be used. However, a conventional lead rubber electrode in a sponge pocket can also be used (sponges do not make as much a mess as contact gel).
- For the stimulating electrode (for asymmetrically compensated pulses, the cathode), a lead rubber electrode is used. The electrode is held so that only one corner of the electrode is in contact with the skin. Don't worry: the therapist feels nothing. Stimulation with small point electrodes (probes) is often perceived by patients as "sharp, stinging."
- Now, with one hand, the therapist holds the stimulating electrode on the patient's forearm, where the relevant motor zone is suspected. The other hand is on the intensity control of the device. The therapist watches the patient. The intensity is carefully increased until the patient feels a distinct current sensation. If lucky (or skilled), a slight contraction is already visible. If not, the stimulating electrode is moved over the muscle to be stimulated until a contraction is elicited (in the correct muscle, of course). The stimulation points recorded in most electrotherapy books are very imprecise (Gobbo et al. 2011, 2014). The stimulation zone is usually in the proximal third of the muscle belly.
- If only a single muscle is to be stimulated, a small adhesive electrode can be placed at this point (possibly trimmed); if several muscles (or muscle groups) are to be stimulated in succession, manual stimulation is continued.
- Now the current is turned down again and the patient is again informed about the intended therapy. There are many possibilities here: the patient should focus only on the movement, imagine the movement as a function, or try to actively participate in the movement or resist it. It is definitely useful to involve the contralateral side.
- Where possible, the activity should be incorporated into a meaningful function. For example, the patient can be asked to grasp something, and NMES can be used to support release, or the gripping function can be supported by stimulating the flexors.
- The patient is told when the current is coming, and then the intensity is slowly increased over 2–3 s until a contraction is elicited. The intensity must be ramped up; the contraction should look "physiological": rise in 2–3 s, hold for a few seconds, fade in 1–2 s: in other words, like a ramped current. Contractions should not last longer than about 5 to a maximum of 10 s. Strong contractions elicit more cortical activity.
- Each contraction is followed by a pause. The duration of the pause depends on the patient; usually, no more than 4–6 contractions are elicited per minute.
- The contraction strength is regulated by the intensity and adapted to the patient's abilities. If the patient has activity, only a slight increase is needed, possibly even just sensory, so that the patient perceives the muscle. If the sense of movement is no longer present, a somewhat stronger contraction is usually required. There are many possibilities. For example, 2 or 3 times relatively strong, then only once weak, so that the patient's activity can be assessed.
- Of course, if you own a suitable device, the sequence could be programmed into the device. However, this restricts flexibility during treatment too much and is not recommended by the author.

Since this application is not about strengthening therapy, but about facilitation, the contraction phases should sensibly be alternated with active movement exercises, preferably functional or, for example, with PNF techniques. The method works excellently in patients who "can no longer find" their quadriceps postoperatively.

4.6.7 General Information on NMES

The clear advantage of NMES in rehabilitation is the ability to activate muscles in situations where the patient cannot or is not allowed to do so themselves.

Disadvantages include the lack of coordination training, the unphysiological, mostly rather isometric contraction, and the considerable sensory burden caused by the current. The reversal of the contraction sequence does not necessarily have to be a disadvantage.

It is clear that NMES can never replace active training in a healthy muscle-nerve complex, but it is certainly a very useful supplement. For example, a patient who can only weakly contract their quadriceps postoperatively uses only their type I muscle fibers. If this patient additionally stimulates (perhaps) their type II fibers with NMES, the training effect is certainly greater.

The compensated pulse forms used in TENS are excellent for eliciting muscle contractions, especially the biphasic rectangular pulses. The phase duration can usually be freely selected between 100 and 400 µs, and the frequency can also be conveniently set even on smaller devices. The advantage over medium-frequency currents is that with frequencies below 50–60 Hz, HFF is avoided. The phase duration does not seem to play a major role in force development. Giroux et al. (2018) compared force development and subjective perception during supramaximal stimulation of the quadriceps with phase durations of 200 and 1000 µs in healthy subjects and found no difference using a dynamometer.

A "strength training" protocol can be designed as in Russian Stimulation "10–50–10" or similar protocols can be used. For example, 10–20–30: ramp up for 10 s to a strong contraction, hold for 20 s, at least 30 s rest. If the muscle fatigues, the tension phase is shortened or the rest is extended. This process is repeated 15 to 20 times. To optimize muscle fiber recruitment and avoid local exhaustion, the stimulation parameters and especially the electrode placement should be varied during training.

Since fatigue resistance is also trained with this application, a separate "endurance training" is probably not necessary. Nevertheless, an endurance-oriented (oxidative, aerobic) protocol can be programmed on the device with many, not too strong contractions, interrupted by short breaks. The muscle work performed is responsible for the training effect, not the stimulation frequency used.

For smaller muscles, stimulation is performed with a small stimulating electrode over the motor stimulation zone, with the second indifferent electrode placed nearby. The motor stimulation zone is usually located in the proximal third of the muscle. The simplest approach is to use the clinical device in CV mode, not turn the current up too high, and then search for the stimulation zone. For larger muscles, correspondingly large electrodes are used, ensuring that as many stimulation zones as possible are reached.

It is clear that NMES can never replace active training in a healthy muscle-nerve complex, but it is a very useful supplement. A patient who trains actively and uses NMES trains more than one who "only" trains actively. But what would happen if this patient replaced the NMES time with active training (Lieber et al. 1996)?

A few comments on the studies on NMES available so far:

- The method is almost always applied to healthy subjects; our knowledge about patients is rather limited.
- When active performance could be controlled via feedback (EMG), active training was just as effective as NMES.
- Control groups were often not used.

- As a rule, it was found that active training combined with NMES is more effective than just (equally long) active training or NMES alone.
- Battery-powered devices are just as good as mains-powered devices.
- NMES for atrophy prophylaxis is better than doing nothing.

4.6.8 Indications

- Muscle training to maintain or improve kinesthetics in situations where normal muscle activity is not ensured.
- Prevention and/or elimination of inactivity atrophy after/during prolonged immobilization.
- Muscle training after operations and function disorders due to trauma or medical causes.
- Intention training for coordination disorders after peripheral paralysis or central neurological conditions.
- Scoliosis in young CP patients.

4.6.9 Contraindications

See Low Frequency/TENS, especially the explanations in Sect. 3.12.3 on the topic of "pacemakers".

Of course, local structural stability must be taken into account during muscle stimulation. It is expressly recommended to contact the responsible surgeon and, if necessary, obtain written confirmation of the referral.

4.7 Muscle Stimulation with Medium-Frequency Alternating Currents

In addition to low-frequency, TENS-like pulse currents, medium-frequency alternating currents, also called kilohertz currents, are used to stimulate innervated muscles. The use of this current form became very popular after the allegedly great successes of so-called Russian Stimulation were reported in the 1970s. The method was said to be not only particularly effective but also more pleasant than NF stimulation (Andrianowa et al. 1974).

The impulses used in an MF current are very short (125 µs at 4000 Hz, 200 µs at 2500 Hz), so only an intact nerve-muscle complex can respond. The stimulation occurs at the nerve ("indirect"), which transmits the action potentials to the muscle. In the case of a peripheral nerve lesion, these currents are ineffective; here, longer triangular pulses are needed, and the stimulation then occurs at the muscle ("direct"). There is no evidence to support claims that MF currents have a "direct" effect on the muscle.

4.7.1 BMAC, Russian Stimulation

Various terms are used to describe these kilohertz currents. The best known are the tetrapolar exogenous interference according to Nemec and the bipolar endogenous interference, also called premodulated interference. The classic tetrapolar version should really no longer be used for strengthening, as it is completely impossible to achieve targeted stimulation with it. The reasons for this can be found in the chapter on interferential current (Sect. 3.10.6). Premodulated IF is not effective for strength development, as part of the impulses in the sinusoidal burst remain subthreshold and ineffective (Fig. 4.5D). In Russian Stimulation (RS), on the other hand, a continuous sinusoidal 2500 Hz alternating current is broken into 10 ms bursts; the frequency at which these bursts are delivered can be set on the device. All pulses in the burst have the same intensity (= amplitude), which is why this method is

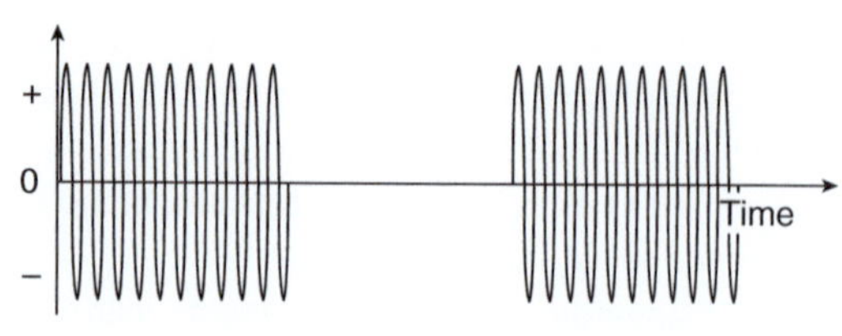

Fig. 4.5 Russian Stimulation or BMAC. From Ward 2009, with kind permission

significantly more effective than the two previously mentioned (Fig. 4.5, see also Fig. 3.7). This is a frequency-modulated medium-frequency alternating current, the most common term being Burst Mode Alternating Current (BMAC) (Ward et al. 2004; Ward 2009; Ward and Chuen 2009).

Russian Stimulation became popular in the 1970s due to the allegedly very good results of Dr. Yakov Koz (also spelled "Kotz" or "Kots"), then Professor of Physical Culture at the State Academy of Moscow. Dr. Koz administered electrical stimulation to his athletes and cosmonauts in addition to normal training and claimed to achieve strength gains of around 40% in 3 weeks with his method. These claims could not be confirmed during an exchange program in Canada in 1977 (Ward and Shkuratova 2002).

His reasoning for combining active training with EMS was as follows: At that time, training focused mainly on volume and strength. In terms of muscle fiber type, this training mainly targeted the slow-twitch motor units—units that fatigue slowly and are innervated by Aα2 neurons. It was already known that electrical stimulation primarily stimulates the fast-twitch motor units—that is, the units used for controlling rapid, precise movements and innervated by Aα1 motoneurons. By combining both methods, both types of motor units could be activated.

Koz originally used a low-frequency 50 Hz rectangular pulse current, phase duration 1 ms, i.e., neofaradically. After many trials, he found that a 10–50–10 mode was optimal for training: 10 s maximum contraction, 50 s rest, repeat 10 times, once a day (Andrianowa et al. 1974). Koz initially did not use medium-frequency currents; these were only introduced later and had a somewhat different effect on fatigue. The current and training form found makes physiological sense: At a stimulation frequency of 50 Hz, the causes of fatigue lie in the depletion of neurotransmitter reserves and conduction problems in the T-tubule system, i.e., not the type of fatigue that leads to improved training status. It is therefore sensible to avoid fatigue, hence the 50 s rest.

Later, other scientists used a medium-frequency pulse current instead of Koz's current form (Andrianowa et al. 1974). This MF current, broken into 50 Hz bursts with a base frequency of 2500 Hz, causes relatively rapid fatigue via these very mechanisms and therefore cannot be as effective as the form used by Koz. However, the higher frequencies are indisputably much more pleasant for training. Stimulation occurs either directly at the muscle (over the motor stimulation zones), with Andrianova finding that frequencies around 2500 Hz were optimal, or "indirectly" at the nerve with frequencies around 1000 Hz. The distinction is purely academic, as the very short impulses always only stimulate the nerve. Koz's claim that the training was not painful due to the frequencies used must be put into perspective: His users, elite athletes in the former USSR, were used to enduring a lot to be among the world's best. This should be seen in the context of the spirit of the times. Incidentally, Bergquist et al. (2012) found that stimulation of the quadriceps via the femoral nerve recruits more motor units than conventional muscle stimulation. However, since stimulation via the nerve is somewhat impractical (the stimulating electrode shifts with each contraction) and only about 30% of MVC was achieved, the investigators see its use more as a supplement to normal stimulation rather than a replacement.

4.7.2 BMAC, Aussie Stimulation

For many years, a group of Australian researchers led by Alex Ward has been working on RS and has tried to optimize stimulation in terms of tolerability and effectiveness. They found that a 1000 Hz alternating current, applied in 2–4 ms bursts, was optimal (Ward 2009). The current quickly became known as Aussie Stimulation, in reference to RS. Since other researchers later continued to investigate with different parameters but still used the same term, the expression Burst Mode Alternating Current was introduced to avoid confusion: BMAC (Fig. 4.5). This term is preferable because it precisely expresses what is meant, and each researcher can use

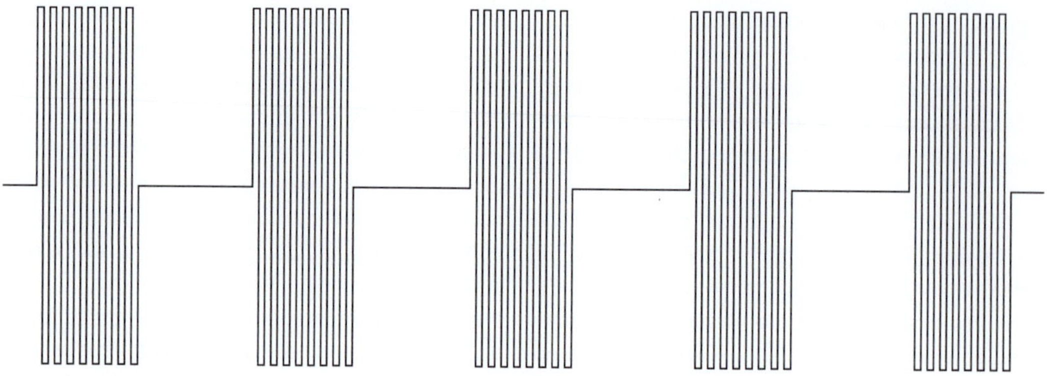

Fig. 4.6 BMBPC: Burst Modulated Biphasic Pulsed Current, rectangular pulses

their preferred parameters—as long as these are reported correctly, of course. A few years ago, a new current form was added, Burst Modulated Biphasic Pulsed Current or BMBPC (Fig. 4.6). In BMAC, bursts consist of sinusoidal single pulses, as in RS. BMBPC forms bursts from an alternating current consisting of rectangular pulses. The 1000 Hz BMAC and 1000 Hz BMBPC appear to be equally effective for strength development and are significantly more effective than 2500 Hz BMAC (= Russian Stimulation) (Adams et al. 2018). Whether BMAC is more effective for strength development than NF stimulation is somewhat controversial, although "conventional" NF stimulation seems to have the edge. Da Silva et al. (2015) found no difference, Scott et al. (2015) found NF stimulation more effective for strength development, and Szecsi and Fornusek (2014) favor BMAC. Medeiros et al. (2017) found BMAC and NF equally effective for stimulating the M. quadriceps, provided the same phase duration (250 μs) is used (and equally unpleasant). Stimulation with longer phases (500 μs), however, was more effective for strength development. Modesto et al. (2019) found no difference in results with BMAC (2500 Hz, 250 μs) or NF stimulation (100 Hz, 200 μs) in their soccer players. The subjects found NF more pleasant and therefore considered this method better. Vaz and Frasson found in their review (2018) no reasons to prefer BMAC over NF stimulation.

4.8 Motor Points or Muscle Stimulation Points

Almost all electrotherapy books contain illustrations intended to show where a particular muscle is most easily stimulated. However, many colleagues have tried in vain to locate specific points based on these illustrations, only to end up desperately moving the stimulating electrode around until they could elicit a strong contraction. The reason? The drawings are too imprecise. First, there are no stimulation points, but rather stimulation zones. Second, larger muscles have several stimulation points (for example, 7 if you want to stimulate the entire quadriceps, Lim et al. 2021). Third, there is a difference between nerve entry points and motor stimulation zones, and these rarely coincide in terms of location. The nerve entry site (NES) corresponds to the point where the motor nerve terminal penetrates the perimysium (Botter et al. 2011). The motor point (MP) corresponds to the location where a contraction can be elicited with the lowest stimulation intensity (Botter et al. 2011; Gobbo et al. 2011, 2014; Behringer et al. 2014). Unfortunately, these terms are used interchangeably, which can lead to problems with localization. Botter et al. (2011) created an overview of motor stimulation points in the leg and impressively demonstrated the great variation in their localization (Fig. 4.7). Franz et al. (2018) localized MPs in the upper extremity using electrical

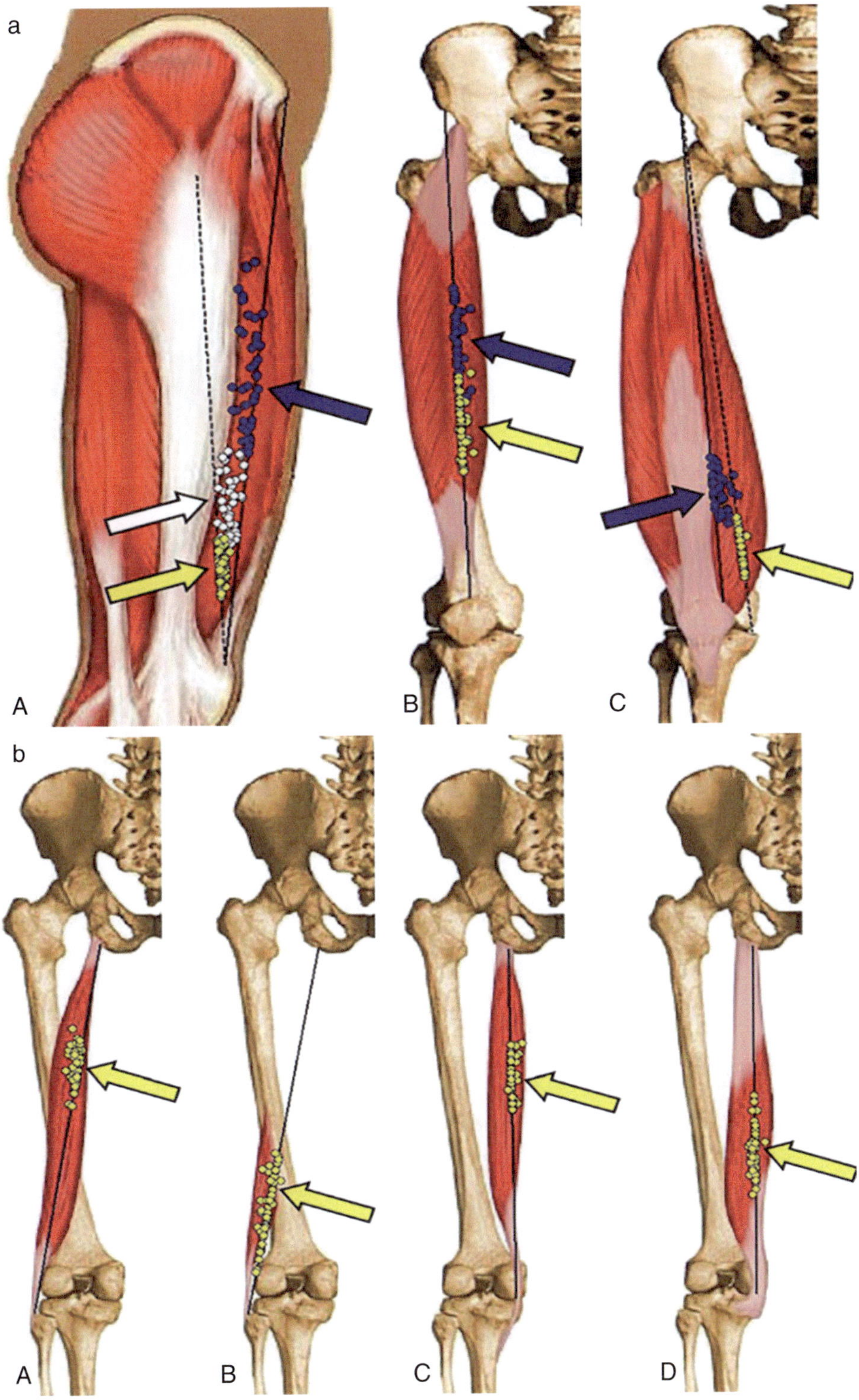

Fig. 4.7 (**a**) Motor points in different areas of the quadriceps muscle in 53 subjects. A: Vastus lateralis, B: Rectus, C: Vastus medialis. Arrows indicate the average area. (**b**) Motor points in the hamstrings. A: Long head, B: Short head, C: Semitendinosus, D: Semimembranosus. (**c**) Motor points in the lower leg. A: Tibialis anterior, B: Peroneus longus, C: Gastrocnemius. From Botter et al. (2011), with kind permission

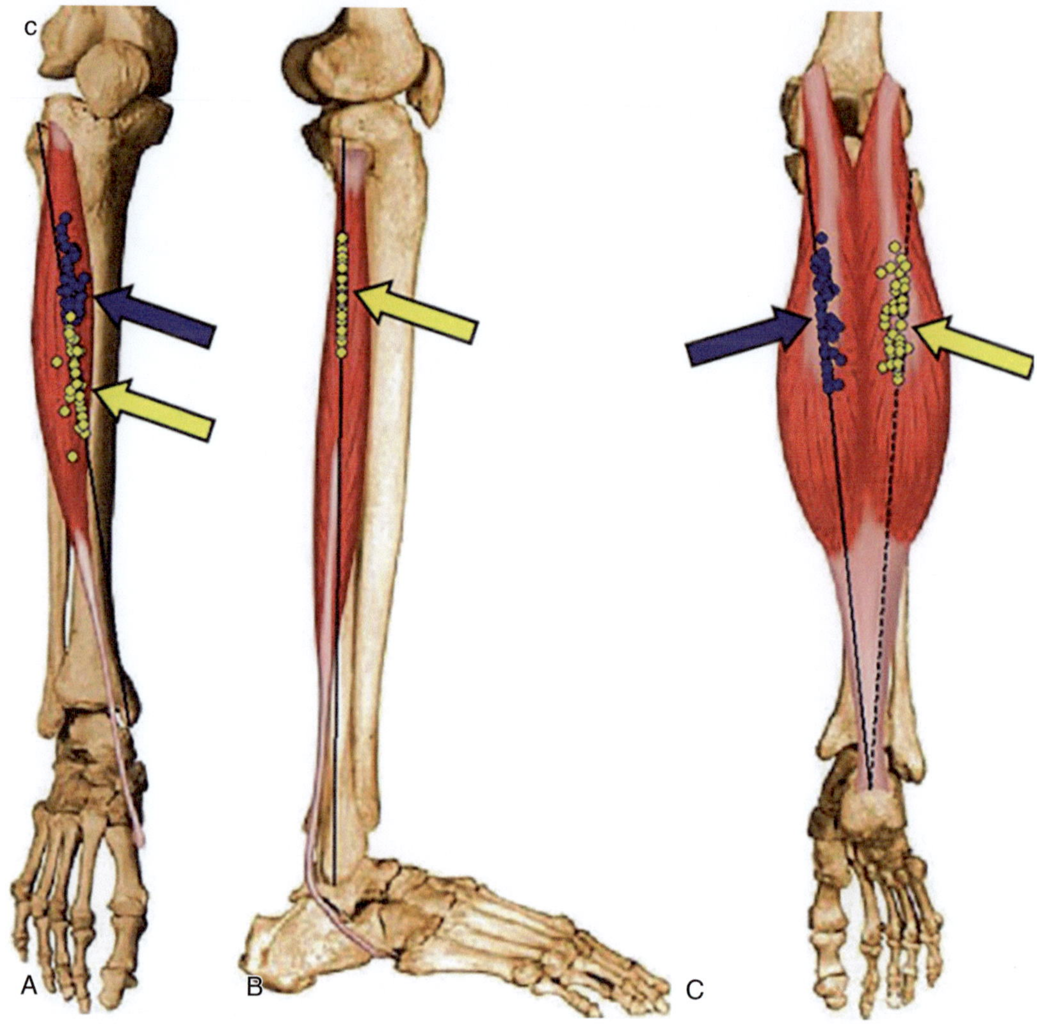

Fig. 4.7 (continued)

stimulation and compared their location with that of NES, found via cadaver studies. Only the locations in the pectoralis minor and descending trapezius matched; the others (biceps, latissimus, pectoralis major, ascending and transverse trapezius) did not. There are comparable studies on muscles such as the tibialis anterior, hip adductors, abdominal muscles, soleus, and many more, and all authors come to the same conclusion: The locations show great variation, but the zones are generally located in the proximal third of the muscle belly. At least that's something.

Localization Test

Gobbo et al. (2014) rightly point out that NMES is clearly less effective if the electrodes are not correctly placed. They mention that many manufacturers include illustrations with their stimulation devices suggesting electrode placement, which are often useless. The authors therefore recommend performing a brief, simple localization test before each application. To do this, a large indifferent electrode is placed on or near the muscle to be stimulated. Using a frequency of 1–2 Hz, a phase duration of 100–200 μs, low intensity, and a small stimulating electrode, the area where the strongest contraction can be elicited is sought in the presumed stimulation area. This spot is marked, and then the actual stimulation can begin. The authors also point out that the MPs migrate caudally or cranially with a change in position of the relevant joint, which must of course be taken into account. In other words: Do not test in full extension and then stimulate in 90° flexion.

For the reasons mentioned above, the author of this book refrains from providing illustrations showing individual motor points. As a general rule, the motor stimulation zone is usually found in the proximal third of the muscle belly. Furthermore, one should definitely heed the recommendation of Gobbo et al.

4.9 Stimulation of Denervated Muscles

The effectiveness of stimulation of denervated muscles is still controversial, as it has not yet been demonstrated in humans that it improves reinnervation. In addition, there is no consensus as to whether stimulation is harmful or not. Animal studies show that NMES not only maintains the physiology and structure of the tissue by preventing changes in connective tissue, but also improves reinnervation.

What do we know?

There are studies in rodents showing that very intensive electrical stimulation lasting 12–24 h daily, possibly even combined with increased activity (hours of treadmill running), impairs reinnervation. Ironton et al. (1978) demonstrated, for example, that 10–12 h of electrical stimulation daily impairs nerve growth. Tam et al. (2001) observed a similar result after one month of 8 h of continuous stimulation daily. Gigo-Benato et al. (2010) found, not surprisingly, that a protocol of 20 contractions at 48-h intervals cannot prevent atrophy. This type of study is often cited by opponents of NMES. It is argued that excessive activation of denervated muscles (electrically or actively) negatively affects the production of certain trophic factors and thus reduces the receptivity for new functional connections (Tam et al. 2001; Willand et al. 2013a, b). Several mechanisms are discussed in this context, such as increased local acetylcholine release, suppression of ACh receptors, reduction of certain growth factors such as IGF (Insulin-like Growth Factor) and Neural Cell Adhesion Molecule (NCAM), and increased local calcium concentration. Be that as it may: It is considered established that moderate stimulation of denervated muscle in vivo does not slow reinnervation (Rozman et al. 2000; Gittins et al. 1999; Willand et al. 2013a, b; Mäkelä et al. 2019), but even improves it (Willand 2015; Willand et al. 2015), probably through increased intramuscular production of BDNF and GDNF.

BDNF and GDNF (Brain-Derived and Glial Cell Line-Derived Neurotrophic Factor) are potent neurotrophic factors that stimulate nerve regeneration after injury. BDNF is one of the most important and is responsible for promoting sprouting and growth of motor and sensory neurons. GDNF promotes the survival of motoneurons and improves myelination after injury, enhances neurite outgrowth, and acts as a synaptotrophin to promote terminal branching at motor endplates and synapses.

In the author's opinion, the most important argument for such stimulation is based on findings from studies on brain plasticity. As already discussed in detail, unused brain areas are "taken over" by neighboring areas after denervation or amputation. Therefore, in patients with surgically treated nerve lesions or after replantations, the affected skin area should be stimulated as often as possible and—very importantly—as variably as possible. It is very likely (but has never been studied) that muscle stimulation has a similar effect on the motor cortex as sensory stimulation does on the sensory cortex. This would also explain why functional outcomes in patients after sensory reinnervation training are better than in those who were not stimulated (Lundborg 2003).

It can still often be observed that atrophy cannot be prevented in vivo with electrical stimulation, but only slowed down. The cause is unclear; perhaps the growth factors mentioned above play a role. It may also be due to the fact that stimulation in humans is usually started relatively late. Many patients for whom stimulation would be indicated have serious injuries that take priority in treatment. By the time these problems are at least partially resolved, so much time has usually passed that significant atrophy has already occurred. This is then difficult to reverse. Effective muscle training with NMES requires strong contractions, and post-traumatically/postoperatively the pain threshold is low. In addition, too low a stimulation intensity is often used out of the unfounded fear that the reinnervation process could be disturbed.

Electrical stimulation is not only about atrophy prophylaxis and maintaining kinesthetics. In a denervated muscle, the amount of fat and collagen increases. Initially, this increase is only relative because the muscle mass decreases, but later it is absolute because more fat and collagen are actually produced: fibrosis can occur. This tissue change naturally impairs muscle function and can even hinder reinnervation. A traumatized or overloaded denervated muscle may fibrose more quickly because the healing processes are disturbed due to denervation; these processes are neurogenically controlled. Consistent stimulation can prevent this fibrosis (Zealear et al. 2000a, b).

It is now assumed that metabolic processes that occur only in denervated muscles play an important role in reinnervation and that certain proteins that are increasingly produced act as "guides". For example, the denervated muscle produces more acetylcholine (ACh) receptors on its membrane. For this reason, such a muscle responds more strongly to certain stimuli. These receptors probably function as targets for regrowing axons. In addition, denervated muscles have increased concentrations of NCAM (Neural Cell Adhesion Molecule). This is a glycoprotein that is present in embryonic muscles before they are innervated. NCAM guides axons toward the not yet innervated muscle. With these processes, the muscle is very likely signaling its denervated state to the nervous system so that reinnervation can take place at all. How else would the nerve fibers know where to go (Brushart 1993; Brushart et al. 1998; Zealear et al. 2002, 2014)?

4.9.1 Practical Implementation

It has recently been clearly shown that stimulation of denervated muscle is useful. Unfortunately, the treatment parameters are unclear. However, it seems wise not to overdo the stimulation: the denervated muscle must remain recognizable to the nervous system as damaged, and one wants to avoid any inhibitory processes as described above. Fortunately, many studies have at least found something in common in this regard: It appears that reinnervation occurs despite sometimes intensive stimulation. The muscle therefore apparently remains an interesting target for the regrowing nerve and contractile despite (or because of) stimulation. Nevertheless, the question of "session frequency" remains open. Our stimulation patients generally require active therapy two to three times a week anyway due to parallel therapies, whether with a physiotherapist or occupational therapist. So why not combine them? The more varied the information for the sensorimotor cortex, the better. Probably.

Tetanic pulse currents are usually more pleasant for the patient than muscle twitches elicited by single pulses. With relatively long triangular pulses and low frequencies, tetanic pulse currents can be constructed depending on the duration of denervation. The lower frequencies can be used because denervated muscle fibers twitch more slowly and tetanic contractions often occur at as low as 10–20 Hz.

Only as many contractions should be elicited as until the first signs of fatigue appear. Denervated muscle is sensitive to overload. It is advisable to carefully explore the performance limit in the first sessions. Even if the patient is able to voluntarily contract the muscle again after a certain time, this does not mean that therapy should be stopped. After consultation with the neurologist, stimulation should be continued, of course combined with active exercise therapy and any additional measures such as sensory training, until an optimal functional result is achieved.

Stimulation of partially denervated muscles is probably unnecessary. In the case of partial denervation, collateral reinnervation occurs fairly quickly via so-called nodal and terminal sprouting. In nodal sprouting, a side branch grows from a node of Ranvier 100–200 μ from a denervated endplate. This branch grows toward the denervated muscle fiber and adopts it. In terminal sprouting, a branch grows from a nerve terminal that already innervates a muscle fiber, which then ensures the innervation of a nearby denervated muscle fiber. The motor units naturally become larger in such cases.

These processes proceed relatively quickly because the new fibers only have to bridge a short distance: they grow from undamaged nerve fibers in the same muscle in a healthy person at a rate of about 1 mm per day. So it is possible to wait and see how things develop. For the prognosis of reinnervation, it should be mentioned that nerve growth is slower in older patients, diabetics, and alcoholics.

4.9.2 Procedure for the Electrical Stimulation of Denervated Muscle

See also "General measures before, after, and during treatment" for low frequency (Sect. 2.11.1 ff).

Adhesive Electrodes

Adhesive electrodes should generally never be used when working with uncompensated impulses, i.e., those with a direct current component (= DC component)—impulses that are typically used for the stimulation of denervated muscles.

A German company once offered single-use electrodes with a special adhesive layer. This adhesive was chemically formulated to buffer, i.e., neutralize, the alkali and acid produced by monophasic (i.e., uncompensated) impulses. Therefore, these electrodes could be used with currents containing a DC component. But only once, of course.

Well, then the requirements for electrodes were changed, the company conducted new tests, which unfortunately led to inconsistent results, and now the company has decided to no longer approve their electrodes for use with uncompensated impulses.

I quote here an employee of the company who kindly explained the matter to me in detail:

> "The coating of the single-use electrodes is indeed designed to buffer ions generated by direct currents or uncompensated currents. Until early 2021, we were able to approve a current density of 1 mA DC per cm^2 of electrode area for use. This was also indicated on the electrode packaging. In the course of adapting the electrodes to the new MDR [Medical Device Regulation] requirements, corresponding tests were repeated, unfortunately this time with inconsistent results. Since further research could not be undertaken, we unfortunately had to decide to exclude the use of direct currents and currents with a DC component. A buffering effect is present, but unfortunately it cannot be reliably quantified. We exclude multiple use of the electrodes. The indeterminable and thus limiting factor is the adhesive strength of the electrodes, which may be impaired after a single use (for example, due to fat or sweat). Here too, unfortunately—even if the electrode would technically allow it in individual cases—we cannot permit multiple use due to the properties no longer being reliably ensured. If the electrode is detached from the patient's skin, the reduced contact area would generate an increased current density."

In theory, one could achieve a kind of regeneration of the buffer by reversing the polarity or swapping the electrodes, since acids and bases formed before the polarity reversal would have reacted with the basic and acidic components of the buffer, respectively. The polarity reversal would thus lead to a simple neutralization of the acids and bases produced by electrolysis.

However, if these "buffer electrodes" are an approved medical device, any non-compliant regeneration would lead to legal issues in the event of patient claims for any damages.

It should therefore be strongly emphasized at this point that the user (the therapist) is liable for any damage (burns) resulting from non-compliant use of these single-use electrodes. The company, of course, assumes no responsibility in such cases.

What should be considered in the practical application of such stimulation?

- Before the first treatment, if desired, an SD curve can be created to roughly assess the condition of the muscle (Stephens 1973; Paternostro-Sluga et al. 2002). As a follow-up control, the curve is worthless, as it can take very different, clinically irrelevant forms in the various phases of denervation and reinnervation. Since the neurologist can clearly make such an assessment more accurately, the value of such a curve must be questioned. The curve is also worthless for determining stimulation values. The optimal phase duration could supposedly be determined from the SD curve: one would take the value at which the triangular impulse curve (DIC) reaches its lowest point. Since this value represents the threshold, it is clearly too low for treatment. For this, stronger contractions must be elicited, which is done with longer impulses and significantly higher intensities (Pieber et al. 2015). The intensity used naturally also depends on the patient.
- The treatment parameters can be very easily estimated without an SD curve as follows:
  - In cases of mild degeneration (rather recent injury, up to a few weeks):

    If single impulses (triangle) are to be used: T = 20–100 ms, R = 1000–2000 ms

    If surge current can be used: for example, T = 10 ms, R = 20 ms, or T = 30 ms, R = 60 ms (ratio 1:2), ramp up about 2 s, hold 2–5 s, pause 10–30 s
- In cases of moderate degeneration (after about 30 days) (Stephens 1973):
  - Here, single impulses (triangle) must be used: T = 100–200 ms, R = 1000–2000 ms
- In cases of severe degeneration (after months):
  - Single impulses, triangle, T = 200–500 ms, R = 1000–2000 ms
- Larger muscles are stimulated bipolarly with 2 electrodes of equal size, which must be adapted to the muscle size. Smaller muscles (hand, forearm) can be stimulated with a single small electrode. The indifferent electrode (usually the anode) is placed nearby. Button electrodes are practical for small hand muscles, but patients often find the impulses rather unpleasant. A rubber electrode with a little ultrasound gel or in a sponge pouch can be conveniently shaped and works very well.
- To capture as many muscle fibers as possible, the electrodes should be placed on the muscle at the proximal and distal ends and must be as large as possible. Caution: If the electrodes are too large, adjacent innervated muscle may also contract (so-called spillover).
- To avoid overstraining the muscle, one should not work against gravity at the beginning. The muscle is not pre-stretched, and relevant joints are positioned in a neutral position comfortable for the patient. Over time, the load can be increased.
- To selectively stimulate the denervated muscle fibers, triangular impulses are used. Intact nerves, unlike denervated muscles, adapt to the gradually increasing long impulses. Therefore, the innervated muscle fibers do not contract.
- By reversing the polarity, one tests which configuration elicits the best contraction: cathode distal or proximal. Usually, better contractions are obtained when the cathode is distal. In denervated tibialis anterior, better contractions seem to occur when the cathode is proximal (Pieber et al. 2015).
- In recent injuries, i.e., in the first 3–4 weeks, tetanizing pulse currents can be set with relatively short impulses. The pauses between individual impulses in a pulse series must not be too short, usually about twice as long as the phase duration; this must be determined experimentally. With a phase duration of 10 ms, this results in a pause of about 20 ms and thus a frequency of about 330 Hz (frequency = 1000 ms ÷ phase duration PLUS_SPI phase interval). A phase duration of 30 ms

requires a pause of about 60 ms. This results in a stimulation frequency of about 11 Hz.

- The contractions must, if tolerated by the patient, be strong, but should not last longer than a few seconds to avoid overstraining the muscle. The pauses between contractions must be long enough to prevent the muscle from fatiguing too quickly, usually up to about 30 s. Sometimes, after a series (8 to 10 times), a longer break (5–10 min) is needed. This time should be used productively.
- To make the contractions less unpleasant for the patient, a surge current is recommended: 1–2 s ramp-up time, 2–4 s hold, 1 s ramp-down.
- If the muscle fatigues, the session is ended. Prolonging the phase duration or increasing the stimulation intensity could damage the muscle. There are no studies on this in humans.

To optimize therapy, the patient should imagine the movement to be performed during the contraction phase and, if possible, participate. The patient should also participate with the contralateral side.

- For long-standing denervations, longer impulses must be used; in this case, contractions can only be elicited with single impulses. Sometimes up to 600 ms phase duration or longer is needed, although longer impulses are not exactly pleasant. Studies in paraplegic patients show that muscle can be successfully stimulated even after years of denervation and that the muscle can improve structurally and thus functionally (Kern et al. 2004, 2005).

Commercially available TENS devices, even if they have NMES programs, are unsuitable for stimulating denervated muscles. The impulses are usually far too short (mostly up to a maximum of 400 μs instead of several hundred milliseconds). However, there are now very good (rental) devices for home therapy. It should be obvious that a patient must be extremely well informed and regularly monitored before such a device is issued.

4.9.2.1 Indications

- Paresis due to lesions of peripheral nerves (e.g., radial nerve palsy, peroneal nerve palsy, facial nerve palsy).
- Paresis due to spinal cord lesions.
- Paresis due to lesions in the CNS.
- Prophylaxis of atrophy during immobilization (e.g., stimulation of the calf muscles after Achilles tendon rupture or quadriceps/hamstring stimulation after knee surgery) falls within the indication area of normal muscle stimulation, as innervation is intact in these cases.

4.9.2.2 Contraindications

- See low frequency Sect. 3.11.
- Special attention: trophic disorders and sensory loss in the treatment area, conditions not stable under load (fractures, nerve, tendon, and ligament sutures).
- Metal implants, pacemakers.

4.9.3 The SD Curve

There are no studies on the clinical relevance of the SD curve (strength-duration curve,). The few relevant publications on the topic are mentioned below.

Creating an SD curve was once mandatory in physiotherapeutic electrotherapy training, but today this aspect has rightly receded into the background, as neurologists have had methods available for many decades that allow a much faster and, above all, significantly more precise and meaningful assessment of a denervated muscle. The physiotherapist can non-invasively and cost-effectively determine chronaxie, rheobase, and the accommodation coefficient in just a few minutes. These determinations even have very good interrater reliability, with a kappa value better than 0.9 (Nelson and Hunt 1981; Schuhfried et al. 2005). The sensitivity of the examination is very good, so it is indeed possible to determine whether a muscle is denervated or not. And that's about it. There is no correlation with the extent or course of denervation (Paternostro-Sluga et al. 2002). Any "kinks" in the curve that may indicate partial denervation or reinnervation must be interpreted with great caution. The SD curve only provides information about the excitability of the muscle fibers in the immediate vicinity of the electrodes, so it is definitely not representative of the entire muscle, unless the muscle is very small. Moreover, many processes occur in the muscle in the first weeks after denervation and during subsequent reinnervation that lead to changes in the curves, which are very resistant to interpretation (Stillman 1967; Paternostro-Sluga et al. 2002) (Fig. 4.8).

Traditionally, electrical stimulation diagnostics also includes testing the ability to be faradised of a muscle. This involves checking whether a muscle can be stimulated with a

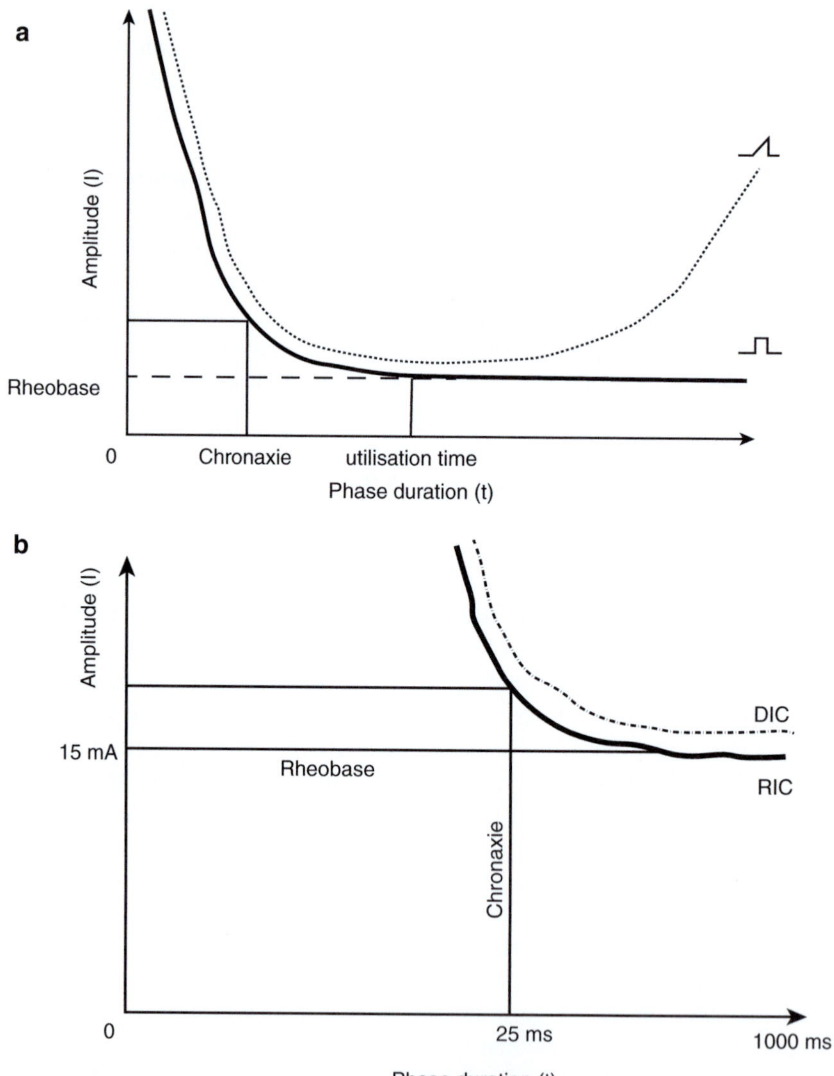

Fig. 4.8 (**a**) SD curve of an innervated muscle, (**b**) SD curve of a denervated muscle, (**c**) SD curve of a partially denervated muscle. The "kinks" or "garlands" arise because, in fact, several SD curves are combined in one graph. RIC: rectangular impulse characteristic. DIC: triangular impulse characteristic

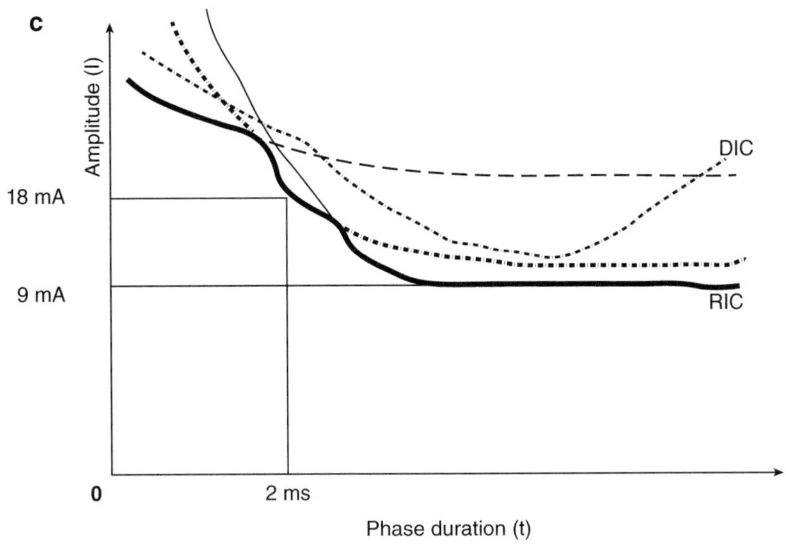

Fig. 4.8 (continued)

(neo-)faradic current, a current form that today consists of uncompensated rectangular impulses of 1 ms duration and 19 ms phase interval, i.e., with a frequency of 50 Hz (there is actually a somewhat older reference for this: Rosenthal and Bernhardt 1884). If the muscle responds promptly, it is not denervated, unless the incident occurred only a few days ago. If it does not respond at all or shows an abnormal way of contracting, "worm-like," one does not know much more either. Such meaningless "diagnostic" tests should finally be abandoned, and the valuable time in teaching and with patients should be used more sensibly.

Below, some terms related to the SD curve are explained, as they frequently appear in the literature and facilitate communication with specialists. A description of the procedure and interpretation of the curve is omitted for the reasons mentioned above.

In an SD curve, the relationship between current strength (I) and impulse or phase duration (t) of a rectangular and triangular impulse is graphically represented in two curves. The aim is to gain insight into the electrical excitability of the muscle. For this, a barely perceptible twitch is elicited in the muscles to be examined using rectangular and triangular impulses of different durations. "Perceptible" here means that the examiner must perceive the contraction, not the patient. The respective intensity (usually the current in mA, sometimes the voltage in V) is recorded together with the phase duration in a pre-printed special graph. The resulting curves are intended not only to allow conclusions about the degree of denervation of the muscle but also about the course of therapy.

The rectangular impulse curve (RIC = rectangular impulse characteristic) shows:

- The rheobase
  - Current strength that a rectangular impulse of "infinite" duration must have to elicit a barely perceptible contraction. For this purpose, a phase duration of 500 ms or 1000 ms is set, with the phase interval being at least twice as long to avoid muscle fatigue. This means stimulation is performed at a frequency of about 0.5–1 Hz. The rheobase value is different for each muscle and normally also varies considerably on the same muscle. This is due, among other things, to electrode pressure, existing edema, skin perfusion, ambient temperature, sweating, skin trophism, and the thickness of

subcutaneous fat tissue. The rheobase is therefore only useful for direct side-to-side comparison. The value decreases after denervation due to increased ACh receptor formation for about 3 weeks (Dobin and Fizzell 1951; Walton 1954).

- The chronaxie
  - Time that a rectangular impulse with double the rheobase intensity needs to elicit a barely perceptible contraction. The value is normally 0.1–1 ms and increases within the first few days after denervation. Values above 1 ms are considered pathological (Paternostro-Sluga et al. 2002), up to 7 ms as "moderately elevated," and 10–100 ms indicate severe damage in total denervation.
- The utilization time
  - Time that a rectangular impulse needs at the *rheobase value* to elicit a barely perceptible contraction. In healthy tissue, this value is about 10 ms and corresponds roughly to the point on the rectangular curve where the "horizontal" begins to rise to the left.

In the triangular impulse curve (DIC = triangular impulse characteristic), the following are assessed:

- The adaptation threshold
  - Current strength that an impulse of "infinite" duration must have to elicit a barely perceptible contraction. This value is determined at a phase duration of 500 ms or 1000 ms, with the 1000 ms impulse being perceived as very unpleasant.
- The optimal phase duration
  - Phase duration that a triangular impulse needs to elicit a barely perceptible contraction in a muscle with the lowest possible current strength. Allegedly, this is the most suitable setting for therapeutic application. There are no studies confirming this. For therapy, rather strong contractions must be elicited. Pieber et al. (2015) in their study on optimal parameters for stimulation of denervated muscles, without regard to an SD curve, elicited "moderately strong" contractions without "unnecessary discomfort" for the patient, with movement being produced in the relevant joints (wrist and ankle). Parameters: 1 Hz, 200 ms, triangular impulse, 30 mm Ø electrodes for the extensor digitorum communis and 50 mm Ø for the tibialis anterior.
- The ratio of the adaptation threshold of the DIC to the rheobase of the RIC yields the accommodation coefficient AC (also AQ) or α. If the values are equal, AC = 1. This means a complete loss of accommodation ability and indicates complete denervation. At 1000 ms, AC is between 2 and 6, at 500 ms between 1.5 and 2.5.

As already mentioned, we should leave such tests to specialists, as they offer no added value for therapy.

References

Adams C, Scott W, Basile J, Hughes L, Leigh J, Schiller A, Walton J (2018) Electrically elicited quadriceps muscle torque: a comparison of 3 waveforms. J Orthop Sports Phys Ther 48(3):217–224

Alamer A, Melese H, Nigussie F (2020) Effectiveness of neuromuscular electrical stimulation on post-stroke dysphagia: a systematic review of randomized controlled trials. Clin Interv Aging 15:1521–1531

Allon EF (2019) The role of neuromuscular electrical stimulation in the rehabilitation of the pelvic floor muscles. Br J Nurs 28(15):968–974

Amaral SL, Linderman JR, Morse MM, Greene AS (2001) Angiogenesis induced by electrical stimulation is mediated by angiotensin II and VEGF. Microcirculation 8(1):57–67

Andersen JL, Gruschy-Knudsen T, Sandri C, Larsson L, Schiaffino S (1999) Bed rest increases the amount of mismatched fibers in human skeletal muscle. J Appl Physiol 86(2):455–460

Andersen JL, Weiss A, Sandri C, Schjerling P, Thonell LE, Pedrosa-Domellof F, Leinwand L, Schiaffino S (2002) The 2B myosin heavy chain gene is expressed in human skeletal muscle. J Physiol 539:29–30

Andrianowa GG, Koz JM, Martjanow WA, Chwilon WA (1974) Die Anwendung der Elektrostimulation für das Training der Muskelkraft. Leistungssport 4(2):138–142

Appell JJ (1992) Elektrotherapie zum Kraftaufbau der Skelettmuskulatur. Morphologische und elektrophysiologische Zusammenhänge. In: Wentzensen A, Schmelz A (Hrsg) Elektromyostimulation in der Traumatologie. Thieme, Stuttgart/New York, S 1–7

Ausoni S, Gorza L, Schiaffino S, Gundersen K, Lømo T (1990) Expression of myosin heavy chain isoforms in stimulated fast and slow rat muscles. J Neurosci 10(1):153–160

Behringer M, Franz A, McCourt M, Mester J (2014) Motor point map of upper body muscles. Eur J Appl Physiol 114(8):1605–1617

Berghmans LC, Hendriks HJ, De Bie RA, van Waalwijk van Doorn ES, Bø K, van Kerrebroeck PE (2000) Conservative treatment of urge urinary incontinence in women: a systematic review of randomized clinical trials. BJU Int 85(3):254–263

Bergquist AJ, Clair JM, Collins DF (2011) Motor unit recruitment when neuromuscular electrical stimulation is applied over a nerve trunk compared with a muscle belly: triceps surae. J Appl Physiol 110(3):627–637

Bergquist AJ, Wiest MJ (1985) Collins DF (2012) Motor unit recruitment when neuromuscular electrical stimulation is applied over a nerve trunk compared with a muscle belly: quadriceps femoris. J Appl Physiol 113(1):78–89

Bickel CS, Gregory CM, Dean JC (2011) Motor unit recruitment during neuromuscular electrical stimulation: a critical appraisal. Eur J Appl Physiol 111(10):2399–2407

Binder-Macleod S, Russ D (1999) Effects of activation frequency and force on low-frequency fatigue in human skeletal muscle. J Appl Physiol 86(4):1337–1346

Björkman A, Rosén B, Lundborg G (2004) Acute improvement of hand sensibility after selective ipsilateral cutaneous forearm anaesthesia. Eur J Neurosci 20(10):2733–2736

Blickenstorfer A, Kleiser R, Keller T, Keisker B, Meyer M, Riener R, Kollias S (2009) Cortical and subcortical correlates of functional electrical stimulation of wrist extensor and flexor muscles revealed by fMRI. Hum Brain Mapp 30(3):963–975

Bossert FP, Jenrich W, Vogedes K (2006) Leitfaden Elektrotherapie: mit Anwendungen bei über 130 Krankheitsbildern. Urban & Fischer Verlag/Elsevier GmbH, München, ISBN-13: 978-3437319235

Botter A, Oprandi G, Lanfranco F, Allasia S, Maffiuletti NA, Minetto MA (2011) Atlas of the muscle motor points for the lower limb: implications for electrical stimulation procedures and electrode positioning. Eur J Appl Physiol 111(10):2461–2471

Brandes R, Lang F, Schmidt RF (2019) Physiologie des Menschen: mit Pathophysiologie, 32. Aufl. Springer-Lehrbuch, Berlin/Heidelberg, ISBN-13: 978-3662564677

Brushart T (1993) Motor axons preferentially reinnervate motor pathways. J Neurosci 13(6):2730–2738

Brushart T, Gerber J, Kessens P, Chen YG, Royall R (1998) Contributions of pathway and neuron to preferential motor reinnervation. J Neurosci 18(21):8674–8681

Burnley M, Jones AM (2018) Power-duration relationship: physiology, fatigue, and the limits of human performance. Eur J Sport Sci 18(1):1–12

Caiozzo V, Baker M, Herrick R, Tao M, Baldwin K (1994) Effect of spaceflight on skeletal muscle: mechanical properties and myosin isoform content of a slow muscle. J Appl Physiol 76:1764–1773

Caiozzo V, Baker M, Baldwin K (1997) Modulation of myosin isoform expression by mechanical loading: role of stimulation frequency. J Appl Physiol 82(1):211–218

Carraro U, Boncompagni S, Gobbo V, Rossini K et al (2015) Persistent muscle fiber regeneration in long term denervation. Past, present, future. Eur J Transl Myol 25(2):4832

Carriker CR (2017) Components of fatigue: mind and body. J Strength Cond Res 31(11):3170–3176

Cattagni T, Lepers R, Maffiuletti NA (2018) Effects of neuromuscular electrical stimulation on contralateral quadriceps function. J Electromyogr Kinesiol 38:111–118

Chan Kwan Kit-lan P (1991) Contemporary trends in electrical stimulation: the frequency-specificity theory. Hong Kong Physiother J 13:23–27

Charlton CS, Ridding MC, Thompson PD, Miles TS (2003) Prolonged peripheral nerve stimulation induces persistent changes in excitability of human motor cortex. J Neurol Sci 208(1–2):79–85

Chipchase LS, Schabrun SM, Hodges PW (2011) Peripheral electrical stimulation to induce cortical plasticity: a systematic review of stimulus parameters. Clin Neurophysiol 122(3):456–463

Collins DF (2007) Central contributions to contractions evoked by tetanic neuromuscular electrical stimulation. Exerc Sport Sci Rev 35(3):102–109

Collins DF, Burke D, Gandevia SC (2001) Large involuntary forces consistent with plateau-like behavior of human motoneurons. J Neurosci 21(11):4059–4065

Collins DF, Burke D, Gandevia SC (2002) Sustained contractions produced by plateau-like behaviour in human motoneurones. J Physiol 538(Pt 1):289–301

Correia GN, Pereira VS, Hirakawa HS, Driusso P (2014) Effects of surface and intravaginal electrical stimulation in the treatment of women with stress urinary incontinence: randomized controlled trial. Eur J Obstet Gynecol Reprod Biol 173:113–118

Del Vecchio A, Casolo A, Negro F, Scorcelletti M, Bazzucchi I, Enoka R, Felici F, Farina D (2019) The increase in muscle force after 4 weeks of strength training is mediated by adaptations in motor unit recruitment and rate coding. J Physiol 597(7):1873–1887

Dempsey-Jones H, Themistocleous AC, Carone D, Ng TWC, Harrar V, Makin TR (2019) Blocking tactile input to one finger using anaesthetic enhances touch perception and learning in other fingers. J Exp Psychol Gen 148(4):713–727

Dirks ML, Wall BT, Snijders T, Ottenbros CL, Verdijk LB, van Loon LJ (2014) Neuromuscular electrical stimulation prevents muscle disuse atrophy during leg immobilization in humans. Acta Physiol (Oxford) 210(3):628–641

Dirks ML, Hansen D, Van Assche A, Dendale P, Van Loon LJ (2015) Neuromuscular electrical stimulation prevents muscle wasting in critically ill comatose patients. Clin Sci (Lond) 128(6):357–365

Dmochowski R, Lynch CM, Efros M, Cardozo L (2019) External electrical stimulation compared with intravaginal electrical stimulation for the treatment of stress urinary incontinence in women: a randomized controlled noninferiority trial. Neurourol Urodyn 38(7):1834–1843

Dobin NB, Fizzell JA (1951) Electrodiagnostic and electromyographic study of muscle denervated by section of the anterior roots. Q Bull Northwest Univ Med Sch 25(4):338–341

Ehrsson HH, Rosén B, Stockselius A, Ragnö C, Köhler P, Lundborg G (2008) Upper limb amputees can be induced to experience a rubber hand as their own. Brain 131(Pt 12):3443–3452

Elmelund M, Biering-Sørensen F, Due U, Klarskov N (2018) The effect of pelvic floor muscle training and intravaginal electrical stimulation on urinary incontinence in women with incomplete spinal cord injury: an investigator-blinded parallel randomized clinical trial. Int Urogynecol J 29(11):1597–1606

Erickson ML, Ryan TE, Backus D, McCully KK (2017) Endurance neuromuscular electrical stimulation training improves skeletal muscle oxidative capacity in individuals with motor-complete spinal cord injury. Muscle Nerve 55(5):669–675

Fahrer H, Rentsch HU, Gerber NJ, Beyeler C, Hess CW, Grünig B (1988) Knee effusion and reflex inhibition of the quadriceps. A bar to effective retraining. J Bone Joint Surg (Br) 70(4):635–638

Filipovic A, Kleinöder H, Dörmann U, Mester J (2011) Electromyostimulation – a systematic review of the influence of training regimens and stimulation parameters on effectiveness in electromyostimulation training of selected strength parameters. J Strength Cond Res 25(11):3218–3238

Filipovic A, Kleinöder H, Dörmann U, Mester J (2012) Electromyostimulation – a systematic review of the effects of different electromyostimulation methods on selected strength parameters in trained and elite athletes. J Strength Cond Res 26(9):2600–2614

Finazzi-Agrò E, Petta F, Sciobica F, Pasqualetti P, Musco S, Bove P (2010) Percutaneous tibial nerve stimulation effects on detrusor overactivity incontinence are not due to a placebo effect: a randomized, double-blind, placebo-controlled trial. J Urol 184(5):2001–2006

Francis S, Lin X, Aboushoushah S, White TP, Phillips M, Bowtell R, Constantinescu CS (2009) fMRI analysis of active, passive and electrically stimulated ankle dorsiflexion. Neuroimage 44(2):469–479

Franz A, Klaas J, Schumann M, Frankewitsch T, Filler TJ, Behringer M (2018) Anatomical versus functional motor points of selected upper body muscles. Muscle Nerve 57(3):460–465

Gandhoke GS, Belykh E, Zhao X, Leblanc R, Preul MC (2019) Edwin Boldrey and Wilder Penfield's homunculus: a life given by Mrs. Cantlie (in and out of realism). World Neurosurg 132:377–388

Gigo-Benato D, Russo TL, Geuna S, Domingues NR, Salvini TF, Parizotto NA (2010) Electrical stimulation impairs early functional recovery and accentuates skeletal muscle atrophy after sciatic nerve crush injury in rats. Muscle Nerve 41(5):685–693

Giroux C, Roduit B, Rodriguez-Falces J, Duchateau J, Maffiuletti NA, Place N (2018) Short vs. long pulses for testing knee extensor neuromuscular properties: does it matter? Eur J Appl Physiol 118(2):361–369

Gittins J, Martin K, Sheldrick J, Reddy A, Thean L (1999) Electrical stimulation as a therapeutic option to improve eyelid function in chronic facial nerve disorders. Invest Ophthalmol Vis Sci 40(3):547–554

Gobbo M, Gaffurini P, Bissolotti L, Esposito F, Orizio C (2011) Transcutaneous neuromuscular electrical stimulation: influence of electrode positioning and stimulus amplitude settings on muscle response. Eur J Appl Physiol 111(10):2451–2459

Gobbo M, Maffiuletti NA, Orizio C, Minetto MA (2014) Muscle motor point identification is essential for optimizing neuromuscular electrical stimulation use. J Neuroeng Rehabil 11:17

Gondin J, Brocca L, Bellinzona E, D'Antona G, Maffiuletti NA, Miotti D, Pellegrino MA, Bottinelli R (2011) Neuromuscular electrical stimulation training induces atypical adaptations of the human skeletal muscle phenotype: a functional and proteomic analysis. J Appl Physiol 110(2):433–450

Graham GM, Thrasher TA, Popovic MR (2006) The effect of random modulation of functional electrical stimulation parameters on muscle fatigue. IEEE Trans Neural Syst Rehabil Eng 14(1):38–45

Gregory CM, Bickel CS (2005) Recruitment patterns in human skeletal muscle during electrical stimulation. Phys Ther 85(4):358–364

de Groat WC, Griffiths D, Yoshimura N (2015) Neural control of the lower urinary tract. Compr Physiol 5(1):327–396

Guo GY, Kang YG (2018) Effectiveness of neuromuscular electrical stimulation therapy in patients with urinary incontinence after stroke: a randomized sham-controlled trial. Medicine (Baltimore) 97(52):e13702

Harkey MS, Gribble PA, Pietrosimone BG (2014) Disinhibitory interventions and voluntary quadriceps activation: a systematic review. J Athl Train 49(3):411–421

Henneman E, Somjen G, Carpenter DO (1965) Excitability and inhibitability of motoneurons of different sizes. J Neurophysiol 28(3):599–620

Henriksson-Larsén K, Fridén J, Wretling ML (1985) Distribution of fibre sizes in human skeletal muscle.

An enzyme histochemical study in m tibialis anterior. Acta Physiol Scand 123(2):171–177

Hong Z, Sui M, Zhuang Z, Liu H, Zheng X, Cai C, Jin D (2018) Effectiveness of neuromuscular electrical stimulation on lower limbs of patients with hemiplegia after chronic stroke: a systematic review. Arch Phys Med Rehabil 99(5):1011–1022.e1

Hopkins JT, Ingersoll CD, Krause BA, Edwards JE, Cordova ML (2001) Effect of knee joint effusion on quadriceps and soleus motoneuron pool excitability. Med Sci Sports Exerc 33(1):123–126

Hopkins J, Ingersoll CD, Edwards J, Klootwyk TE (2002) Cryotherapy and transcutaneous electric neuromuscular stimulation decrease arthrogenic muscle inhibition of the vastus medialis after knee joint effusion. J Athl Train 37(1):25–31

Hortobágyi T, Maffiuletti NA (2011) Neural adaptations to electrical stimulation strength training. Eur J Appl Physiol 111(10):2439–2449

Hortobágyi T, Dempsey L, Fraser D, Zheng D, Hamilton G, Lambert J, Dohm L (2000) Changes in muscle strength, muscle fibre size and myofibrillar gene expression after immobilization and retraining in humans. J Physiol 524(Pt 1):293–304

Hudlická O, Tyler K, Aitman T (1980) The effect of long-term electrical stimulation on fuel uptake and performance in fast skeletal muscle. In: Pette D (Hrsg) Plasticity of muscle. Walter de Gruyter, Berlin, S 401–408

Ironton R, Brown MC, Holland RL (1978) Stimuli to intramuscular nerve growth. Brain Res 156(2):351–354

Jacomo RH, Alves AT, Lucio A, Garcia PA, Lorena DCR, de Sousa JB (2020) Transcutaneous tibial nerve stimulation versus parasacral stimulation in the treatment of overactive bladder in elderly people: a triple-blinded randomized controlled trial. Clinics (Sao Paulo) 75:e1477

Janssen DA, Martens FM, de Wall LL, van Breda HM, Heesakkers JP (2017) Clinical utility of neurostimulation devices in the treatment of overactive bladder: current perspectives. Med Devices (Auckl) 10:109–122

Jiang Y, Wang H, Liu Z, Dong Y, Dong Y, Xiang X, Bai L, Tian J, Wu L, Han J, Cui C (2013) Manipulation of and sustained effects on the human brain induced by different modalities of acupuncture: an fMRI study. PLoS One 8(6):e66815

Joa KL, Han YH, Mun CW, Son BK, Lee CH, Shin YB, Ko HY, Shin YI (2012) Evaluation of the brain activation induced by functional electrical stimulation and voluntary contraction using functional magnetic resonance imaging. J Neuroeng Rehabil 9:48

Jones DA, Bigland-Ritchie B, Edwards RH (1979) Excitation frequency and muscle fatigue: mechanical responses during voluntary and stimulated contractions. Exp Neurol 64(2):401–413

Jubeau M, Gondin J, Martin A, Sartorio A, Maffiuletti NA (2007) Random motor unit activation by electrostimulation. Int J Sports Med 28(11):901–904

Kaas AL, van de Ven V, Reithler J, Goebel R (2013) Tactile perceptual learning: learning curves and transfer to the contralateral finger. Exp Brain Res 224(3):477–488

Kamel DM, Yousif AM (2017) Neuromuscular electrical stimulation and strength recovery of postnatal diastasis recti abdominis muscles. Ann Rehabil Med 41(3):465–474

Karabay İ, Doğan A, Ekiz T, Köseoğlu BF, Ersöz M (2016) Training postural control and sitting in children with cerebral palsy: Kinesio taping vs. neuromuscular electrical stimulation. Complement Ther Clin Pract 24:67–72

Kern H, Chr H, Moedlin M, Forstner C, Vogelauer M, Richter W, Mayer W, Zanin ME, Rossini K, Carraro U (2004) First sound evidence of muscle regeneration in recovery of function of human permanent denervated muscle by a long-lasting functional electrical stimulation training: biopsy findings. Zdrav Vestn 73:II-29-31

Kern H, Rossini K, Carraro U, Mayer W, Vogelauer M, Hoellwarth U, Chr H (2005) Muscle biopsies show that FES of denervated muscles reverses human muscle degeneration from permanent spinal motoneuron lesion. J Rehab Research Dev 42(3 Suppl 1):43–53

Klakowicz PM, Baldwin ER, Collins DF (2006) Contribution of M-waves and H-reflexes to contractions evoked by tetanic nerve stimulation in humans. J Neurophysiol 96(3):1293–1302

Knowles CH, Horrocks EJ, Bremner SA, Stevens N, Norton C, O'Connell PR, Eldridge S, CONFIDeNT study group (2015) Percutaneous tibial nerve stimulation versus sham electrical stimulation for the treatment of faecal incontinence in adults (CONFIDeNT): a double-blind, multicentre, pragmatic, parallel-group, randomised controlled trial. Lancet 386(10004):1640–1648

Kolasinski J, Makin TR, Logan JP, Jbabdi S, Clare S, Stagg CJ, Johansen-Berg H (2016) Perceptually relevant remapping of human somatotopy in 24 hours. elife 5:e17280

La Rosa VL, Ciebiera M, Lin LT, Sleiman Z, Cerentini TM, Lordelo P, Kahramanoglu I, Bruni S, Garzon S, Fichera M (2019a) Multidisciplinary management of women with pelvic organ prolapse, urinary incontinence and lower urinary tract symptoms. A clinical and psychological overview. Prz Menopauzalny 18(3):184–190

La Rosa VL, Platania A, Ciebiera M, Garzon S, Jędra R, Ponta M, Butticè S (2019b) A comparison of sacral neuromodulation vs. transvaginal electrical stimulation for the treatment of refractory overactive bladder: the impact on quality of life, body image, sexual function, and emotional well-being. Prz Menopauzalny 18(2):89–93

Lee JH, Baker LL, Johnson RE, Tilson JK (2017) Effectiveness of neuromuscular electrical stimulation for management of shoulder subluxation post-stroke: a systematic review with meta-analysis. Clin Rehabil 31(11):1431–1444

Lee IS, Jung WM, Lee YS, Wallraven C, Chae Y (2015) Brain responses to acupuncture stimulation in the prosthetic hand of an amputee patient. Acupunct Med 33(5):420–424

Lieber RL, Silva PD, Daniel DM (1996) Equal effectiveness of electrical and volitional strength training for quadriceps femoris muscles after anterior cruciate ligament surgery. J Orthop Res 14(1):131–138

Lim D, Del Castillo M, Bergquist AJ, Milosevic M, Masani K (2021) Contribution of each motor point of quadriceps femoris to knee extension torque during neuromuscular electrical stimulation. IEEE Trans Neural Syst Rehabil Eng. https://doi.org/10.1109/TNSRE.2021.3052853. Epub ahead of print

Lundborg G (2000) Brain plasticity and hand surgery: an overview. J Hand Surg (Br) 25(3):242–252

Lundborg G (2003) Richard P. Bunge memorial lecture. Nerve injury and repair – a challenge to the plastic brain. J Peripher Nerv Syst 8(4):209–226

Lundborg G (2005) Nerve injury and repair, regeneration, reconstruction, and cortical remodeling, 2. Aufl. Churchill Livingstone, London, ISBN-13: 978-0443067112

Lundborg G, Rosén B (2007) Hand function after nerve repair. Acta Physiol (Oxford) 189(2):207–217

Maddocks M, Nolan CM, Man WD, Polkey MI, Hart N, Gao W, Rafferty GF, Moxham J, Higginson IJ (2016) Neuromuscular electrical stimulation to improve exercise capacity in patients with severe COPD: a randomised double-blind, placebo-controlled trial. Lancet Respir Med 4(1):27–36

Maffiuletti NA (2010) Physiological and methodological considerations for the use of neuromuscular electrical stimulation. Eur J Appl Physiol 110(2):223–234

Maffiuletti NA, Gondin J, Place N, Stevens-Lapsley J, Vivodtzev I, Minetto MA (2018) Clinical use of neuromuscular electrical stimulation for neuromuscular rehabilitation: what are we overlooking? Arch Phys Med Rehabil 99(4):806–812

Mäkelä E, Venesvirta H, Ilves M, Lylykangas J, Rantanen V, Ylä-Kotola T, Suominen S, Vehkaoja A, Verho J, Lekkala J, Surakka V, Rautiainen M (2019) Facial muscle reanimation by transcutaneous electrical stimulation for peripheral facial nerve palsy. J Med Eng Technol 43(3):155–164

Mazur-Bialy AI, Kołomańska-Bogucka D, Nowakowski C, Tim S (2020) Urinary incontinence in women: modern methods of physiotherapy as a support for surgical treatment or independent therapy. J Clin Med 9(4):1211

Medeiros FV, Bottaro M, Vieira A, Lucas TP, Modesto KA, Bo APL, Cipriano G Jr, Babault N, Durigan JLQ (2017) Kilohertz and low-frequency electrical stimulation with the same pulse duration have similar efficiency for inducing isometric knee extension torque and discomfort. Am J Phys Med Rehabil 96(6):388–394

Meesen RL, Cuypers K, Rothwell JC, Swinnen SP, Levin O (2011) The effect of long-term TENS on persistent neuroplastic changes in the human cerebral cortex. Hum Brain Mapp 32(6):872–882

Mesin L, Merlo E, Merletti R, Orizio C (2010) Investigation of motor unit recruitment during stimulated contractions of tibialis anterior muscle. J Electromyogr Kinesiol 20(4):580–589

Miller BF, Gruben KG, Morgan BJ (2000) Circulatory responses to voluntary and electrically induced muscle contractions in humans. Phys Ther 80(1):53–60

Minetto MA, Botter A, Bottinelli O, Miotti D, Bottinelli R, D'Antona G (2013) Variability in muscle adaptation to electrical stimulation. Int J Sports Med 34(6):544–553

Miyamoto T, Kamada H, Tamaki A, Moritani T (2016) Low-intensity electrical muscle stimulation induces significant increases in muscle strength and cardiorespiratory fitness. Eur J Sport Sci 16(8):1104–1110

Modesto KAG, de Oliveira PFA, Fonseca HG, Azevedo KP, Guzzoni V, Bottaro MF, Babault N, Durigan JLQ (2019) Russian and low-frequency currents training programs induced neuromuscular adaptations in soccer players: randomized controlled trial. J Sport Rehabil 29:1–25

Moe JH, Post HW (1962) Functional electrical stimulation for ambulation in hemiplegia. J Lancet 82:285–288

Morrissey MC (1988) Electromyostimulation from a clinical perspective. A review. Sports Med 6(1):29–41

Morrissey MC (1989) Reflex inhibition of thigh muscles in knee injury. Causes and treatment. Sports Med 7(4):263–276

Nelson RM, Hunt GC (1981) Strength-duration curve: intrarater and interrater reliability. Phys Ther 61(6):894–897

Nix WA, Vrbova G (Hrsg) (1986) Electrical stimulation and neuromuscular disorders. Springer Verlag, Berlin/Heidelberg, ISBN-13 978-3-642-71339-2

Nuhr M, Crevenna R, Gohlsch B, Bittner C, Pleiner J, Wiesinger G, Fialka-Moser V, Quittan M, Pette D (2003) Functional and biochemical properties of chronically stimulated human skeletal muscle. Eur J Appl Physiol 89(2):202–208

Paternostro-Sluga T, Schuhfried O, Vacariu G, Lang T, Fialka-Moser V (2002) Chronaxie and accommodation index in the diagnosis of muscle denervation. Am J Phys Med Rehabil 81(4):253–260

Penfield W, Boldrey E (1937) Somatic motor and sensory representation in the cerebral cortex of man as studied by electrical stimulation. http://citeseerx.ist.psu.edu/viewdoc/download?doi=10.1.1.873.4232&rep=rep1&type=pdf. Zugegriffen am 20.02.2021

Pérez M, Lucia A, Rivero JL, Serrano AL, Calbet JA, Delgado MA, Chicharro JL (2002) Effects of transcutaneous short-term electrical stimulation on M.

vastus lateralis characteristics of healthy young men. Pflugers Arch 443(5–6):866–874

Peters KM, Carrico DJ, Perez-Marrero RA, Khan AU, Wooldridge LS, Davis GL, Macdiarmid SA (2010) Randomized trial of percutaneous tibial nerve stimulation versus Sham efficacy in the treatment of overactive bladder syndrome: results from the SUmiT trial. J Urol 183(4):1438–1443

Pette D, Staron RS (2000) Myosin isoforms, muscle fiber types, and transitions. Microsc Res Tech 50(6):500–509

Pieber K, Herceg M, Paternostro-Sluga T, Schuhfried O (2015) Optimizing stimulation parameters in functional electrical stimulation of denervated muscles: a cross-sectional study. J Neuroeng Rehabil 12:51

Pogliano C (2012) Penfield's homunculus and other grotesque creatures from the Land of If. Nuncius 27(1):141–162

Popović DB (2014) Advances in functional electrical stimulation (FES). J Electromyogr Kinesiol 24(6):795–802

Porcelli S, Marzorati M, Pugliese L, Adamo S, Gondin J, Bottinelli R, Grassi B (2012) Lack of functional effects of neuromuscular electrical stimulation on skeletal muscle oxidative metabolism in healthy humans. J Appl Physiol 113(7):1101–1109

Prochazka A (2019) Motor neuroprostheses. Compr Physiol 9(1):127–148

Proske U, Gandevia SC (2018) Kinesthetic senses. Compr Physiol 8(3):1157–1183

Qi YC, Niu XL, Gao YR, Wang HB, Hu M, Dong LP, Li YZ (2018) Therapeutic effect evaluation of neuromuscular electrical stimulation with or without strengthening exercise on spastic cerebral Palsy. Clin Pediatr (Phila) 57(5):580–583

Ramírez-García I, Blanco-Ratto L, Kauffmann S, Carralero-Martínez A, Sánchez E (2019) Efficacy of transcutaneous stimulation of the posterior tibial nerve compared to percutaneous stimulation in idiopathic overactive bladder syndrome: randomized control trial. Neurourol Urodyn 38(1):261–268

Rice DA, McNair PJ (2010) Quadriceps arthrogenic muscle inhibition: neural mechanisms and treatment perspectives. Semin Arthritis Rheum 40(3):250–266

Ridding MC, Brouwer B, Miles TS, Pitcher JB, Thompson PD (2000) Changes in muscle responses to stimulation of the motor cortex induced by peripheral nerve stimulation in human subjects. Exp Brain Res 131(1):135–143

Rodriguez-Falces J, Place N (2013) Recruitment order of quadriceps motor units: femoral nerve vs. direct quadriceps stimulation. Eur J Appl Physiol 113(12):3069–3077

Roig M, Reid WD (2009) Electrical stimulation and peripheral muscle function in COPD: a systematic review. Respir Med 103(4):485–495

Rosén B, Chemnitz A, Weibull A, Andersson G, Dahlin LB, Björkman A (2012) Cerebral changes after injury to the median nerve: a long-term follow up. J Plast Surg Hand Surg 46(2):106–112

Rosenthal J, Bernhardt M (1884) Elektrizitätslehre für Mediziner und Elektrotherapie, 3. Aufl. Verlag August Hirschwald, Berlin. https://ia800907.us.archive.org/17/items/elektrizittsle00rose/elektrizittsle00rose_bw.pdf. Zugegriffen am 15.02.2021

Rozman J, Zorko B, Seliskar A (2000) Regeneration of the radial nerve in a dog influenced by electrical stimulation. Pfluegers Arch – Eur J Physiol 439(3 Suppl):R184–R186

Sanjuán Vásquez M, Montes-Castillo ML, Zapata-Altamirano LE, Martínez-Torres S, Vázquez-Mellado J, López López CO (2019) Combining Russian stimulation with isometric exercise improves strength, balance, and mobility in older people with falls syndrome. Int J Rehabil Res 42(1):41–45

Scaldazza CV, Morosetti C, Giampieretti R, Lorenzetti R, Baroni M (2017) Percutaneous tibial nerve stimulation versus electrical stimulation with pelvic floor muscle training for overactive bladder syndrome in women: results of a randomized controlled study. Int Braz J Urol 43(1):121–126

Schiaffino S, Reggiani C (2011) Fiber types in mammalian skeletal muscles. Physiol Rev 91(4):1447–1531

Schnizer W, Manert W, Kleinschmidt J, Magyarosy I, Drexel H (1980) Die Wirkung verschiedener elektrotherapeutischer Verfahren auf Durchblutung und Venenkapazität der unteren Extremität. Z Phys Med 9:85

Schuhfried O, Vacariu G, Paternostro-Sluga T (2005) Reliability of chronaxie and accommodation index in the diagnosis of muscle denervation. Phys Med Rehab Kur 15(3):174–178

Scott W, Adams C, Cyr S, Hanscom B, Hill K, Lawson J, Ziegenbein C (2015) Electrically elicited muscle torque: comparison between 2500-Hz burst-modulated alternating current and monophasic pulsed current. J Orthop Sports Phys Ther 45(12):1035–1041

Seyri K, Maffiuletti N (2011) Effect of Electromyostimulation Training on Muscle Strength and Sports Performance. Strength Cond J 33(1):70–75

da Silva VZ, Durigan JL, Arena R, de Noronha M, Gurney B, Cipriano G Jr (2015) Current evidence demonstrates similar effects of kilohertz-frequency and low-frequency current on quadriceps evoked torque and discomfort in healthy individuals: a systematic review with meta-analysis. Physiother Theory Pract 31(8):533–539

Smerdu V, Karsch-Mizrachi I, Campione M, Leinwand L, Schiaffino S (1994) Type IIX MHC transcripts are expressed in type IIb fibers of human skeletal muscle. Am J Phys 267(6 Pt 1):C1723–C1728

Smith GV, Alon G, Roys SR, Gullapalli RP (2003) Functional MRI determination of a dose-response relationship to lower extremity neuromuscular electrical stimulation in healthy subjects. Exp Brain Res 150(1):33–39

Spector P, Laufer Y, Elboim Gabyzon M, Kittelson A, Stevens Lapsley J, Maffiuletti NA (2016) Neuromuscular electrical stimulation therapy to restore quadriceps muscle function in patients after orthopaedic surgery: a novel structured approach. J Bone Joint Surg Am 98(23):2017–2024

Spencer JD, Hayes KC, Alexander IJ (1984) Knee joint effusion and quadriceps reflex inhibition in man. Arch Phys Med Rehabil 65(4):171–177

Staron R, Hagerman F, Hikida R, Murray T, Hostler D, Crill M, Ragg K, Toma K (2000) Fiber type composition of the Vastus Lateralis muscle of young men and women. J Histochem Cytochem 48:623–630

Stein C, Fritsch CG, Robinson C, Sbruzzi G, Plentz RD (2015) Effects of electrical stimulation in spastic muscles after stroke: systematic review and meta-analysis of randomized controlled trials. Stroke 46(8):2197–2205

Steinacker JM, Wang L, Lormes W, Reissnecker S, Liu Y (2002) Strukturanpassungen des Skelettmuskels auf Training. Dtsch Z Sportmed 12:354–360

Stephens WGS (1973) The assessment of muscle denervation by electrical stimulation. Physiotherapy 59(9):292–294

Stewart F, Berghmans B, Bø K, Glazener CM (2017) Electrical stimulation with non-implanted devices for stress urinary incontinence in women. Cochrane Database Syst Rev 12(12):CD012390

Stillman BC (1967) Some aspects of the theory, performance, and interpretation of the strength duration test. Aust J Physiother 13(2):62–71

Szecsi J, Fornusek C (2014) Comparison of torque and discomfort produced by sinusoidal and rectangular alternating current electrical stimulation in the quadriceps muscle at variable burst duty cycles. Am J Phys Med Rehabil 93(2):146–159

Tam SL, Archibald V, Jassar B, Tyreman N, Gordon T (2001) Increased neuromuscular activity reduces sprouting in partially denervated muscles. J Neurosci 21(2):654–667

Tan K, Wells CI, Dinning P, Bissett IP, O'Grady G (2019) Placebo response rates in electrical nerve stimulation trials for fecal incontinence and constipation: a systematic review and meta-analysis. Neuromodulation. https://doi.org/10.1111/ner.13092. Epub ahead of print. Zugegriffen am 12.02.2021

Thériault R, Boulay MR, Thériault G, Simoneau JA (1996) Electrical stimulation-induced changes in performance and fiber type proportion of human knee extensor muscles. Eur J Appl Physiol Occup Physiol 74(4):311–317

Thrasher A, Graham GM, Popovic MR (2005) Reducing muscle fatigue due to functional electrical stimulation using random modulation of stimulation parameters. Artif Organs 29(6):453–458

Thrasher TA, Popovic MR (2008) Functional electrical stimulation of walking: function, exercise and rehabilitation. Ann Readapt Med Phys 51(6):452–460

Vanderthommen M, Duchateau J (2007) Electrical stimulation as a modality to improve performance of the neuromuscular system. Exerc Sport Sci Rev 35(4):180–185

Vaz MA, Frasson VB (2018) Low-frequency pulsed current versus kilohertz-frequency alternating current: a scoping literature review. Arch Phys Med Rehabil 99(4):792–805

Veldman MP, Gondin J, Place N, Maffiuletti NA (2016) Effects of neuromuscular electrical stimulation training on endurance performance. Front Physiol 7:544

Vieira PJ, Chiappa AM, Cipriano G Jr, Umpierre D, Arena R, Chiappa GR (2014) Neuromuscular electrical stimulation improves clinical and physiological function in COPD patients. Respir Med 108(4):609–620

Vromans M, Faghri PD (2018) Functional electrical stimulation-induced muscular fatigue: effect of fiber composition and stimulation frequency on rate of fatigue development. J Electromyogr Kinesiol 38:67–72

de Wall LL, Heesakkers JP (2017) Effectiveness of percutaneous tibial nerve stimulation in the treatment of overactive bladder syndrome. Res Rep Urol 9:145–157

Walløe L, Wesche J (1988) Time course and magnitude of blood flow changes in the human quadriceps muscles during and following rhythmic exercise. J Physiol 405:257–273

Walton JN (1954) The value of electrodiagnostic methods in the investigation of neuromuscular disease. Physiotherapy 40(3):76–84

Wand BM, Stephens SE, Mangharam EI, George PJ, Bulsara MK, O'Connell NE, Moseley GL (2014) Illusory touch temporarily improves sensation in areas of chronic numbness: a brief communication. Neurorehabil Neural Repair 28(8):797–799

Ward AR (2009) Electrical stimulation using kilohertz-frequency alternating current. Phys Ther 89(2):181–190

Ward AR, Chuen WL (2009) Lowering of sensory, motor, and pain-tolerance thresholds with burst duration using kilohertz-frequency alternating current electric stimulation: part II. Arch Phys Med Rehabil 90(9):1619–1627

Ward AR, Shkuratova N (2002) Russian electrical stimulation: the early experiments. Phys Ther 82(10):1019–1030

Ward AR, Robertson VJ, Ioannou H (2004) The effect of duty cycle and frequency on muscle torque production using kilohertz frequency range alternating current. Med Eng Phys 26(7):569–579

Watanabe K, Kouzaki M, Ando R, Akima H, Moritani T (2015) Non-uniform recruitment along human rectus femoris muscle during transcutaneous electrical nerve stimulation. Eur J Appl Physiol 115(10):2159–2165

Wesche J (1986) The time course and magnitude of blood flow changes in the human quadriceps muscles following isometric contraction. J Physiol 377:445–462

Willand MP (2015) Electrical stimulation enhances reinnervation after nerve injury. Eur J Transl Myol 25(4):243–248

Willand MP, Holmes M, Bain JR, Fahnestock M, De Bruin H (2013a) Electrical muscle stimulation after immediate nerve repair reduces muscle atrophy without affecting reinnervation. Muscle Nerve 48(2):219–225

Willand MP, Zhang JJ, Chiang CD, Borschel GH, Gordon T (2013b) Electrical muscle stimulation increases early reinnervation following nerve injury and immediate repair. In: 6th International IEEE/EMBS conference on Neural Engineering (NER), San Diego, S 315–318

Willand MP, Chiang CD, Zhang JJ, Kemp SW, Borschel GH, Gordon T (2015) Daily electrical muscle stimulation enhances functional recovery following nerve transection and repair in rats. Neurorehabil Neural Repair 29(7):690–700

Willand MP, Borschel GH, Gordon T (2016a) Electrically stimulating nerve and muscle to enhance regeneration and reinnervation following peripheral nerve injury. IFESS 2016 – La Grande Motte, France. https://ifess2016.inria.fr/files/2016/02/IFESS_2016_paper_49.pdf. Zugegriffen am 10.02.2021

Willand MP, Rosa E, Michalski B, Zhang JJ, Gordon T, Fahnestock M, Borschel GH (2016b) Electrical muscle stimulation elevates intramuscular BDNF and GDNF mRNA following peripheral nerve injury and repair in rats. Neuroscience 334:93–104

Zealear DL, Billante CL, Chongkolwatana C, Herzon GD (2000a) The effects of chronic electrical stimulation on laryngeal muscle reinnervation. ORL J Otorhinolaryngol Relat Spec 62(2):87–95

Zealear DL, Billante CR, Chongkolwatana C, Rho YS, Hamdan AL, Herzon GD (2000b) The effects of chronic electrical stimulation on laryngeal muscle physiology and histochemistry. ORL J Otorhinolaryngol Relat Spec 62(2):81–86

Zealear D, Rodriguez R, Kenny T, Billante M, Cho Y, Billante C, Garren K (2002) Electrical stimulation of a denervated muscle promotes selective reinnervation by native over foreign motoneurons. J Neurophysiol 87(4):2195–2199

Zealear DL, Mainthia R, Li Y, Kunibe I, Katada A, Billante C, Nomura K (2014) Stimulation of denervated muscle promotes selective reinnervation, prevents synkinesis, and restores function. Laryngoscope 124(5):E180–E187

Zoladz JA (2018) Muscle and exercise physiology, 1. Aufl. Elsevier, Academic Press, London, ISBN: 9780128145937

5 Ultrasound Therapy

5.1 Definition of Sound

Sound consists of mechanical vibrations in a medium, that is, rapid movements of molecules and atoms. Frequencies below 20 Hz are referred to as subsonic or infrasound, while frequencies above 20 kHz (20,000 Hz) are called ultrasound. This definition of sound is based on human hearing. It was arbitrarily established.

Ultrasound therapy refers to the medical application of acoustic energy with a frequency of more than 20 kHz. In practice, sound frequencies between 0.7 and 3 MHz are used. This is a compromise between acceptable penetration depth and not too much divergence (scattering). Lower frequencies penetrate deeper but diverge more, while higher frequencies penetrate less deeply into a homogeneous medium but exhibit less divergence.

Infrasound can, under laboratory conditions, stimulate or inhibit the growth of various human cells and those of rodents, depending on the conditions. To date, there are no scientifically proven therapeutic applications, so this will not be discussed further here.

Sound waves require a medium for transmission (gas, liquid, solid matter). The action of sound causes the particles in a medium to oscillate rapidly around their resting position. When a molecule is set in motion, its immediate neighbors are also moved, until the movement is transmitted through the entire material or the kinetic energy is converted into thermal energy.

A sound wave is thus acoustic energy that is passed from one molecule or atom to another. In the direction of propagation, there are periodic compressions when the particles approach each other (compressions), and rarefactions when they move away from each other (expansions); in this context, these are called longitudinal waves. This results in alternating pressure states in the tissue (Fig. 5.1).

P. van Kerkhof, *Evidence-Based Electrotherapy*, https://doi.org/10.1007/978-3-662-73019-5_5

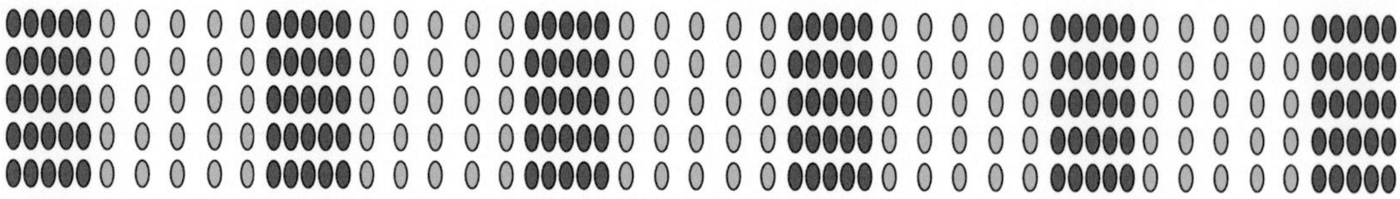

Fig. 5.1 Compressions (overpressure) and expansions (underpressure) in the ultrasound beam (schematic)

5.2 Behavior of Sound

There are six ways in which sound behaves when it encounters an obstacle. Ultrasound behaves in the same way as audible sound.

1. Reflection
2. Absorption
3. Scattering
4. Refraction
5. Diffraction
6. Focusing

5.2.1 Reflection

Reflection occurs when sound encounters a medium with a different acoustic impedance. The acoustic impedance or wave resistance of a medium is a value that indicates how sound propagates in that medium. During reflection, part of the sound is reflected at the interface between the two media, and part penetrates into the other medium (transmission). The greater the difference in acoustic impedance between two media, the more sound is reflected. The penetrating sound energy is converted into thermal energy, generating heat.

On a smooth surface, such as a metal implant, sound is reflected like a mirror. Since osteosynthesis material is usually convex, the sound is scattered (Arnold 1983). Due to the very different acoustic impedances of water (in tissue) and steel, ultrasound is almost completely reflected. If the surface is very irregular, as with bone, diffuse and uneven reflection occurs.

The angle of incidence equals the angle of reflection. The laws of reflection known from optics for flat, convex, and concave mirrors apply here. Concave surfaces focus (concentrate) the sound, convex surfaces scatter it. Flat and concave surfaces that could be reached by ultrasound do not exist in the human body. Osteosynthesis material is always convex, so incident sound waves are always scattered in all directions.

5.2.2 Standing Waves

Between tissue layers with different acoustic impedances, so-called standing waves can occur due to reflection: A sound wave striking perpendicularly is reflected and meets the incoming sound wave. As a result, the sound waves are repeatedly superimposed by reflections, and interference can occur.

Due to these interference phenomena, at certain points the sound waves can partially or completely cancel each other out or reinforce each other. Such a standing wave can only occur with continuous sound (= continuous wave) and with static application. Areas where the sound waves reinforce each other are called hotspots. Due to the normal, construction-related inhomogeneity of a sound beam, hotspots also occur; this phenomenon is discussed in Sect. 5.2.9 on the beam non-uniformity ratio (BNR). Especially when the tissue layer above the bone is thin (patella, wrist area, malleoli), extremely painful periosteal irritation due to heat can occur.

It is therefore important to move the ultrasound transducer during treatment. This distributes the sound energy more evenly in the tissue and largely prevents the formation of hotspots due to such interference phenomena.

5.2.3 Absorption

When sound waves encounter a medium, the waves are either completely or partially absorbed or reflected, depending on the medium. The degree of sound absorption depends on the sound frequency, the angle of incidence, and, of course, the medium. The greater the difference in acoustic impedance between adjacent tissues, the more sound is reflected and the less sound penetrates. During absorption, the sound energy is converted into heat in the tissue by friction.

Denser tissue such as collagen and bone absorbs more sound energy than less dense tissue such as fat or muscle. This is because more molecules must be moved in denser tissue, which requires more energy. For this reason, sound penetrates less deeply into denser tissue, but causes more friction, and therefore more heat is generated in this tissue and at the interface. The surrounding tissue is subsequently heated more by conduction. Normally, this heat is carried away by the blood circulation.

Sound with a frequency of 3 MHz penetrates less deeply into a homogeneous medium than sound with a lower frequency such as 1 MHz. The molecules, forced to move more rapidly at 3 MHz, absorb more energy. Therefore, higher frequencies heat the tissue more quickly than lower ones. Several investigators have shown with in vivo measurements that 3 MHz ultrasound heats the tissue more deeply than expected; more on this later.

The depth at which the sound energy has been reduced by half due to absorption is called the half-value depth (HVD). In a water tank or in a tissue phantom, this energy decrease is measurable, and thus the HVD for homogeneous media can be calculated. Interestingly, Draper in 1995 showed that the temperature increase during insonation with 1 MHz at depths of 2.5 and 5 cm was the same after a certain period. Apparently, the energy delivery in inhomogeneous human tissue in vivo is not comparable to that in a water tank or tissue phantom. This raises doubts about the clinical significance of the HVD.

5.2.4 Diffraction and Refraction

Diffraction refers to the phenomenon where the original propagation direction of a sound source is altered (bent) by an object or in an inhomogeneous medium. Refraction of sound refers to the change in direction of sound waves when passing between two media of different density. How bizarre such refractions can be in human tissue was demonstrated by Frye et al. (2007). In three subjects, blisters appeared anteriorly on the lower leg, 6 h after insonation was performed dorsally on the calf with 1 MHz, 1.5 W/cm^2, continuously for 10 min. The blisters were located exactly opposite the treatment area, at a distance of about 10 cm. Medical causes were ruled out; the investigators suspect a technical cause.

5.2.5 Frequency

Frequency indicates how many oscillations occur per unit of time. The greater the number of oscillations per unit time, the higher the pitch for audible sound. Applying ultrasound at a frequency of 3 MHz means forcing the tissue to undergo 3,000,000 oscillations per second. The higher the frequency, the faster the movement imposed on the molecules, the greater the friction, and the greater the heating. The faster the movement, the higher the energy loss over a certain distance, so less energy remains to penetrate deeper into the tissue.

5.2.6 Pressure Changes in Tissue

Of particular physical interest are the enormous pressure changes that occur in tissue. Since the direction of movement changes very rapidly (at 1 MHz, 1,000,000 times per second), the particle acceleration is very high: about 1,000,000 m/s^2, that is, 100,000 times the acceleration due to gravity! This results in a high alternating sound pressure: alternating phases of overpressure and underpressure, with maximum values differing by about 2 bar (about 20 m water column). Due to reflections in the tissue and interference within the sound waves, the pressure conditions shift from place to place, leading to large pressure differences between the particles. This pressure difference can be about 8–9 bar/mm. For comparison: car tire pressure is about 2.5 bar. The pressure fluctuations at 1 W/cm^2 and 1 MHz are 1.7 bar. With a wavelength of 1.5 mm, this means a pressure gradient of 3.4 bar over a distance of 0.75 mm.

5.2.7 Generation of Ultrasound

In 1880, the French physicists Pierre and Jacques Curie discovered the piezoelectric effect (Curie and Curie 1880; Fig. 5.2). When pressure is applied to a crystal, electrical charges are generated on the surface of the piezoelectric material. This is also the principle behind the operation of the pickup in a record player and the pickup for stringed instruments: Small sensor plates, attached in the bridge of a guitar beneath the strings, pick up the vibrations produced by the strings and convert them into electrical signals. At that time, the Curie brothers used tourmaline, quartz, topaz, cane sugar, and sodium potassium tartrate; today, certain polycrystalline materials such as lead zirconate titanate, barium titanate, or silicon acetate are used.

In a piezoelectric crystal, the positive and negative charges are separated. The charges are balanced. The displacement of ions in crystals due to mechanical stress shifts the centers of negative and positive charge relative to each other, resulting in electrical polarization and thus a measurable electrical voltage difference at the surfaces of the crystal.

These piezoelectric effects also occur in the human body, especially in bone tissue, collagen fibers, and proteins. It is quite possible, though not proven, that these phenomena are involved in the biological effects of ultrasound. One theory assumes that under the influence of sound pressure, a mechanical deformation of enzymes occurs, which either stimulates ("switches on") or inhibits ("switches off") the activity of these

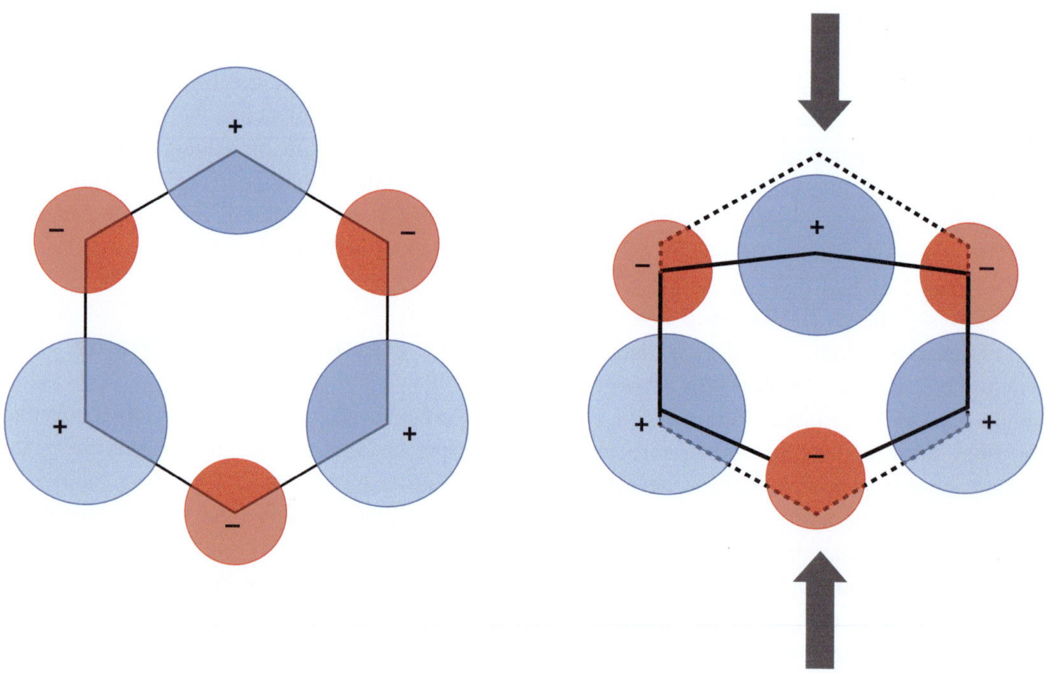

Fig. 5.2 Piezoelectric effect. Left: initial state, right: charge displacement due to mechanical deformation

enzymes (Johns 2002). This theory is supported, among others, by Francis et al. (1992). The investigators were able to show that improved fibrinolysis with therapeutically relevant doses (1 MHz, 1 W/cm^2) was not temperature-dependent and could not be explained by mechanical destruction (cavitation). They assume that the enzymes responsible for fibrinolysis are mechanically "potentiated."

The French-Luxembourgish physicist and inventor Gabriel Jonas Lippmann mathematically demonstrated in 1881 that this piezoelectric effect is reversible (Lippmann 1881), and the Curies immediately confirmed this experimentally. This means: If the piezoelectric material is exposed to an alternating voltage, the material undergoes a change in shape, corresponding to the frequency of the alternating voltage and the resonance frequency of the piezoelectric material, provided the thickness of the crystal is correct.

When an external electric field is applied to the crystal, the ions in each unit cell are displaced by electrostatic forces so that the entire crystal deforms. If the frequency of the alternating voltage is 1000 Hz, the crystal, if the thickness is correct, vibrates at a frequency of 1000 Hz and produces a tone with f = 1000 Hz = sound. If the applied alternating voltage is 1 MHz, sound with a frequency of 1 MHz is generated. In this way, sound with very high frequencies can be produced.

Paul Langevin, a friend of the Curies, especially of their sister Marie, applied this principle in 1917 together with Constantin Chilowski to construct the ASDIC (Anti Submarine Division Investigation Committee), a submarine detection system and the precursor of sonar (Sound Navigation and Ranging).

He was allegedly also the first to observe biological effects of ultrasound. He exposed fish in an aquarium to high ultrasound intensities: 1 kW/cm^2. The animals first aligned themselves in the direction of the sound and, after briefly moving very vigorously, floated belly up. The cause of death was not determined: embolism? Cooked brain? Langevin also reportedly described that it was extremely painful to put his hand in the water. Unfortunately, the reference for these statements cannot be found; the author only copied it from elsewhere. The first devices suitable for humans were constructed around 1938 and successfully used to treat sciatica, back pain, plexus neuralgia, and myalgia.

An ultrasound device essentially consists of an alternating current generator that produces the high-frequency alternating current necessary to set the piezoelectric element mounted in the transducer into vibration.

Two fields can be distinguished in the ultrasound beam (Fig. 5.5):

1. the near field, also called the Fresnel zone, and
2. the far field, the Fraunhofer zone.

Since a piezoelectric element does not usually vibrate uniformly, the energy output is also not uniform. The front of a transducer, where the sound emerges, does not vibrate as a unit. One must imagine the front surface as a large number of individual points emitting sound. The outgoing sound waves influence each other. The near field is therefore characterized by interference phenomena in the sound beam, which lead to considerable intensity fluctuations, so-called hotspots, and by a slight convergence of the sound beam. Intensities can occur that are 5 to 10 times, sometimes up to 30 times, the set value. The locations of these areas do not always occur at the same place in the beam. Because the insonated tissue is not homogeneous and therefore many different reflections occur, the hotspots move during insonation. It is therefore not possible to predict where in the beam these energy peaks will occur.

The convergence is the direct result of the aforementioned destructive and constructive interference phenomena. The therapeutic effects mainly take place in the near field. In the far field, these interference phenomena are absent and the sound beam is more scattered. Most of the sound energy is emitted around the central axis of the sound beam; toward the edge of the transducer, the sound energy decreases significantly (Fig. 5.3 and 5.4). The diameter of this

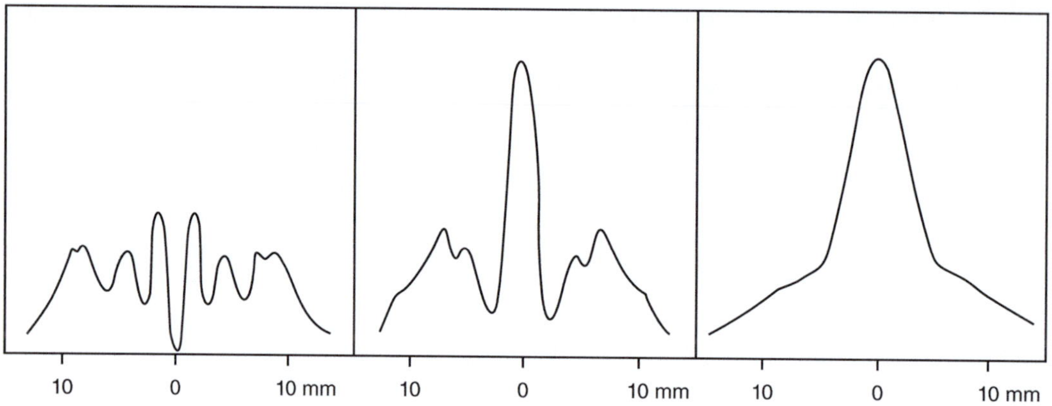

Fig. 5.3 Distribution of sound energy in cross-section (various transducers). Note the energy peaks in the center. © Enraf-Nonius B.V. Delft, Netherlands, with kind permission

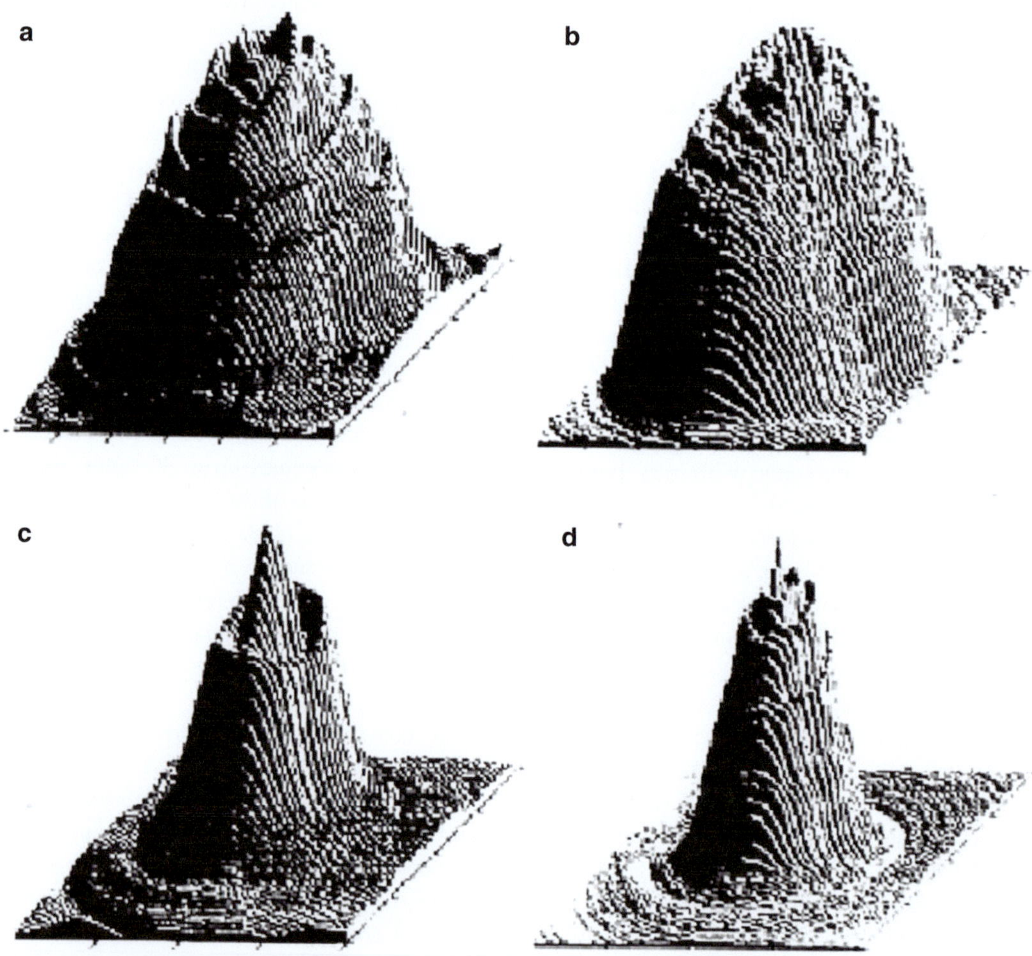

Fig. 5.4 Energy distribution over the transducer. **a**: Large head 1 MHz, **b**: large head 3 MHz, **c**: small head 1 MHz, **d**: small head, 3 MHz. © Enraf-Nonius B.V. Delft, Netherlands, with kind permission

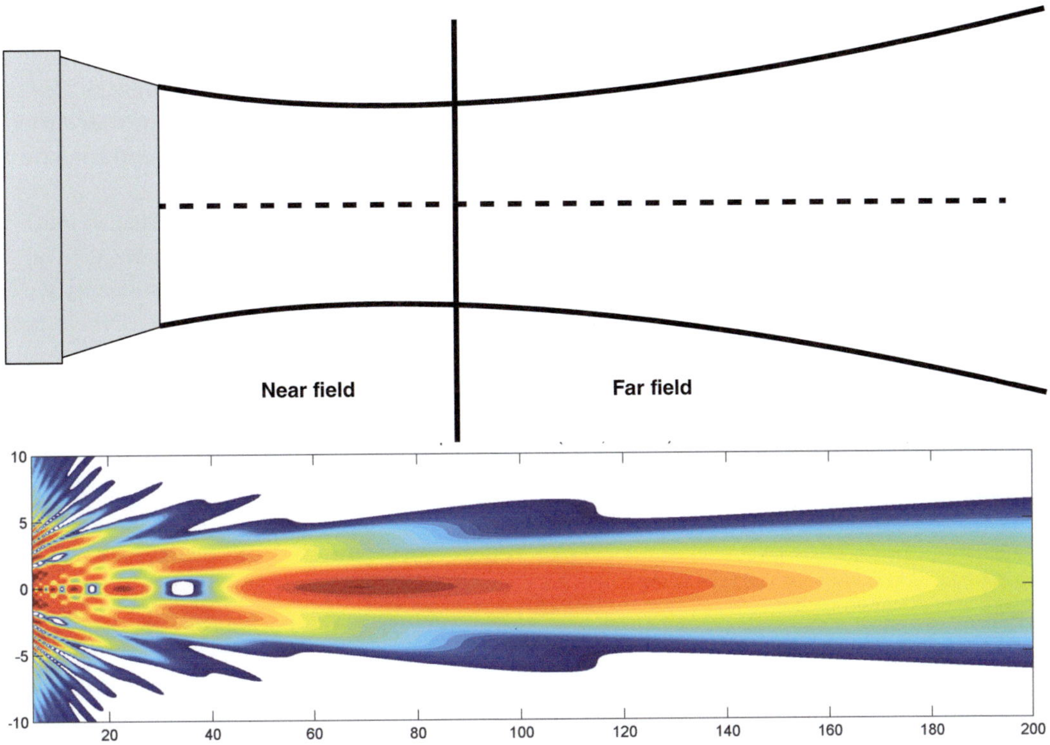

Fig. 5.5 Sound pressure in water, 4 MHz. Note the chaotic conditions in the first 40 mm. © Michael Lenz, Wikimedia Commons, licensed under CreativeCommons License by-sa-2.0-de, URL: http://creativecommons.org/licenses/by-sa/2.0/de/legalcode

central axis varies from transducer to transducer, and thus the energy output in this area also varies. Johns et al. (2007a, b) suspect that this is one of the causes of the sometimes quite different temperature measurements in tissue (Fig. 5.5).

The length of the near field depends on the diameter of the transducer and the wavelength, and for a 5 cm^2 head and 1 MHz is about 10 cm, for a 1 cm^2 transducer and 1 MHz about 2 cm. The length of the near field at 3 MHz is three times as long, because the wavelength is proportionally shorter.

The length of the near field is calculated using the formula $r^2 \div \lambda$. Here, "r" is the radius of the sound element and λ the wavelength. Example calculation: 25 mm head, 3 MHz: $12.5^2 \div 1.5 = 10$ cm near field length.

The wavelength of the emitted ultrasound depends on the thickness of the piezo element. At 3 MHz, the wavelength is 0.5 mm, at 1 MHz 1.5 mm. The thickness of the element is half the desired wavelength, so for 1 MHz it is 0.7 mm and for 3 MHz it is 0.25 mm. Very thin and sensitive, therefore. This is why transducers cannot withstand rough handling. This element is excited to vibrate by high-voltage pulses and thus produces the desired sound frequency.

5.2.8 Effective Radiating Area (ERA)

Sound emerges from the front of the transducer. But not everything you see at the front produces sound. The housing in which the piezo element is located has a certain thickness, and therefore the diameter of the piezo element is somewhat smaller than the outer surface of the transducer. The area that actually produces sound is called the ERA: the effective radiating area. A

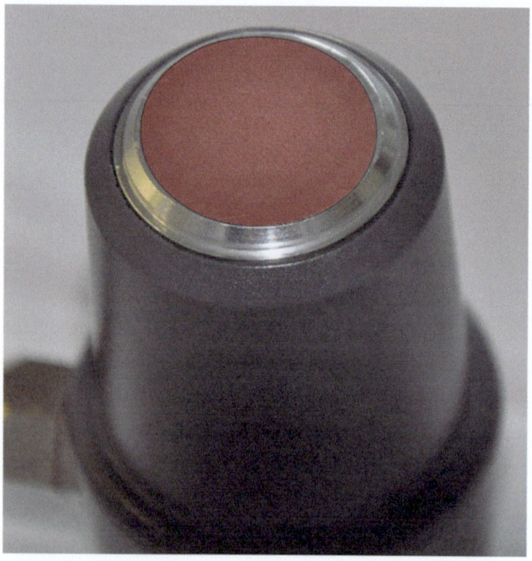

Fig. 5.6 An older transducer. The ERA is red

transducer may have an area of 5 cm^2, but the ERA in such a case may be 4–4.5 cm^2. The size of the ERA must be taken into account when determining dosage parameters (Fig. 5.6).

5.2.9 Beam Nonuniformity Ratio (BNR)

It is common knowledge, then, that the ultrasound beam is not homogeneous. The "Beam Nonuniformity Ratio" (BNR), indicated on the transducer, specifies how high the peak value in the beam is relative to the set intensity. More technically expressed: The BNR is the ratio of the maximum emitted energy to the average emitted energy.

Sometimes the BNR is not marked on the transducer itself, but on a plastic strip that is attached to the transducer cable. These adhesive strips have the tendency to disappear quickly.

With a BNR of 5:1 and a set intensity of 1.5 W/cm^2, the **normally** occurring peak value is therefore $5 \times 1.5 = 7.5$ W/cm^2. When and where in the ultrasound beam this value occurs is unpredictable.

The BNR can be considered a quality characteristic. The higher the BNR, the higher the energy peaks. Transducers with a BNR above 8:1 are not approved for medical applications. When inquiring with an electrotherapy device distributor about the BNR of a particular device, the response was that their devices do not have a BNR. Professional expertise …

BNR values of 5:1 to 6:1 are normal; ideally, a BNR = 1:1 would be desirable, but this value is technically unattainable. Even with very well-designed modern transducers, the BNR is usually between 2:1 and 5:1, so *peaks* must *always* be expected!

This amplification of ultrasound energy differs from the amplification caused by reflection at interfaces and **cannot** be prevented by moving the transducer. However, moving the transducer does prevent local overheating, as the ultrasound energy is better distributed over the treatment area. The phenomena likely influence each other.

It is clear that this phenomenon has consequences for dosing. This will be discussed in more detail below. Due to the uneven distribution of ultrasound energy, there is also an uneven occurrence of so-called acoustic cavitation (see below, Sect. 5.3.2). Since cavitation also generates heat, this could likewise explain the occurrence of hotspots.

The energy value in watts/cm^2 displayed on the device refers to the average energy delivered over the entire transducer surface. This is called the "spatial average intensity." Some devices display the value in watts per cm^2, while others allow the display of the total energy emitted by the entire transducer.

For example, the display on a 5 cm^2 transducer set to 1 W/cm^2 may show a value of 5 W. This is not the intensity per cm^2; please do not confuse this and always pay attention to the device settings!

The energy peaks that occur due to the (normal!) inhomogeneity are referred to as "spatial peak intensity." These peaks are not displayed on any screen.

For pulsed ultrasound, the average energy delivered over a certain period is called the "temporal average," while the energy peaks are called the "temporal peak"—this is the

Table 5.1 Ultrasound Technical Terms

Spatial Average Temporal Average, SATA	Average energy output in the ultrasound beam over a certain period
Spatial Peak Temporal Average, SPTA	Maximum energy output in the ultrasound beam over a certain period
Spatial Peak Temporal Peak, SPTP	Maximum energy output during an ultrasound pulse in the beam
Spatial Average Temporal Peak, SATP	Average energy output during the ultrasound pulses

Table 5.2 Ultrasound Glossary

Wavelength	Distance between two identical zones of compression or rarefaction in the material ($\lambda = c/f$)
Sound pressure	Alternating pressure resulting from the oscillation of particles in a medium = acoustic streaming = "sonic wind"
Acoustic impedance	Obsolete: sound wave resistance = acoustic impedance = sound wave impedance. Defined by the ratio of sound pressure to particle velocity ($R = p/v$). Another, physically less meaningful term is sound hardness
Absorption coefficient	Describes the absorption rate. Along with reflection, it significantly determines the propagation of ultrasound in tissue
Half-value thickness, half-value depth	Distance after which the ultrasound intensity has been reduced by half. In "soft body tissue" at 1 MHz supposedly about 3–4 cm, at 3 MHz supposedly about 2.5 cm. However, this is not correct
Penetration depth	The greatest depth at which a therapeutic effect can still be expected. This is the point where 10% of the delivered energy remains
ERA = effective radiating area	Effective radiating area of the transducer
BNR (Beam Nonuniformity Ratio)	Indicates how high the peak value in the beam is relative to the set intensity. Must not exceed 8, usually around 4–5

maximum energy delivered during an ultrasound pulse. This means, for example, that in pulsed mode, you set the device to 1 W/cm^2 (this is the effective energy of a pulse), but since you are operating in pulsed mode, only 20% of this is delivered over the set time—depending on the pulse setting. The various technical terms result in some interesting word combinations (Table 5.1). For further technical terms, see Table 5.2.

A SATA of 0.5 W/cm^2 can be achieved by setting 0.5 W/cm^2 in continuous mode or by setting 1 W/cm^2 in pulsed mode at 50% pulsing. If the treatment duration is the same with these settings, exactly the same amount of ultrasound energy reaches the tissue. Draper et al. demonstrated in 2004 that this leads to the same degree of heating in the insonated tissue.

This means that with the same SATA, pulsed ultrasound produces the same thermal effects as continuous ultrasound. If you want to prevent these thermal effects with pulsed ultrasound, you must be sure to take the SATA into account.

5.3 Effects of Ultrasound

As outlined above, sound vibrations require a medium for their propagation; sound cannot travel in a vacuum. Thus, the first effect that occurs in tissue is mechanical in nature. The vibrations cause compression and expansion in the tissue at the same frequency as the ultrasound. This leads to pressure fluctuations in the tissue and changes in the volume of body cells. The rapid movements in the tissue generate heat through friction. The higher the sound frequency, the faster the movements, and the more rapid the heating.

The sound pressure causes a flow in the tissue, referred to as "acoustic streaming," or more poetically as "sonic wind." Acoustic streaming contributes to the improved transport of particles in tissue by ultrasound. The mechanical effect is of great therapeutic importance, as it is likely responsible for all the effects of ultrasound. These effects occur with both continuous and pulsed ultrasound. In this sense, the thermal effects can be considered secondary to the mechanical effects.

5.3.1 Demonstration of Functionality

When ultrasound is applied, the patient usually feels local warmth. Especially when treating structures close to the periosteum, it can, if one is not careful, become quite painful for a short time. The patient thus notices that something is happening. Depending on the dosage, the patient may feel nothing. It is therefore useful to show the patient in the first session that "something is happening" nonetheless. In any case, patients should be fully informed about the therapy to be used. The simplest way to do this is as follows (note: this method is *not* suitable for function control!):

Drip some water onto the carefully held horizontal ultrasound head and turn up the intensity. The water begins to move under the influence of the sound waves, and often concentric circles form. If the intensity is increased, the movement becomes more vigorous, and a mist forms—not steam: the water is not boiling. The water now splashes up, and the droplets are mechanically flung away. This is, incidentally, how an ultrasonic nebulizer works. This can be demonstrated most clearly in pulsed mode.

There is a second, somewhat more elaborate method, which is, however, extremely impressive and very suitable for training purposes. To do this, spread some contact gel on the ultrasound head and place the head on the (own) supinated back of the hand, slightly medial or lateral to the third metacarpal. Make a hollow with your hand and pour some water into it. You can hold the ultrasound head between your knees to have one hand free, or have a student assist you.

If you now turn up the intensity (or have it turned up) and carefully move the ultrasound head or your hand back and forth a little, you can "aim" the sound between the metacarpals. You will then see the water in your hand being agitated. Depending on the intensity, distinct eddies and waves form. This provides an impressive demonstration of sound penetration. Caution: If you stay in the same spot for too long, it can become extremely painful due to periosteal irritation! However, the learning effect is enormous.

5.3.2 Cavitation

The probably most important mechanical effect is acoustic cavitation (ter Haar et al. 1982; ter Haar 1999; O'Brien 2007). Cavitation is the process by which bubbles are formed in a liquid due to the action of external forces. Ter Haar demonstrated that cavitation bubbles can occur in vivo at therapeutically relevant intensities (ter Haar et al. 1982). This was in a guinea pig thigh, and ultrasound was not applied dynamically, but at least it was in vivo. Frequency 0.75 MHz, intensity 0.68 W/cm^2, ultrasound head diameter 2.5 cm, insonated subaqueously, so quite low dosed. There are two physical explanatory models for the occurrence of cavitation. Both interpretations assume that bubbles can form in a liquid when pressure changes occur:

1. **Water is mechanically torn apart**

Liquids are held together by cohesion. This cohesive force determines the tensile strength of the liquid. For example, when a ship's propeller rotates at high speed through water, this cohesive force is overcome and the water is literally torn apart, resulting in cavities: bubbles. Bubbles can also form in water flowing rapidly over rocks in this way.

As soon as these bubbles reach a certain size and the internal pressure of the bubble becomes less than the water pressure, the bubbles collapse. Such implosions can release forces so great that the ship's propeller corrodes; this is called cavitation erosion. In an ultrasound application, the alternating pressure of the longitudinal sound wave causes compressions and expansions (= dilatations) in the liquid. The tensile forces during the expansion phase (the phase between two successive compressions) can, similar to the rotating ship's propeller, tear the liquid apart, resulting in the formation of

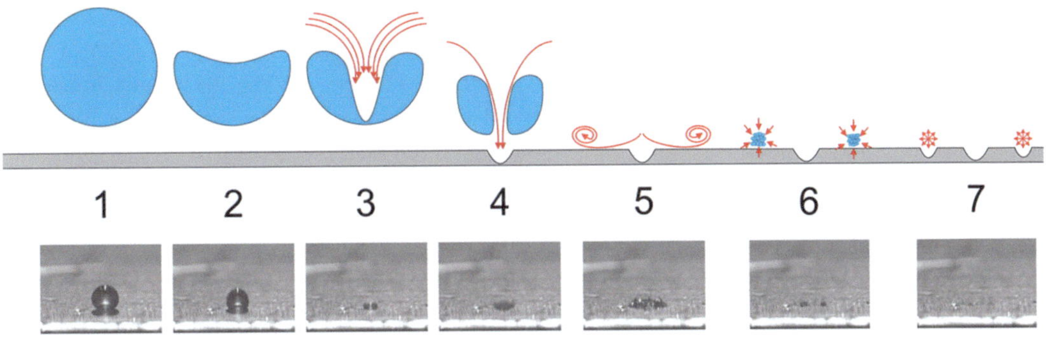

Abb. 5.7 Inertial (transient, unstable) cavitation. 1–7: The bubble collapses and a microjet is formed. The force of the microjet damages the surface nearby. Below: images of the process. From Dular et al. 2019, with kind permission

cavities (cavitas)—bubbles form, depending on the sound frequency, up to a size of about 150 µm, so not as dramatic as with the ship's propeller. The bubbles are either empty or filled with gas or vapor.

2. **Water evaporates at body temperature**

Water normally evaporates at an air pressure of 1013.25 hPa (millibar) at 100 °C. If the pressure drops, for example, to about 56 hPa, water evaporates at 35 °C, and even lower, for example, to 31 hPa at 25 °C. For this reason, water boils faster in a mountain hut at 2000 m, but only gets to about 93 °C.

Between the compression and expansion phases during an ultrasound application, there are, as is well known, strong pressure fluctuations: at 1 W/cm^2 about 1.7 bar = 1722 hPa. In the negative pressure phases, the pressure drops so much that water can evaporate at body temperature, and bubbles form during evaporation.

Various processes occur during cavitation. Bubbles already present in the liquid can pulsate or grow, new bubbles can form, and interactions between different gas bubbles can occur. Two different types of cavitation are known: stable and transient (= inertial) cavitation. In stable cavitation, the gas bubbles pulsate for a certain short time without collapsing. In inertial cavitation, the bubbles grow until they reach a certain critical size and then implode. This happens when the internal pressure of the bubble is less than the pressure of the liquid. The evaporation process stops and the vapor bubbles collapse. Such events last only a few microseconds but still have a mechanical impact on the surrounding cells (van Warmel et al. 2006). These implosions can generate pressure surges with shock waves of extremely high peaks (up to several thousand bar), and these can trigger pressure waves at a speed of 10^3 m/s. If such implosions occur near a solid object—a ship's propeller, a cell wall, or a kidney stone—liquid jets, called microjets, are formed. These microjets can reach speeds of 100 m/s (Figs. 5.7 and 5.8).

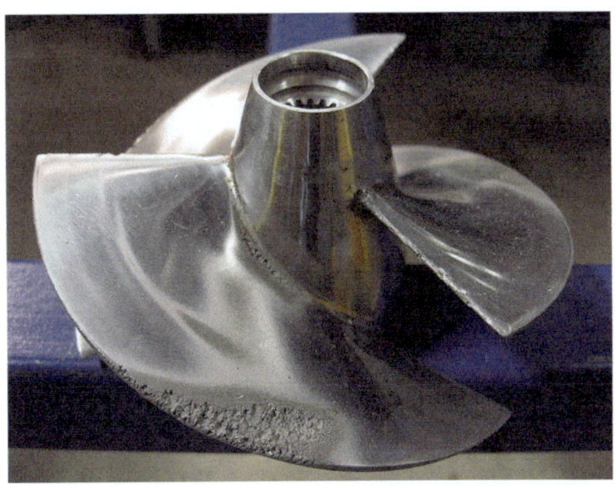

Abb. 5.8 Cavitation erosion on a ship's propeller. Note the greater damage at the outer edge, where the speed is greatest. © Axda0002, Wikimedia Commons, licensed under CreativeCommons License by-sa-2.0-de, URL: http://creativecommons.org/licenses/by-sa/2.0/de/legalcode

Under the influence of therapeutic ultrasound, the gas bubbles expand and contract without reaching a certain critical size. Due to the high frequencies (around 1 MHz), the sound pulses are so short that the time during which the bubbles can grow is also very short. The pulsing of the ultrasound probably has the same effect: no sound energy can accumulate, so the bubbles can return to their original size during the "off" phase. These bubbles grow and shrink, i.e., alternate between compression and expansion phases, and as long as the internal pressure of the bubble remains above the liquid pressure, they remain stable and pulsate in the rhythm of the (ultra)sound wave. This is called "stable cavitation" (noninertial cavitation). All the processes described above lead to mechanical destabilization of the structure in which cavitation occurs. For example, reversible openings are formed in the stratum corneum, making it more permeable (Fig. 5.9). This improvement in permeability, supported by sound pressure, enables the delivery of drugs, also known as sonophoresis or phonophoresis (Mitragotri et al. 1995a, b).

The occurrence of cavitation under the influence of ultrasound is frequency-dependent; the threshold at which cavitation occurs in liquids with therapeutic ultrasound is 2.5 W/cm^2. Mitragotri et al. (1995a, b) found in vitro a 13-fold increase in skin permeability for estradiol when using 1 MHz, 2 W/cm^2 continuous ultrasound. When using 3 MHz, 2 W/cm^2, the improvement was only about 2-fold; with pulsed ultrasound (1 MHz, pulse 2 ms, 100 Hz, 2 W/cm^2), no improvement was detectable. According to the authors, the destabilization of the phospholipid bilayer of the skin and cells caused by cavitation is responsible for the improvement in permeability. The size of the cavitation bubbles is also frequency-dependent. Lower frequencies (20 kHz) cause bubbles up to a maximum of 150 μm. Higher frequencies, for example 1 MHz, produce much smaller bubbles up to 1 μm. The bubble size determines where in the tissue these bubbles can occur. In the skin, the bubbles cannot grow much, so cavitation effects with physiotherapeutically common frequencies and intensities probably occur only in the skin (Mitragotri et al. 1995a, b). The larger bubbles that occur when using ultrasound at a frequency of 20 kHz are probably responsible for the fact that this frequency is particularly effective for the sonophoresis of larger molecules such as insulin, which has a molar mass of 5808 g/mol. The inertial cavitation that occurs, with its microjets and shock waves, causes a stronger destabilization of the lipid bilayers compared to the effects that occur when using 1 MHz ultrasound (Wolloch and Kost 2010). For comparison: the estradiol mentioned above has a molar mass (M) of 272 g/mol.

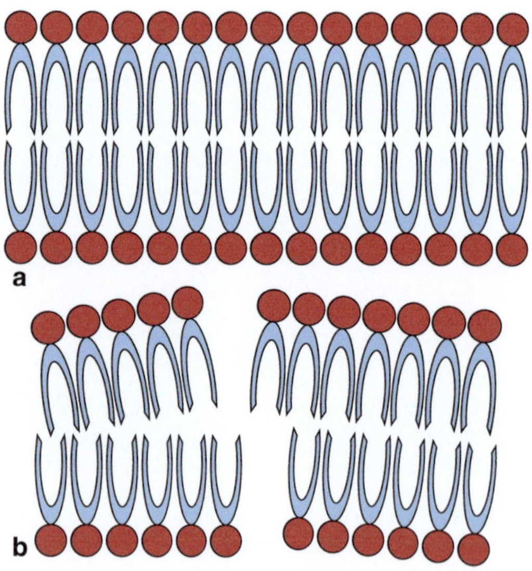

Abb. 5.9 **a** Intact lipid bilayer of a cell membrane, **b** cell membrane destabilized by cavitation

The bubble activity enhances the effect of sound pressure. The physiological effects of this membrane destabilization impact membrane permeability. The permeability of the skin and cell membranes increases, which is manifested, for example, in an increase in intracellular Ca concentration in chondrocytes, an immediate decrease in potassium concentration in thymocytes (precursors of T-lymphocytes), and increased uptake of calcium in cartilage and bone cell cultures (see also the section on sonophoresis, Sect. 5.9). The increased intracellular

Ca concentration, for example, influences protein synthesis. However, this increased protein production could also occur as a reaction to primary tissue damage due to unstable cavitation.

5.3.3 Microstreaming, Small Scale Streaming

In the fluid around the pulsating bubbles, turbulence, eddies, and flows form, which, in addition to the sound pressure, represent a significant mechanical stress for the cell wall, leading to mechanical destabilization of the cell wall. This results in improved permeability and has been demonstrated in vitro, for example, by an increased intracellular calcium concentration (Mortimer and Dyson 1988). The microscopic circulation (the eddies and vortices) is referred to as "microstreaming" (Elder 1959) or, according to Kolb and Nyborg (1956), "small scale streaming."

It is not certain whether unstable cavitation occurs at the usual therapeutic dosages. Tezel and Mitragotri (2003) assume that with so-called low frequency ultrasound (20–100 kHz), unstable cavitation occurs directly on the skin surface at the boundary to the stratum corneum. Due to this unstable (inertial) cavitation, microjets would be formed. The combination of implosions and microjets would increase the permeability of the stratum corneum. These researchers have calculated that about 1–10 such jets are formed per cm^2, with the fluid being accelerated to 50–150 m/s (180–540 km/h!). Unstable cavitation can, as has already been demonstrated histologically and macroscopically in vitro by Frenkel and colleagues in 1999 in fish, lead to cell destruction at sufficiently high dosages. Frenkel et al. worked with 1 MHz ultrasound, applied statically subaqueously, ERA 10 cm^2, 0.5–1.0 W/cm^2, distance between ultrasound head and fish head 15 cm (Frenkel et al. 1999). After 90 s of insonation at 0.75 W/cm^2, minor microscopic damage was detectable in the uppermost skin layer. A thermal effect was ruled out; when degassed water was used, the effects did not occur, so cavitation was involved. Considering these results in light of the measurements by Ward and Robertson (1996a, b, see Sect. 5.6.2), the question arises as to how much sound energy actually reached the fish after 15 cm and to what extent the scalp of a fish is comparable to human skin.

5.3.4 Histamine

Ultrasound can trigger mast cell degranulation and consequently the release of histamine (Fyfe and Chahl 1984). This causes vasodilation and plasma extravasation, thus influencing the local inflammatory response. This reaction has been observed in rats, but can certainly also occur in humans. Fyfe and Chahl believe that this histamine may be involved in the healing processes stimulated by ultrasound.

It is unclear whether the sound acts directly on the mast cells. The release can very well occur indirectly in connection with a local inflammatory response. The TRPV1 receptors responsible for this neurogenically controlled reaction normally respond to temperatures around 43 °C. If a local inflammatory reaction is present, these receptors are sensitized by various inflammatory mediators (prostaglandins, bradykinin). The receptors now fire at body temperature or below: a reason for resting pain in inflammatory processes. Even a temperature increase of 0.5–1 °C leads to additional irritation of the affected nerve fibers. These release their neuropeptides, and the released substance P triggers the release of histamine from the mast cells.

It is therefore possible to trigger histamine release with ultrasound. This may be desirable in the case of a chronic inflammatory reaction, but in the case of a fresh injury with a normally progressing inflammatory response, it could disrupt healing and undesirably prolong the inflammatory reaction. Therefore, one must carefully consider whether to use thermal dosing in the case of an inflammatory reaction.

5.3.5 Heat

The rapid movements in the tissue generate frictional heat. The special feature of heat development is the selective heating of boundary layers, for example at the transitions between subcutaneous fat tissue and muscle fascia, between loose connective tissue and tendons or joint capsule, and at the bone. In particular, reflection at the bone: around 30% of the sound energy causes pronounced heating of structures close to the bone, such as muscle insertions, joint capsules, and ligaments. If the temperature increase is large enough and lasts long enough, various secondary effects are triggered by the heating.

The proven effects include:

- Heating with all its consequences: an increase in metabolic activity, pain relief, relaxation, improved extensibility of collagen, improved blood circulation (Mense 1978; Lehmann 1990; Baker and Bell 1991; Draper et al. 1995; Rose et al. 1996; Draper et al. 1998a, b; Hardy and Woodall 1998; Cruz et al. 2016)
- Improved particle transport through acoustic streaming (Tezel and Mitragotri 2003; Dalecki 2004; Joshi and Raje 2002; Polat et al. 2011; ter Haar 2007)
- Improved permeability through cavitation (Joshi and Raje 2002; Merino et al. 2003; Alvarez-Román et al. 2003; Rich et al. 2014; ter Haar 2007; Tezel and Mitragotri 2003; Ueda et al. 2009; Wolloch and Kost 2010)
- Microstreaming through cavitation (Joshi and Raje 2002; Polat et al. 2011; Smith 2007; Wolloch and Kost 2010)
- Influence on nerve conduction (Halle et al. 1981; Kramer 1987)
- Increased histamine release (Fyfe and Chahl 1984; Dyson and Luke 1986)
- Increased vascularization (Young and Dyson 1990; Huang et al. 2014; Nazer et al. 2015)
- Accelerated fibrinolysis (Francis et al. 1992; Everbach and Francis 2000; Sakharov et al. 2000)

These effects only occur at temperatures between 40 and 45 °C, with the elevated temperature needing to be maintained at this level for 5–30 min (Lehmann 1990).

How long it takes to reach a certain temperature has been investigated several times in vivo in humans and animals (Adair and Levine 2019; Draper et al. 1993, 1995; Hynynen et al. 1990; Levine et al. 2001; Montgomery et al. 2013). Based on the results of these studies, it is possible to calculate quite precisely how long one must insonate to reach a certain temperature. How exactly this is done is explained further below in Sect. 5.8.

For a long time, the thermal effect was the only effect proven in vivo. To what extent the various biological effects are specifically mechanical or actually secondary to the temperature increase is still debated today.

5.4 Application

A distinction is made between "continuous" or "continuous wave" ultrasound and "pulsed" ultrasound. Normally, the ultrasound head is placed on the skin and moved over the tissue to be treated at a speed of 2–4 cm/s (about as fast as an ant walks), sometimes up to 8 cm/s, whereby the speed does not affect the temperature increase as long as one works carefully (Weaver et al. 2006). The more one is distracted, the more one leaves the relevant treatment area (Grey 2003).

Continuous ultrasound is insonation delivered without interruption at constant intensity. With pulsed ultrasound, the sound is delivered in pulses. This reduces the thermal effect, while the mechanical effect is maintained.

Pulsed is not synonymous with athermal! Pulsed ultrasound with a 50% pulse setting (duty cycle), 3 MHz, 1.0 W/cm^2, 10 min heats the tissue just as much as continuous ultrasound, 3 MHz, 0.5 W/cm^2 for 10 min, namely almost a 3 °C increase at a depth of 2 cm in the calf muscle of 16 healthy volunteers (Gallo et al. 2004).

5.5 Site of Insonation

Normally, treatment is performed locally. Indirect insonation aims to achieve effects by treating nerves, nerve roots, and segmental connections. Various approaches are possible, such as radicular, paravertebral treatment, segmental insonation of hyperalgesic zones (Head zones), direct insonation of peripheral nerves, and gangliotropic treatment (the stellate ganglion) for circulatory problems in the arm (Raynaud, CRPS). The effectiveness of these treatments has never been clearly proven. Publications from the 1950s describe that treatment of the stellate ganglion with ultrasound produced results comparable to a nerve block. A study from 2014 on the same topic could not demonstrate any effect (0.5 W/cm^2 and 3 W/cm^2, 1:4 pulse, 1 cm^2 ERA, 5 min, 20 treatments) (Askin et al. 2014). There are also publications from that time about successful treatments of radicular pain and postherpetic pain. Unfortunately, the dosage parameters used are unclear. However, it is known that heating affects nerve conduction velocity (Mense 1978; Halle et al. 1981; Kramer 1985, 1987), and perhaps the effects can be explained in this way (overview in Lehmann 1990).

The so-called neural therapeutic setup described in some electrotherapy books, based on connective tissue massage, lacks any scientific basis.

5.6 Coupling Media

5.6.1 Direct Coupling

In order for sound to be transmitted to the tissue at all, a coupling substance is required. Otherwise, the sound would be 100% reflected at the transducer-air interface (the acoustic impedance of aluminum is 34,600 times greater than that of air). Typically, a special substance is used (e.g., Aquasonic®), which also conducts electricity. This makes it possible, if desired, to combine ultrasound with various electrotherapies, so-called simultaneous procedures. However, there is neither a physiological basis nor clinical evidence that this method is more effective than the separate application of ultrasound and, for example, TENS (Royer et al. 2018; Sangtong et al. 2019). Therefore, this procedure will not be discussed further.

Pharmaceutical gels are also suitable for coupling. In so-called sonophoresis (see Sect. 5.9), a medication is locally delivered through the skin using ultrasound. For this, the medication can be mixed 1:1 with regular ultrasound gel (Myrer et al. 2001) or only the pharmaceutical gel can be used (Cage et al. 2013). Ointments, due to their high fat content, absorb a great deal of sound and are therefore completely unsuitable as coupling agents (Ashton et al. 1998; Cameron and Monroe 1992; Cage et al. 2013). If ultrasound is to be used for local heating, a standard ultrasound gel should definitely be used. Naturally, the coupling agent should be at a comfortable temperature.

The temperature of the coupling agent is not unimportant! Oshikoya et al. found that gel that was too cold (18 °C) or too warm (39 °C) had a rather negative effect on the in vivo measured temperature increase (Oshikoya et al. 2000). The measurements were conducted on 18 healthy young men. A temperature probe was inserted 5 cm deep into the calf. The best result was achieved with a gel at 25 °C (temperature increase to 39.8 °C after 10.63 min at 5 cm depth, 1 MHz, BNR 4:1, ERA 4.1 cm^2, device was calibrated). With the 18 °C gel, using the same device, a temperature of 38.9 °C was reached after 12.96 min, and with the 39 °C gel, the tissue was warmed to 38.82 °C after 11.12 min. Thus, both too cold and too warm slowed the temperature increase. Not by much, but still.

5.6.2 Water

Water is often used as a medium for indirect coupling in so-called subaqueous ultrasound applications, especially when the treatment field is uneven or small, such as with hand patients or around the upper ankle joint. The problem, however, is that water does not conduct nearly as well as one might think (Robertson and Ward 1995a, b; Draper et al. 1993). If you still wish to use this method, there are several things to consider.

As Robertson and Ward did (1995a, b; 1996), take several pork knuckles and place them under precisely defined conditions in a water container, insert a thermocouple into the knuckles, and apply ultrasound. The fact that this involves dead tissue is irrelevant; the cooling effect of circulation would only have made the result more pronounced. Result: If the temperature increase in the tissue measured at 0 cm treatment distance (i.e., direct contact) is taken as 100%, the temperature increase in the tissue with the transducer at a 1 cm distance is 69% of that, at 2 cm it is 56%, and at 4 cm only 44% of the initial value (Ward and Robertson 1996a). The authors therefore recommend using a dosage factor to determine the desired intensity. The intensity should be increased by this factor: by 1.3 at 1 cm, 1.59 at 2 cm, and 2.07 if treating at 4 cm distance. Or, more simply: direct contact = 0 cm = no adjustment, 1 cm distance = 30% higher, 2 cm = 55% higher, and at 3 cm = 80% higher dosage. Treatment at a 4 cm distance is discouraged, as the high settings required quickly lead to cavitation bubbles forming on the transducer, which greatly hinder energy delivery. One could use boiled and sealed, cooled water. However, if the water is not kept sealed, it will reabsorb gases (nitrogen, oxygen, etc.), making the effort pointless. In a second study, the authors clearly confirmed the accuracy of these factors (Ward and Robertson 1996a, b).

Anyone who has ever treated subaqueously knows how difficult it is to maintain a constant distance to the target tissue.

Draper et al. conducted temperature measurements at a depth of 3 cm in the calf of 20 subjects during an ultrasound application (1.5 W/cm^2, 1 MHz, 10 min, device was calibrated, ERA 5 cm^2) (Draper et al. 1993). In 10 subjects, the transducer was applied directly to the skin with gel, while in the other 10, subaqueous treatment was performed with a constant transducer-calf distance of 1 cm. The gel group reached an average temperature of 40.3 °C after 10 min, while the subaqueous group reached only 37.5 °C. The initial temperature was 35.5 °C. Almost a 4 °C difference due to 1 cm! According to Robertson, the intensity should have been increased to 1.95 W/cm^2: 30% more.

It should also be noted that metal basins reflect sound, while plastic basins absorb sound. In 1995, Robertson was able to show that the temperature in the aforementioned 45 mm thick piece of pork increased by 50% more when using a metal basin compared to ultrasound in a plastic basin (2 cm distance, 1 MHz, ERA 5 cm^2, 1 W/cm^2, treated statically for 40 min). This is most likely due to the many reflections in the metal basin. The dosage factors mentioned above were determined in plastic basins. This means that the dosage must somehow be adjusted when using a metal basin, but unfortunately, data on this is lacking. So please use plastic basins.

For the therapist, it is advisable not to keep the hand in the water (for too long). Over time, this can lead to unpleasant sensations, and some colleagues even develop real pain in their fingers. To avoid such irritation, a thick kitchen glove can be worn. The air in the glove prevents sound penetration. Thin, tight-fitting latex gloves can conduct sound.

5.6.3 Gel Pads

A rather elegant method of coupling is the use of special gel pads (Merrick et al. 2002). These single-use pads, 1–2 cm thick and made of polyacrylamide, are used in situations where direct contact should be avoided, for example in wound treatment. Of course, they can also be used in uneven areas such as the MCP joints. When treating wounds, applying some sterile physiological saline or sterile ultrasound gel between the pad and the wound improves sound transmission. It is essential to avoid the formation of air bubbles. In a standard treatment, a little gel is applied between the skin and the pad and between the pad and the transducer as usual, i.e., skin-gel pad-gel-transducer (Bishop et al. 2004).

Sound transmission with pads is not the same as with regular gel. For example, Bishop et al. found that at a depth of 1 cm posterolateral to the ankle, halfway between the lateral malleolus and the Achilles tendon, after 10 min of ultrasound, the temperature increase was 7.72 °C with gel, 4.98 °C with the pad without gel, and 6.68 °C with the gel pad-gel combination (1 W/cm^2, 3 MHz, ERA 4 cm^2, BNR 3:1, n = 18, 3 measurements each).

5.6.4 Latex Gloves

Lima et al. investigated whether water-filled latex and nitrile gloves are suitable as cost-effective pads for ultrasound treatment (Lima et al. 2017). In the laboratory, they examined how much sound energy passed through gloves made of latex and nitrile filled with degassed, demineralized water. Unfortunately, the investigators did not mention whether they used ultrasound gel between the transducer and the glove. Nevertheless, the results were very good; the energy loss was never more than 0.5 W/cm^2. The gloves used had a thickness of 12 µm, i.e., 0.012 mm. Of course, water-filled condoms can also be used. These come in various thicknesses, from 45 to 105 µm, thus significantly thicker than the gloves mentioned.

To prevent air bubbles from forming due to cavitation, the water must be boiled beforehand, and as much air as possible should be squeezed out of the glove before sealing, as air greatly impedes sound energy transmission. This requires some skill and should be practiced before doing it in the presence of a patient. Plastic bags with so-called zip-lock closures are easy to seal, but may be too thick. There is no literature on this.

Steiss and Adams investigated how much air between the transducer and the skin impedes penetration (Steiss and Adams 1999). The authors measured the temperature increase during ultrasound treatment in the biceps femoris muscle of dogs at depths of 5 and 10 cm. Parameters: intensities ranging from 0.5–2.0 W/cm^2, 10 min, 1 MHz, continuous ultrasound. Results: Temperature increase at 5 cm depth in shaved treatment areas > 1.6 °C. Unshaved: increase at 5 cm depth between 0.4 °C and 0.7 °C, depending on hair length. In the fur, increases of 8.3 °C (short hair) up to 22.2 °C (long hair) were measured! Hair is hollow and contains air. Please shave, not just for dogs.

When treating wounds with this method, the wound should be moistened with sterile saline or sterile gel to improve coupling. To optimize transmission, ultrasound gel should be applied between the transducer and the glove (or condom). For intact skin, gel is applied to the skin. The transducer is then pressed against the glove with enough pressure to leave about 1 cm between the head and the skin. The head can now be moved without sliding over the glove, simply by deforming the assembly, or the transducer can be moved over the surface as usual. It is essential to ensure that the head is always held perpendicular to the tissue, otherwise the sound will be reflected!

5.7 Application Technique

Normally, treatment is performed dynamically: To ensure even energy distribution and to avoid hotspots, the transducer is moved in a controlled manner over the area to be treated, at a speed of about 2–4 cm per second. Whether you move in circles, figure eights, or back and forth is irrelevant, as long as you keep in mind that most of the energy is delivered in the center of the sound beam. This is where the tissue is heated the most. Therefore, it makes sense to overlap the treated areas.

Grey has shown how important it is to move the transducer extremely evenly over the treatment area, without leaving the area to be treated (Grey 2003). As soon as therapists are distracted by casual conversation, etc., the boundaries of the treatment area are constantly crossed, and this must be compensated for by adjusting the treatment time!

Conclusion
The author believes that templates, as used in many studies, are very useful. Perhaps our device manufacturers could come up with something?

Rotating around a central axis is pointless and even dangerous: Most of the ultrasound energy is delivered in the center of the transducer. Therefore, this central rotation would only lead to very strong heating in the center and certainly not to a better distribution of the ultrasound energy.

5.8 Treatment Technique, Dosage

The first question, as with any application, is whether ultrasound is indicated or not. The following scheme can be used to answer this question (Fig. 5.10):

1. Are there any **contraindications**? See below for more information.
2. What is your **treatment goal**?
   - Do you want to stimulate metabolic processes or (re)activate an inflammatory response to accelerate healing?
   - Do you want to achieve pain relief or improve blood circulation?
   - Do you want to improve the extensibility of shortened or scarred structures?
   - Do you want to deliver a medication?

If there is neither inflammation nor pain nor scarring, ultrasound is not indicated.

3. What **tissue** do you want to treat: collagen or muscle? Keep in mind that collagen heats up about 2 to 3 times faster than muscle (see below)! If the target tissue is unknown, treatment should not be performed.
4. How large is the **treatment area**? It should not be larger than about 2 to 3 times the ERA.
5. How **deep** is the problem located? About 5 cm is the limit.

After you have answered these questions and concluded that ultrasound is a meaningful

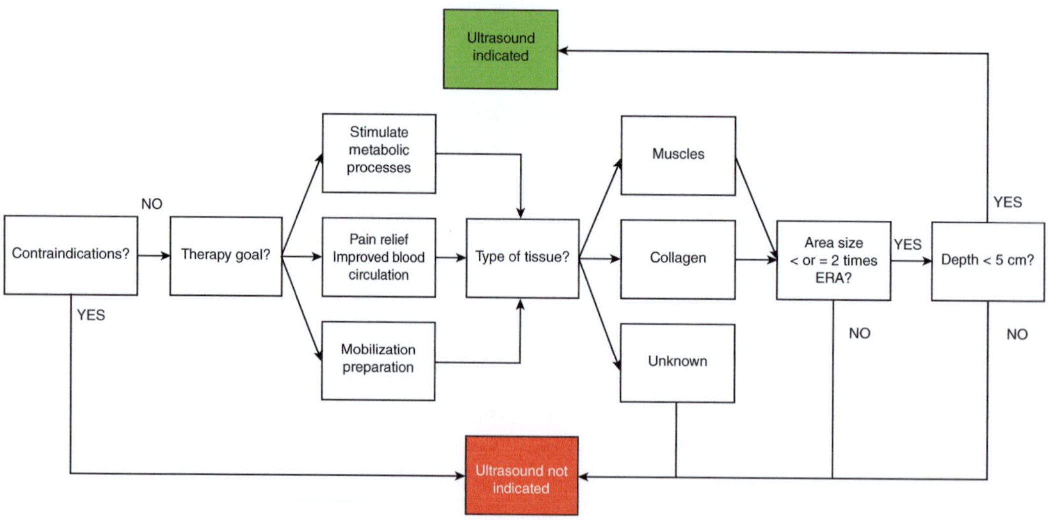

Fig. 5.10 Decision aid for the use of ultrasound

addition to your treatment, the question of dosage arises. The following discusses considerations for dosage in the thermal use of ultrasound.

5.8.1 Treatment Area

The size of the treatment area is of crucial importance. If the area to be treated is too large, the treatment will take too long, and while one part is being treated, the tissue elsewhere will cool down again (Garrett et al. 2000). Keep in mind that, depending on the indication, it takes several minutes to reach the desired temperature in the tissue. After that, this temperature must be maintained at this level for at least 5 min or longer. If the treatment is stopped too early, it was pointless and time and money have been wasted. The following dosage recommendations are based on studies in which an area of 2 × ERA was treated and whose effectiveness has been confirmed in patient studies.

These treatments usually lasted around 10–15 min. Now one might ask how to dose for smaller areas, for example, in a mobility-restricted acromioclavicular joint that is to be prepared for mobilization. The treatment area corresponds to about one ERA of 5 cm^2. In practice, you will quickly find that this is not a problem. If the transducer is carefully and evenly moved over the joint, you are essentially treating an area of 2 × ERA. Please note that most of the ultrasound energy is delivered in the central area of the treatment field: the edges receive significantly less (Miller et al. 2008), so the target tissue should be in the center of the treatment area.

5.8.2 Dosage

Dosage in ultrasound is somewhat challenging, but not impossible.

Older dosage recommendations, as found in older electrotherapy books, will not be discussed. These suggestions do not take into account the target tissue, the therapeutic goal, or the size of the treatment area (van Kerkhof 2011; Draper 2014).

In the past 25 years, various researchers have conducted studies with the aim of establishing the basics for ultrasound dosage. Draper and his colleagues were particularly thorough and productive, and, for example, investigated in vivo, mostly in the calf muscle, how intramuscular temperature increases at different depths, with different intensities and frequencies. They also studied the effects of pre-treatments with ice or hot packs, subaqueous treatment, treatment with gel and gel pads, the influence of subcutaneous fat thickness, and the heating of collagen tissue. Everything was meticulously documented to provide a foundation for the sound use of ultrasound. Other researchers addressed similar topics and found that Draper's results were sometimes not reproducible despite comparable parameters. The cause was soon clear: What is set on an ultrasound device is very often not what actually comes out of the transducer—in short: there is a lack of output. This is not a new finding.

In the USA, Australia, and Europe, studies on this topic were already conducted in the 1970s and 1980s, always with very depressing results. The oldest accessible publication on this topic is by Stewart et al. from 1974, in which the authors found, for example, that in 85% of the 64 ultrasound devices examined, the intensity deviated by more than 20% from the set value (Stewart et al. 1974). Not that much has changed since then. For example, Pye and Milford found 20 years later, in 1994, that of 85 ultrasound devices used daily in one region of Scotland, 69% had an energy output that deviated by more than 30% from the set value (Pye and Milford 1994). Some devices did not work at all. At the time of writing (2021), the most recent publication on this topic dates from 2016 (Gange et al. 2018). The authors compared the output of two devices from different manufacturers and found that with one device, the desired tissue temperature could not be achieved using research-based parameters, and the treatments were correspondingly ineffective. The list of publications on this topic is unfortunately long, and all studies report large deviations in brand-new devices and different outputs from transducers, new and old, between and within manufacturers. Not least, they report the frustration of researchers who complain about the futility of research because the devices are not interchangeable in terms of output. How are we supposed to use Draper et al.'s parameters when legislators allow ultrasound device manufacturers error margins that can cumulatively deviate up to 150% from the set values (Johns et al. 2007a, b; Straub et al. 2008)? No wonder, then, that the results of clinical studies and treatments in daily practice are often disappointing. This is despite the fact that we now have good measurement methods available and that in German-speaking countries, various laws regarding medical devices unequivocally require regular performance and safety checks of the devices used. Ultimately, it is a question of quality management and ethics (Roman 2017). Manufacturers should provide data from their devices that enable users to use correct treatment parameters.

The following explanations are based on the results of measurements by Draper et al. (1993, 1995), Rose et al. (1996), Chan et al. (1998), Gallo et al. (2004), and Miller et al. (2008). The investigators used ultrasound devices that produced reproducible results for other researchers as well. In device tests, the transducers from these manufacturers always showed the smallest deviations. The book by Justus Lehmann (1990) is the reference for temperature-related biological effects in tissue.

Dosage parameters are:

- Intensity,
- Treatment duration,
- Treatment interval,
- Size of the treatment series.

5.8.3 Thermal Effect

The thermal effect of continuous ultrasound has been demonstrated in many studies.

Under the influence of heat (Lehmann 1990)

- muscle tone is reduced (Mense 1978),
- blood circulation is improved (Baker and Bell 1991),
- permeability is increased (Sundaram et al. 2003; ter Haar 2007),
- pain relief occurs (Williams et al. 1987; Mardiman et al. 1995), and
- the extensibility of collagen is improved (Lehmann et al. 1970; Warren et al. 1971).

Many studies have consistently found that the desired effects only occur after the temperature has been maintained at a higher level for 5–30 min (Lehmann 1990).

Unfortunately, the reported values for the targeted therapeutically effective temperature differ among investigators. In Justus Lehmann's classic *Therapeutic Heat and Cold* from 1990, it is unequivocally stated that therapeutically effective temperatures are between 40 °C and 45 °C. This temperature range is supported by many studies. Lehmann uses the term "vigorous heating" for a treatment in which the tissue temperature is increased up to the tolerance limit without damaging the tissue, i.e., close to 45 °C. However, a very productive researcher like David Draper also refers to an increase of 3–4 °C, citing Lehmann, as "vigorous heating." Starting from an intramuscular temperature of 34–36 °C (triceps surae at 3 cm depth), a 3 °C increase may mean that the desired 40 °C is not reached in some cases.

However, this somewhat lower temperature is sufficient to stimulate metabolic processes. Abramson et al. (1958) were able to show that an intramuscular temperature increased to 38 °C by a 45 °C arm bath led to a significantly increased oxygen consumption and improved blood flow in the forearm.

If you want to affect the extensibility of collagen, the collagen must be heated to a temperature of 40–45 °C for at least 5 min to make it more stretchable. An Achilles tendon normally has an intratendinous temperature of about 30°. According to Draper's definition, a temperature increase of > 4 °C would be sufficient for "vigorous heating" to improve the extensibility of the tendon. In this case, the temperature must increase by at least 10 °C. This is confusing and has already been addressed by several authors; one should follow Lehmann. This improved extensibility, by the way, lasts for a maximum of about 3–5 min after sonication. Draper and Rose refer to this 3–5 min period as the "stretching window" (Draper et al. 1995; Rose et al. 1996).

The time it takes to reach a therapeutically effective temperature with ultrasound has been measured in vivo for muscle tissue and tendons.

5.8.4 Temperature Increase in Muscle Tissue

Draper et al. implanted temperature probes at various depths in the medial triceps surae of 12 subjects to measure temperature changes with 1 MHz ultrasound at 2.5 cm (the theoretical half-value depth for 1 MHz ultrasound) and 5.0 cm (double the HVD), as well as with 3 MHz ultrasound (in 12 other individuals) at 0.8 cm (theoretical HVD for 3 MHz ultrasound) and 1.6 cm depth (double the HVD). Each person received a total of four ten-minute ultrasound treatments, each at 0.5, 1.0, 1.5, and 2.0 W/cm^2, continuously. The temperature was measured every 30 s, the ERA was 4.5 cm^2, the treatment area corresponded to 2 × ERA and was precisely maintained using a template, the BNR was an impressive 1.8:1, and the device was calibrated (Draper and Ricard 1995).

No difference was found in the temperature increase at the various depths, meaning the tissue was heated homogeneously (!). As expected, 3 MHz ultrasound heated the tissue significantly faster than 1 MHz ultrasound, although not three times as fast as theoretically expected (Table 5.3).

Table 5.3 Temperature increase in the medial triceps surae at 1.6 cm and 2.5 cm depth

Temperature increase per minute with 1 MHz	Temperature increase per minute with 3 MHz
0.04 °C at 0.5 W/cm^2	0.3 °C at 0.5 W/cm^2
0.16 °C at 1.0 W/cm^2	0.58 °C at 1.0 W/cm^2
0.33 °C at 1.5 W/cm^2	0.89 °C at 1.5 W/cm^2
0.38 °C at 2.0 W/cm^2	1.4 °C at 2.0 W/cm^2

In an earlier study, Draper (Draper et al. 1993) showed that the thickness of the subcutaneous fat layer does not significantly affect the temperature increase. With 4–30 mm of fat, the increase at a depth of 3 cm in the calf remained nearly the same.

The values can be found in Tables 5.4 and 5.5. These tables allow for an estimation of the temperature increase in muscle tissue, though precise calculations are, of course, not possible.

5.8.5 Temperature Increase in Tendons

Tendons, like scars, have a different density than muscle tissue due to their higher collagen content. Because of this higher density, this tissue heats up more quickly than muscle tissue (Chan et al. 1998; Draper et al. 2010). Chan et al. treated the patellar tendons of 18 subjects in vivo with 3 MHz ultrasound, 1 W/cm^2 continuous, ERA 4.5 cm^2, treatment area 2 × ERA, template for control, BNR 1.8:1, and the device was calibrated. The thermocouple was placed "in the middle of the tendon," about 1 cm distal to the patella, so not very deep. After 4 min, the

Table 5.4 Temperature increase in muscle per minute with 1 MHz continuous ultrasound at a depth of 2.5 and 5 cm. ERA = 4.5 cm^2, treatment area = 2 × ERA (Draper et al. 1995)

	1′	2′	3′	4′	5′	6′	7′	8′	9′	10′
0.5 W/cm^2	0.04 °C	0.08 °C	0.12 °C	0.16 °C	0.20 °C	0.24 °C	0.28 °C	0.32 °C	0.36 °C	0.40 °C
1.0 W/cm^2	0.16 °C	0.32 °C	0.48 °C	0.64 °C	0.80 °C	0.96 °C	1.12 °C	1.28 °C	1.44 °C	1.60 °C
1.5 W/cm^2	0.33 °C	0.66 °C	0.99 °C	1.32 °C	1.65 °C	1.98 °C	2.31 °C	2.64 °C	2.97 °C	3.30 °C
2.0 W/cm^2	0.38 °C	0.76 °C	1.14 °C	1.52 °C	1.90 °C	2.28 °C	2.66 °C	3.04 °C	3.42 °C	3.80 °C

Table 5.5 Temperature increase in muscle per minute with 3 MHz continuous ultrasound at a depth of 0.8 and 1.6 cm. ERA = 4.5 cm^2, treatment area = 2 × ERA, red = potentially damaging (> 45 °C) (Draper et al. 1995)

	1'	2'	3'	4'	5'	6'	7'	8'	9'	10'
0.5W/ cm^2	0.3°C	0.6°C	0.9°C	1.2°C	1.5°C	1.8°C	2.1°C	2.4°C	2.7°C	3.0°C
1.0W/ cm^2	0.58°C	1.16°C	1.74°C	2.32°C	2.9°C	3.48°C	4.06°C	4.64°C	5.22°C	5.80°C
1.5W/ cm^2	0.89°C	1.78°C	2.67°C	3.56°C	4.45°C	5.34°C	6.23°C	7.12°C	8.01°C	8.90°C
2.0W/ cm^2	1.40°C	2.80°C	4.20°C	5.60°C	7.00°C	8.40°C	9.80°C	11.2°C	12.6°C	14.0°C

temperature had increased by 8–9 °C at a rate of just over 2 °C per minute. This is almost 3.5 times faster than muscle tissue is heated with the same settings! After about 4 min, the temperature had already dropped below the therapeutic range, meaning the therapeutic "window" had closed again (see below). Incidentally, the investigators also measured the temperature increase when using the same parameters but with a treatment area of 4 × ERA. As expected, the increase here was only 5 °C, i.e., 1.3°/min, still considerable.

Draper et al. repeated this in 2010, this time on the Achilles tendon. The aims of the study were to measure the temperature increase in the tendon and to compare the ultrasound conductivity of ultrasound pads and ultrasound gel. Result: Pads conduct ultrasound well, but not as well as gel; 2 cm thick pads conduct less well than 1 cm pads. Treatment parameters: calibrated device, 10 min, 3 MHz, ERA 4.2 cm^2, BNR 3.9:1, treatment area 2 × ERA (template), measurement at 1 cm depth in the tendon. Ultrasound was applied laterally to the tendon. Peak temperature increase with gel after 10 min was 13.3 °C (total 42 °C), 1 cm pad 9.3 °C (37.8 °C), 2 cm pad 6.5 °C (34.8 °C).

Conclusion

What do these results tell us? First, that tendons and scars heat up significantly faster than muscle, and this has consequences for treatment parameters. A therapeutically effective tissue temperature is reached more quickly in a scar, tendon, joint capsule, or muscle insertion than in muscle tissue. The different rates of increase observed by Chan (2 °C/min) and Draper (1.3 °C/min) vividly demonstrate the influence of reflections from bone. Draper's subjects lay prone and their Achilles tendons were insonated from lateral to medial, while Chan's subjects lay supine and the ultrasound was applied ventrally to the patellar tendon. Draper had no interfering reflections from bony structures, while Chan had plenty.

Draper's results also show that treatment with pads cannot be recommended without reservation. Merrick et al. (2002) studied the temperature increase in the calf with gel and pads and 1 MHz ultrasound, 1.5 W/cm^2 for 7 min, and achieved significantly better results. Perhaps it was due to their parameters or the ultrasound head, despite calibration. Johns et al. (2007a, b) explain how the conventional, legally required measurement methods unfortunately provide an incomplete picture of the exact output of an ultrasound head, especially of the three-dimensional energy field. In other words: the energy distribution in the acoustic field can vary enormously, and this cannot be measured with simple methods that only describe the ERA or the BNR. Qureshi et al. (2015) developed a temperature-sensitive plate based on liquid crystals that immediately shows the heat distribution directly at the ultrasound head. Unfortunately, it is only one-dimensional, but suitable for quick daily checks (Žauhar et al. 2019), and also cost-effective. Here, manufacturers are once again called upon.

5.8.6 Treatment Examples

Quite generally: If you do not regularly check the performance of your ultrasound transducers, you cannot know how much ultrasound energy is being emitted. This renders the following dosage information completely meaningless.

Conclusion

So: Please arrange for performance checks! Legislators in German-speaking countries are unequivocal on this: Operators of medical devices are required to have their equipment regularly checked for performance. The relevant regulations are freely available online.

The information provided is based on the aforementioned research findings, so please take into account the ERA, BNR, and the size of the treatment area. By the way: Calculations with decimal points are pointless. These are approximate values; the output of your ultrasound device may differ from the reference devices. Of course, the individual course must always be considered, and if therapy results are disappointing, the parameters should be individually adjusted before you throw in the towel.

Trigger points in the descending part of the trapezius muscle at a depth of 1–2 cm (see also Draper 2010)

Whatever is happening in a trigger point: We are dealing with a muscular problem with local pressure pain and a local metabolic issue (Moraska et al. 2013). With ultrasound, we can reduce pressure tenderness (Mardiman et al. 1995; Draper 2010), influence muscle spindle activity (Mense 1978), improve blood flow (Lehmann 1990), and stimulate metabolic processes (van't Hoff rule, Abramson et al. 1958). The depth is irrelevant here; between 0.5 and 2.5 cm, 3 MHz will heat the tissue evenly, while 1 MHz reaches up to 5 cm, but much more slowly (Draper et al. 1993, 1995). The treatment area is about 10 cm^2; with a 5 cm^2 transducer, this corresponds to about 2 × ERA. Please note that the ERA is always smaller than the "outer area" of the transducer. Target tissue: muscle. Treatment goal: pain relief before the "actual" manual trigger point treatment; we will also likely want to stimulate metabolic processes. What happens to the muscle spindles and how this affects the trigger point is unclear. Target tissue temperature: about 40 °C, meaning that starting from an initial temperature of 35–36 °C, we want to achieve about a 4 °C increase.

With 1 MHz ultrasound, this temperature is reached at 2 W/cm^2 after about 10 min. The temperature should then be maintained at this level for at least 5 min, which makes for a long session! Since the trigger points are not deep in the tissue, 3 MHz US can be used very effectively here; 3 MHz actually heats deeper than generally assumed (Draper et al. 1995; Hayes et al. 2004; Franson et al. 2014). At 1.5 W/cm^2, the target temperature is reached after about 5 min. If the patient tolerates this well, you could even treat with 2 W/cm^2, reaching the temperature after about 3 min. The patient should be instructed to report if the treatment becomes uncomfortable. This again highlights the importance of sensitivity testing and good patient instruction.

Maintaining temperature in the therapeutic range

Now comes a very important step! It is not enough to heat the tissue by 4–5 °C; you must absolutely maintain the temperature at this level for at least 5 min (Lehmann 1990). If you were to stop therapy now, the treatment would very likely be pointless. But if you continue with the same settings, the tissue temperature could rise so much that local burns occur (of course, the patient would report discomfort before this happens). To prevent this, you have three strategies available:

1. Switch the device to 50% pulsed ultrasound at the same intensity and frequency (= 1:2 on some devices). As already explained above, pulsed ultrasound is not synonymous with athermal treatment. If you switch to 50% at the same frequency and intensity, this halves the ultrasound energy, and the temperature increase over the next 5 min is only about 2 °C.
   At 3 MHz and 1.5 W/cm^2 in 50% pulsed mode, the temperature increases by about 2 °C after 5 min (50% × 0.89 × 5). At 1.0 W/cm^2, 1:2 pulsed, the temperature increases by 50% × 0.58 × 5 = about 1.5 °C, and at 2 W/cm^2 by a good 2 °C.
2. Reduce the initial 2 W/cm^2 to 1 W/cm^2 at the same frequency. After 5 min, the temperature at 2 W/cm^2 would have increased by another 5 × 1.4 °C, i.e., 7 °C, which could mean a final temperature of around 43 °C. This 43 °C is certainly not too high, but local pain sensitivity may mean the patient cannot tolerate it. By halving the intensity, the temperature increases only slowly and the targeted therapeutically relevant temperature remains between 40 and 45 °C, without overheating the tissue.
3. As a third alternative, you can switch from 3 MHz to 1 MHz. At 1 MHz and 2.0 W/cm^2, the temperature increase is about 0.4 °C/min, so over the next 5 min, the temperature rises from about 40 °C to about 42 °C, still within the therapeutic range.

Moving the transducer faster is pointless, and enlarging the treated area is too imprecise.

The second method—halving the intensity—was tested by Burr et al. in 2004 and unfortunately proved disappointing (Burr et al. 2004). The investigators performed the required measurements at a depth of 3 cm with 1 MHz ultrasound, and reducing from 2.4 W/cm^2 to 1 W/cm^2 initially led to a slight decrease in the achieved temperature. After about 3 min, the temperature was back at the desired level. The authors state that a reduction to 1.5 W/cm^2 might have been more effective in maintaining the target temperature. Why the temperature did not increase as expected by 0.16°/min after switching is unclear. Possibly, the factors mentioned by Johns et al. (2007a, b) played a role, or the cooling effect of improved blood flow was "to blame."

Mobilization of a post-traumatically or post-surgically movement-restricted wrist (after Draper 2010)

The treatment area is located on the volar and dorsal sides of the wrist, each about 1 × ERA (5 cm^2) in size. The structures to be treated are mainly very superficial collagenous tissue such as ligaments, joint capsules, and possibly scar tissue, with the bony structures also being very superficial, so reflections are to be expected. The goal is to prepare the shortened, scarred collagen tissue for mobilization treatment. To do this, the tissue must be heated to a temperature above 41 °C and the elevated temperature maintained at this level for at least 5 min. The following special conditions must be considered:

1. There are two treatment areas, one volar and one dorsal. It makes sense to choose one of the two in a therapy session. Treating both sides adequately is impossible. For example, if you reach the desired temperature volarly and then treat dorsally, by the time the required time for dorsal is up, the therapeutic window (see point 3) for volar has closed again. So, address either flexion or extension. In one session, for example, treat only dorsally and then perform your mobilization treatment as you have learned. The follow-up assessment will show whether the decision was correct.
2. The target tissue is collagen, and this tissue has different acoustic properties than muscle. In particular, collagen heats up 2 to more than 3 times faster than muscle (Draper et al.

2010; Chan et al. 1998). This has consequences for the treatment duration.
3. The desired temperature is 41–45 °C. In this temperature range, changes in the physiological properties of collagen allow for plastic adaptation to stretching (Lehmann et al. 1970). Interestingly, there is a so-called "therapeutic window." Draper et al. (1995) and Rose et al. (1996) have shown that after ultrasound treatment is stopped, the tissue remains at the desired therapeutic temperature of over 40 °C for only about 3–5 min. Only during this time can the collagen tissue be plastically deformed (Lehmann et al. 1970; Warren et al. 1971). After this time has passed, no further plastic adaptation occurs; the window is closed.

It therefore makes sense to begin gentle stretching during the ultrasound treatment! And it is thus completely pointless to perform an ultrasound treatment in the electrotherapy department to prepare for mobilization (or have it performed…), after which the patient has to wait half an hour for the treating therapist to perform the subsequent mobilization.

The initial temperature is 30 °C (Schmidt et al. 2011), the target temperature is about 10 °C higher. With 3 MHz and 1 W/cm^2—due to proximity to bone—a temperature increase of 2 °C/min (Chan et al. 1998) means the target temperature of > 40 °C is reached after 5–6 min, with 1.5 W/cm^2 after just 4–5 min. You can start with 1.5 W/cm^2 and, if the patient experiences pain, reduce the intensity to 1 W/cm^2. After this time, switch to pulsed mode as in the example above and continue treatment for at least 5 min. To make optimal use of the therapeutic window, mobilization treatment should begin during the ultrasound session, ideally as soon as the temperature is in the therapeutic range.

Subacute local overuse problem, for example at the lateral elbow

Assume the target tissue is the muscle insertion, a mixed tissue. The treatment goal is to stimulate metabolic processes, and for this, you want to increase the local temperature. The van't Hoff rule states that a temperature increase of 10 °C can double or triple the activity of metabolic processes; each degree means about 10% more activity. Thus, it seems irrelevant how high the local temperature rises, as long as you stay below 45 °C to avoid tissue damage. An overuse problem is usually locally painful, so you do not want the temperature to rise too much. You also want to keep the treatment within a reasonable time frame. Therefore, for our patient, we choose a local temperature increase of about 4 °C. Starting from a local temperature of about 33 °C, this means about 37–38 °C. Abramson (1958) measured a temperature of just over 35 °C at a depth of 3 cm in the brachioradialis; our muscle insertion will be somewhat cooler. The collagen in this mixed tissue will heat up faster than the muscle tissue, so the treatment parameters are a compromise. Experience shows it is better to base the dosage on the collagen, so this tissue is not overheated, especially due to proximity to bone and local sensitivity. The muscle tissue will be heated anyway by convection (via the blood) and conduction (thermal diffusion).

With 3 MHz and 1 W/cm^2, the target temperature is reached after 3–4 min; remember, we are treating tendon tissue. After reaching the target temperature, switch to 1:2 (50%) pulsed mode and continue ultrasound for 5 min (or longer!).

For thermal applications, you can assume that to warm up tissue with a transducer with an ERA of 5 cm^2, treatment times of at least about 10 to a maximum of 15 min are appropriate for an area up to 10 cm^2. This naturally limits the indications for ultrasound. Nevertheless, when treating trigger points and most insertional tendinopathies, the area to be treated is usually not much larger. Depending on depth and frequency used, the tissue has about 3–8 min to be heated, and the elevated temperature is maintained for at least 5 min. For larger treatment areas, ultrasound treatment takes too long, and shortwave therapy with a coil should be used as an alternative. Garrett et al. have impressively shown that for larger areas (200 cm^2 on the lower leg), shortwave therapy (27.12 MHz) is clearly superior to ultrasound treatment (Garrett et al. 2000). SW, pulsed, average energy output 48 W, 20 min, 3 cm depth: temperature increase 3–4 °C; ultrasound 1 MHz, 1.5 W/cm^2, 20 min: 0.09–0.17 °C (40 × ERA!).

When considering dosage, always take into account the target temperature and the current local temperature. To heat an Achilles tendon with a normal intratendinous temperature of about 30 °C to 41 °C, you must dose differently than for an intramuscular scar at a depth of 3 cm. Here, the scar tissue has the same temperature as the muscle tissue, i.e., around 35 °C. An adherent surgical scar up to 1 cm deep has the same temperature as the surrounding tissue, between 31 and 34 °C in the extremities (Schmidt et al. 2011), possibly even less in the hands.

Regarding movement speed

There are different recommendations regarding the speed at which the transducer should be moved over the treatment area. Weaver et al. investigated how different speeds affect temperature development at a depth of 3 cm in the calf muscle (Weaver et al. 2006). Parameters: 1 MHz, 1.5 W/cm^2, ERA 5 cm^2, area 2 × ERA (template), BNR 2.1:1. Speeds: 2–3 cm/s, 4–5 cm/s, 7–8 cm/s, controlled with a metronome. Result: Speed has no effect on the temperature increase. Except perhaps that 7–8 cm/s might make you a bit nervous. Device manufacturers are once again reminded of the template mentioned above.

Regarding treatment pressure

As with speed, there are different recommendations regarding the pressure with which the transducer should be held against the tissue. Gann answered this question in the lab, and Krasinski et al. addressed this issue in vivo (Gann 2003; Krasinski et al. 2013). Parameters: 3 MHz, ERA 4.1, area 2 × ERA (template), BNR 4.5:1, 1.5 cm depth in the calf, intensities 0.5–2.0 W/cm^2. Pressure: 200 g, 600 g, and 800 g, with the transducer weighted. The time to reach a temperature increase of 2 °C was measured. Result: The difference was not significant, although with 600 g pressure, the 2 °C was reached somewhat faster. The reason is unclear. The investigators suggest that perhaps the cooling circulation was interrupted by the pressure, or that tissue compression reduced the distance between the transducer and the thermocouple. But then 800 g pressure should have shown these effects even more, which was not the case. Let us note that pressure has no significant effect on the treatment outcome.

Regarding half-value depth

Theoretically, depending on the depth of the pathology, you should adjust the intensity on the device. However, the average half-value depths (HVD) are assessed very differently in the literature. The HVD at 1 MHz varies by author from 2.5 cm to about 4 cm, the HVD at 3 MHz between 0.8 and about 2.5 cm. These are rough estimates. Depending on the thickness of the subcutaneous fat layer (HVD 50 mm and 16.5 mm at 1 and 3 MHz, respectively), this should vary: A trigger point deep in the gluteal region would therefore require a different setting than a TP in the dorsal forearm. However, Draper and Sunderland have shown in vivo that the thickness of the subcutaneous fat layer, at least from 4 to 30 mm, has no significant effect on heating with 1 MHz ultrasound at a depth of 3 cm in the calf (Draper and Sunderland 1993).

Interestingly, another study by Draper and Ricard (1995) showed that the temperature increase at the theoretical HVD and at twice the HVD with 1 MHz and 3 MHz ultrasound was the same after a certain time! Demmink et al. (2003) found in their thermographic studies on pork shanks with and without bone no differences in penetration depth with 2 W/cm^2 and 0.86, 2, and 3 MHz ultrasound. These results show that dose calculations that attempt to account for the penetration depth of ultrasound are impossible in practice. The reasons?

- First, due to design, there are irregular interference phenomena with energy peaks in the ultrasound beam, with the BNR indicating their magnitude.
- Second, the three-dimensional energy distribution in the ultrasound beam varies from transducer to transducer, measurable with the so-called Schlieren method (Johns et al. 2007a, b; Straub et al. 2008).
- Third, the energy output measured over the transducer is not uniform (Quan et al. 1989).
- Fourth, unpredictable reflections and interferences occur in the tissue at boundaries and at bone.
- Fifth, the transducer may be damaged because it was dropped and no one said anything.

This is not to say that there is no decrease in energy and thus less heating deeper in the tissue. However, calculations in this regard are futile.

Regarding 3 MHz or 1 MHz

The common rule of thumb “superficial = 3 MHz and deep = 1 MHz” is untenable. For physical reasons, 3 MHz should heat tissue more superficially and 1 MHz more deeply. Hayes et al. (2004) surprisingly found that 3 MHz ultrasound at **2.5 cm depth** produced a temperature increase of 4 °C after just 3.35 min (± 1.23 min), with 40 °C reached after 4.13 ± 1.69 min. Parameters: ERA unknown (< 5 cm^2), BNR 5.5:1 (not verified), area 2 × ERA (with template), 1.5 W/cm^2. The comparative 1 MHz treatment did not even come close to this increase after 10 min (about 1.5 °C increase), but possibly the transducer was defective. The result means that 3 MHz ultrasound can be used effectively at least up to double the (theoretical) HVD, and not, as always claimed, only for very superficial pathologies at 0.3–1.5 cm depth. Franson et al. (2014) also measured the temperature increase with 3 MHz at 3 cm and 3.5 cm in the calf and found that after 8 min, the temperature at 3 cm depth had increased by 4 °C (from 36.51 °C to 40.15 °C). At 3.5 cm, it was still 3.18 °C. Parameters: 1.4 W/cm^2, ERA 4.2 cm^2, BNR 3:1, area 2 × ERA (again, this template …). It is clear that for many indications in physical and occupational therapy, 3 MHz can be used efficiently. The desired temperature is clearly reached more quickly, especially since the target tissue in many cases is scar tissue, which heats up 2 to more than 3 times faster than muscle tissue. For larger areas in muscle, inductive SW therapy is recommended.

5.8.7 Pulsed Ultrasound

The pulsed mode is intended to prevent or reduce the thermal effects of ultrasound while preserving the mechanical effects. The pause prevents the accumulation of heat, as the blood circulation can carry it away. In pulsed mode, the continuous sound is briefly interrupted, i.e., pulsed, depending on the settings. The settings on the device can mean different things depending on the manufacturer. For example, 1:4 can mean that ultrasound is applied for 1 ms, followed by a 4 ms pause, or the same setting can mean that after 2 ms of ultrasound, there is an 8 ms pause. In both cases, the total output of sound energy is reduced to 25%. Other manufacturers indicate these values in percentages, where, for example, 50% means that only half of the sound energy is delivered. However, the energy peaks remain the same! If 1 W/cm^2 is set, for example, 1 W/cm^2 is actually delivered during the 2 ms, and the pauses ensure that the power is reduced over the entire treatment time. More on this can usually be found, more or less clearly explained, in the operating manual.

Pulsed ultrasound is often referred to as “athermal ultrasound.” This is incorrect. There is always a thermal component (see Gallo et al. 2004).

Whether this pulsing is useful is controversial. Many authors consider ultrasound to be a fairly effective and convenient local heat application. Nevertheless, effects occur in the tissue that are not, or not primarily, temperature-dependent and are due to purely mechanical effects, with acoustic cavitation being a good candidate for explanation. Lennart Johns describes in his 2002 publication how mechanical ultrasound energy is absorbed by proteins and how this can lead to structural changes. As a result, the function of an enzyme or enzyme complex could be altered, thereby influencing certain intracellular processes. He calls his original theory the "Frequency Resonance Hypothesis," and his publication is quite interesting. All mechanical effects are difficult to measure in vivo, and our knowledge is limited to results from laboratory studies on cell cultures and animal experiments. The major problem with cell cultures lies in the implementation of dosing. Among other reasons, we still do not have clear treatment guidelines on when, how, and whether ultrasound should be used after an injury. Robertson and Baker published a review on the effectiveness of ultrasound in 2001. Of the many publications they reviewed, 10 were scientifically acceptable and were further analyzed. Reports included continuous and pulsed ultrasound with 5 different frequencies, with intensities between 0.02 and 2.6 W/cm^2 and durations of 2–15 min. And this for the treatment of 9 different indications. The quality or calibration of the ultrasound devices used was not considered.

What the clinician needs are precise details about the pathology, including stage, dosage, and hardware used. In addition, we would like the manufacturer to provide exact information on heating rates at various depths in muscle and tendon, on ERA and BNR. And if it's not too much to ask, please provide a method to quickly and accurately check the output of my device in daily practice. Thank you!

Laboratory investigators are somewhat more consistent. Most often, ultrasound is applied for 10 min at 1 MHz or 3 MHz with intensities of 0.1–1.5 W/cm^2 (Johns 2002). The often-used argument that one cannot extrapolate from the petri dish to patients is not entirely correct. If the stimulus is appropriate, that is, if a certain threshold is exceeded, a cell will respond—whether it is in a petri dish or in the human body. Below is an incomplete list of laboratory-proven effects of ultrasound:

- Ultrasound stimulates the production of interleukin-1β, interleukin-8, vascular endothelial growth factor, basic fibroblast growth factor, fibroblast growth factor, and collagen in osteoblasts and monocytes (Doan et al. 1999; Reher et al. 1999).
- Ultrasound stimulates the growth of fibroblasts and osteoblasts (Harvey et al. 1975; Webster et al. 1980; Doan et al. 1999; Reher et al. 2002).
- Cavitation (ter Haar et al. 1982), together with the associated microstreaming, improves permeability, enabling the delivery of drugs (including Mitragotri et al. 1995a, b; ter Haar 2007).
- Ultrasound stimulates the formation of new blood vessels (Young and Dyson 1990; Reher et al. 1999; Nazer et al. 2015).
- Pulsed ultrasound supports wound healing in rats, chickens, miniature pigs, and humans (Byl et al. 1992; Gan et al. 1995; Emsen 2007; Taradaj et al. 2008).
- Pulsed 1 MHz and 3 MHz ultrasound causes arterial vasodilation in healthy humans via stimulation of the arterial endothelium (Cruz et al. 2016; Hauck et al. 2019).

In this sense, ultrasound is not anti-inflammatory, but rather stimulates inflammation and growth, and this property is particularly valuable in the treatment of fresh injuries and wounds (ter Haar 1999; Ennis et al. 2016).

This raises the question of dosage—a chicken tendon is not a human Achilles tendon. Let's look at some data:

- Emsen (2007) treated his skin-grafted rats daily for "at least 5 min" with pulsed ultrasound (2 ms on, 8 ms off), 1 MHz and 3 MHz, 0.1 W/cm^2 and 0.18 W/cm^2, and was successful with both settings, i.e., fewer necroses than in the control group. He achieved better results with the slightly higher dosage.

- Gan et al. (1995) performed tenotomy and reconstruction of the flexor digitorum profundus tendon in Leghorns. One group of chickens was not treated with ultrasound, one group was treated starting on the 7th postoperative day, and one group starting on the 42nd postoperative day. Direct ultrasound was applied with a 0.5 cm^2 head (sic), 3 MHz, 0.8 W/cm^2, 3 min, 25% pulsed. The treated chickens showed a more regular scar structure and less inflammatory infiltrate, with the early-treated group having the better results. The tensile strength was the same in both treated groups and not less than in the untreated chickens. Incidentally, chicken tendons are comparable in composition to human tendons (Turner et al. 1989).
- Taradaj et al. (2008) observed accelerated healing of leg ulcers in vivo with the following treatment parameters: 0.5 W/cm^2, pulse 2 ms, pause 8 ms, 1 MHz, subaqueous, distance head-ulcer 2 cm. A 5 cm^2 ulcer received 5 min of ultrasound, and for each additional cm^2 the treatment duration was extended by 1 min. Ulcers larger than 20 cm^2 were treated in two stages. Treatment was daily, 6 times per week, for 7 weeks. The results in the ultrasound group were better than in the untreated control group and comparable to a group of patients who underwent surgery. Treating operated patients with ultrasound proved to be pointless.
- Young and Dyson (1990) found more blood vessels in skin sections of rats after 5 days when treated with ultrasound, 5 min daily, 0.75 MHz and 3.0 MHz, 0.1 W/cm^2. After 7 days, the difference between treated and untreated was no longer visible.
- Byl et al. (1992) treated ear injuries in miniature pigs with 1 MHz ultrasound, 2:8 pulsed, 10 min, 3 days at 0.5 W/cm^2 and then 2 days at 1.5 W/cm^2. Despite the fact that ultrasound was applied through the dressing, the treated ears were more tensile after one week than the untreated ones, and more degranulated mast cells were counted in the treated wounds.
- Reher et al. (1999) worked with mice and found that 3 MHz US, 1:4 pulsed, 0.1 W/cm^2 strongly stimulated the osteoblasts present in bone. Higher intensities, 0.75–2 W/cm^2, inhibited activity.
- Doan et al. (1999) used a standard therapeutic ultrasound device with settings of 1 MHz, 2:8 pulsed, and intensities of 0.1, 0.4, 0.7, and 1.0 W/cm^2. The higher intensities (0.7 and 1.0 W/cm^2) showed the greatest increases in DNA synthesis. Reher et al. (1999) also used a standard ultrasound device and achieved the best results with 1 MHz and 0.1 and 0.4 W/cm^2, 2:8 pulsed (2 ms sound, 8 ms pause). Both research groups continuously calibrated their devices.
- Cruz et al. (2016) and Hauck (2019) studied in humans how ultrasound affects the endothelium of an artery. Their parameters: conventional therapy device, calibrated, ERA 5 cm^2, 0.4 W/cm^2, 5 min, continuous and 2:8 pulsed, 1 MHz, the diameter of the brachial artery was measured by the FMD method on the upper arm. They found a significant dilation of the artery, which lasted for 20 min. A thermal component was excluded.

Very complex processes occur during injuries, so it makes sense to interfere with these processes as little as possible. This does not mean that therapy is not indicated. In the animal experiments, healthy, well-nourished animals were used, so it can be assumed that wound healing processes in these animals would proceed optimally even without "therapy." Nevertheless, better results were achieved with ultrasound than in the untreated control animals. In this sense, ultrasound can also be used to optimize these processes in healthy individuals, as is common in sports physiotherapy. In the presence of an underlying disease, where normal healing is delayed, such as in diabetes, therapeutic intervention is clearly indicated. In this case, it is advisable to dose as high as necessary but as low as possible. In any case, pulsed ultrasound appears to be better suited for stimulating wound healing than continuous ultrasound, since the processes mentioned above are not temperature-dependent. In addition, this avoids the potentially harmful effects of continuous ultrasound (Pan et al. 2005).

It is clear that to develop treatment guidelines, we need standardization of research methods. In general, however, it is evident that stimulation of biological processes involved in wound healing tends to be achieved with lower dosages such as 0.5–1 W/cm^2, 2:8 pulsed, after just a few minutes. The frequency appears to be irrelevant. This is logical, since in the studies mentioned above, penetration depth was unimportant.

Another area of application for pulsed ultrasound is the delivery of drugs, known as sonophoresis.

5.9 Sonophoresis

(Ultra-)sonophoresis, also called phonophoresis, refers to the delivery of drugs through intact skin using ultrasound. That the method works is undisputed. How it works is also fairly clear: cavitation in the stratum corneum leads to improved permeability, and the sound pressure "drives" the drug through the resulting "channels" deeper into the tissue (Nyborg 1982; Meidan et al. 1995; Mitragotri et al. 1995a, b; Wolloch and Kost 2010). Cagnie et al. elegantly demonstrated that sonophoresis can deliver about 10 times as much ketoprofen into the synovial membrane of the knee as a standard topical application (Ballerini et al. 1986; Cagnie et al. 2003). Pulsed ultrasound was more effective here than continuous application (1 MHz, 1.5 W/cm^2, ERA 5 cm^2, area 2 × ERA, 20% pulsed, 5 cm Fastum® gel, 5 min). Other researchers came to similar results, sometimes in humans (Ebrahimi et al. 2012), sometimes in rats (Asano et al. 1997). Rosim and colleagues were very original and treated two areas of 225 cm^2 (!) each on the backs of 14 subjects with 1 MHz ultrasound, 0.5 W/cm^2 continuous sound, and then immediately applied 2.5 g of a commercial diclofenac gel per area (Rosim et al. 2005). Blood samples were taken and analyzed before, and 1, 2, and 3 h after. The same procedure was repeated a month later with the same subjects, but this time with the device switched off, i.e., as with a normal topical gel application. Result: 1 and 2 h after pretreatment with ultrasound, the diclofenac concentration in the serum was 2.4 and 1.4 times higher, respectively! Pulsed ultrasound appears to be more effective for sonophoresis, although it is unclear why. Ebrahimi and Asano prefer pulsed ultrasound because it allows them to work with higher intensities without producing significant thermal effects, thus providing more "sound pressure." According to the authors, heating would not only be uncomfortable for the patient but could also destroy the drug. It is also known that the improvement in permeability is frequency-dependent (Meidan et al. 1995; Mitragotri et al. 1995a, b; ter Haar 2007; Wolloch and Kost 2010), with lower frequencies such as 20 kHz often achieving better results. One can speculate whether pulsed 1 MHz ultrasound has similar properties to 20 kHz ultrasound. However, frequency is not the only parameter at play; the physicochemical properties of the drug used also play a very important role in sonophoresis. Beetge et al. (2000) and Mitragotri et al. (1995a, b) explain how, above all, the lipophilic and hydrophilic properties of a substance play an important role in determining whether a drug can be successfully delivered or not.

Of the substances listed in Table 5.6, positive results from clinical studies in humans are available. This means that the use of these substances had a positive effect on the condition studied compared to a control group. Not listed are drugs for which no effect could be demonstrated, and studies for which the parameters could not be determined. If the results of different studies for a particular drug were comparable, the methodologically better study was listed.

There are a large number of studies on sonophoresis, but unfortunately most are unusable because the treatment parameters are not traceable. The studies listed in the table are certainly not highlights of physiotherapy-related research,

Table 5.6 Substances for which usable results from clinical studies are available

Substance	Studies
Ketoprofen 2.5%	CTS 1:4 pulse, 1 MHz, 1 W/cm^2, ERA 5 cm^2, 15 min. Better than placebo and splint only (Yildiz et al. 2011) Osteoarthritis/arthritis of the knee: 1 MHz, 1.5 W/cm^2, 8 min, ERA 5 cm^2, better than control group, but same result as SWD and ultrasound without drug (Boyaci et al. 2013)
Diclofenac	Lateral epicondylitis: 1 MHz, continuous, 2 W/cm^2, 7 min. Better than control group, questionably better than with LLLT (Faisal et al. 2013) CTS: 3 MHz, continuous, 1.5 W/cm^2, ERA 5 cm^2, better than control group (Soyupek et al. 2012) Knee osteoarthritis/arthritis: 1 MHz, 1.5 W/cm^2 continuous or 1:5 pulse, ERA 5 cm^2, area 2 × ERA, 5 min. Phono better than control group, pulse/continuous same result (Deniz et al. 2009) Knee osteoarthritis/arthritis: ERA 4 cm^2, 1 MHz, 1 W/cm^2, 5 min, continuous. Better than ultrasound without drug (Akinbo et al. 2007)
Dexamethasone	Knee osteoarthritis/arthritis 1 MHz, continuous, 1 W/cm^2, 10 min. Better than ultrasound without drug (Said Ahmed et al. 2019) CTS ERA 5 cm^2, 1 W/cm^2, 1 MHz, 20% pulse, 5 min, better than ionto (Bakhtiary et al. 2013)
Betamethasone 0.1%	CTS 1 MHz, 1 W/cm^2, continuous, 10 min. Better than control group (Gurcay et al. 2012)
Ibuprofen 5%	Knee osteoarthritis/arthritis 1 MHz, 1 W/cm^2, 5 min, continuous. Gel better than cream better than control group (Benlidayi et al. 2018) Psoriatic arthritis of the hand: 1 MHz, 1.5 W/cm^2, 5 min, continuous. Better than topical and placebo US (Abd el Baky and Waked 2011)
Indomethacin 1%	Temporomandibular joint: 1 MHz, 0.8–1.5 W/cm^2, ERA 3.4 cm^2, 15 min, continuous. Better than placebo (Shin and Choi 1997)

as there are also criticisms of these publications—usually the sample sizes are small and the technical details of the devices are incomplete. Not a single author mentions, for example, whether the device used was calibrated, and one has to guess the size of the treatment area. Nevertheless, the listed publications may provide the reader with some guidance for dosing.

Consequences for the Use of Sonophoresis, Risks and Side Effects

There are several things to consider with sonophoresis:

- First, as outlined above, not every substance is suitable for sonophoresis. Experience shows (caution: second-lowest level of evidence!) that colleagues sometimes use interesting substances for sonophoresis. The author vividly remembers a patient for whom a colleague used an ointment containing a certain snake venom (made in the USA). The patient had brought this remedy back from a trip and wanted his tennis elbow treated with it. The local reaction was impressive, despite the fact that ointments allow little sound to "pass through." It is essential to perform an allergy test on an inconspicuous area beforehand, unless the patient has already (credibly) used the product without problems.
- Second, not every product is suitable as a coupling medium. Ointments contain too many fatty substances and therefore absorb too much sound; gels are better suited for coupling. Homemade coupling agents with ointments and ultrasound gel do not work or work very poorly (Casarotto et al. 2004; Cage et al. 2013).
- Third, physiotherapists and their equipment are a significant vector in the spread of nosocomial infections (Crowcroft et al. 1996; Schabrun and Chipchase 2006; Sprat et al. 2014). Most commonly, this involves nonspecific microorganisms in the ultrasound gel, but unfortunately, methicillin-resistant Staphylococcus aureus (MRSA) is sometimes also found. In our own investigation at a large hospital, we found Burkholderia

cepacia, a multidrug-resistant microorganism that everyone has on their shoe soles and which can cause very serious complications, especially in patients with cystic fibrosis, in the ultrasound gel. It turned out that in the hospital's central laboratory, all departments using ultrasound (orthopedics, rheumatology, gynecology) were supplied from a large stock canister of ultrasound gel, and this canister was contaminated. It goes without saying that there was a rapid switch to the somewhat more expensive purchase of small bottles. The myth that therapeutic ultrasound heads must not be cleaned with 70% alcohol unfortunately persists. This only applies to heads used for echography. These have a structure at the front that can be damaged by alcohol. For these heads, there are special wipes.

- Fourth, when using an anti-inflammatory agent, the therapeutic goal must be carefully considered. In vitro studies clearly show that ultrasound stimulates the growth of cells involved in wound healing; in this sense, ultrasound is pro-inflammatory. Li et al. (2007) studied the effect of LIPUS (Low Intensity Pulsed Ultrasound) and celecoxib (an NSAID) in rats with a stress fracture. Result: LIPUS stimulated bone healing, celecoxib had a significantly inhibitory effect on osteoblast activity. So, for example, if you apply sonophoresis with diclofenac to a patient with a fresh ankle sprain, you are certainly not doing them any favors.
- Fifth: We can deliver drugs in two ways: with ultrasound and with electricity. That iontophoresis works is proven; more on this in the relevant Sect. 2.13. However, iontophoresis has two major disadvantages: first, it does not reach deep layers (Panus et al. 1999), and second, due to the very long treatment duration, there is always a risk of skin electrolysis, which can cause unsightly burns. With sonophoresis, deeper layers can be reached in a short time without the risk of burns. Incidentally, the study by Rosim et al. shows that it is quite sensible to locally massage in the gel used after sonophoresis to take advantage of the improved permeability (Fig. 5.11).

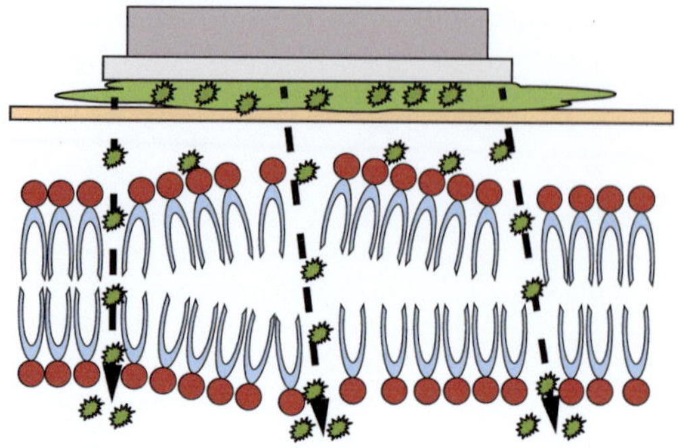

Fig. 5.11 Sonophoresis. The permeability improved by cavitation facilitates the delivery of active substances (green) with sound pressure

5.10 Ultrasound and Wound Healing

Ultrasound has been used for decades in the treatment of poorly healing wounds. Despite a multitude of publications on this topic, there is no consensus regarding the exact procedure or its effectiveness. One important reason for this is, firstly, the poor quality of the studies, as shown by two Cochrane reviews (Cullum and Liu 2017; Kavros and Coronado 2018). The authors conclude that there are too few good studies to definitively assess the effectiveness of ultrasound in the treatment of venous and arterial ulcers. The heterogeneity of the cases studied further complicates matters. A pressure ulcer in a paraplegic patient has a different etiology than a leg ulcer with a venous, arterial, or diabetic background, or even a combination of arterial occlusive disease with diabetic neuropathy. Secondly, in many studies, the dosage and application are unclear, and treatment times are often determined arbitrarily. We have also seen how the performance of ultrasound devices can vary in everyday practice. Nevertheless, from the many publications, it is possible to distill the parameters that most frequently lead to success. Generally, low doses are used, with intensities of 0.5 W/cm^2 up to a maximum of 1 W/cm^2, and a 2:8 pulsed mode is common (2 ms on, 8 ms off). 1 MHz appears to be more effective than 3 MHz, and a treatment duration of 1–3 min per cm^2 is considered appropriate. Both the wound itself and the wound edges are treated. It is not necessary to move the ultrasound head through the open wound. In 2007, Poltawski and Watson investigated whether ultrasound for wound treatment can be applied through dressing material and found that there are a variety of film dressings that conduct ultrasound excellently. The complete list can be found in the publication, which is freely available for download on the internet (Poltawski and Watson 2007). Of course, care must be taken to ensure that there are no air bubbles under the dressing material, as the ultrasound would otherwise be completely reflected.

5.11 High Power Pain Threshold Ultrasound (HPPTUS)

A rather specialized way of using ultrasound is HPPT ultrasound. This method is used in the treatment of myofascial trigger points and was briefly described by Travell and Simons in part 1 of their classic work on trigger points (Travell and Simons 1999, Vol. 1, p. 146). The first systematic clinical investigation dates from 2004 (Majlesi and Ünalan 2004), followed by publications reporting successful outcomes by Bahadir et al. (2009) and Kim et al. (2014a, b). An intensity of 1.5 to 2 W/cm^2 and a frequency of 1 MHz are used. The ultrasound head is held stationary on the trigger point until the patient's pain tolerance threshold is reached. After enduring pain for 4–5 s, the ultrasound head is moved over a larger area for 15–30 s until the pain subsides. This process is then repeated two more times. Majlesi and Ünalan note that the method requires great concentration and good communication between patient and therapist. Kim et al. found better effects with HPPTUS than with conventional ultrasound (1 MHz, continuous, 1 W/cm^2, 5 min), interestingly not in older patients (around 70 years old), where the application produced the same results as conventional ultrasound (1 MHz, 1 W/cm^2, continuous, 5 min) (Kim et al. 2014a, b). Bahadir et al. were able to demonstrate with EMG that the so-called LTR (Local Twitch Response) decreased after HPPTUS. The HPPTUS group combined with active movement therapy had better results than the dry needling group with the same movement therapy. The mechanism of action is unclear. A thermal component is unlikely due to the short duration; perhaps there is a brief but intense increase in permeability that affects the local metabolic state. Pain relief in the sense of DNIC could also be a possibility.

5.12 Extracorporeal Shock Wave Therapy (ESWT)

Extracorporeal shock wave therapy (ESWT) is considered a special type of ultrasound, with some of the same processes being stimulated. It is a treatment in which mechanical stimuli with different frequencies and intensities are transmitted to the tissue, and a distinction must be made between shock waves and pressure waves (Fig. 5.12). "True" ultrasound waves are mechanical waves that act on the tissue for a certain period with constant intensity and equally sized positive and negative pressure phases. A shock wave has a very short wavelength of about 1.5 mm (like ultrasound) and a very rapidly increasing positive pressure phase (< 1 ns), followed by a rather weak negative "rebound phase" (Fig. 5.12). A pressure wave has a significantly longer wavelength of 15 cm to 1.5 m and a somewhat slower rise in intensity (up to 5 μs); the pressure in the tissue can increase up to 1 MPa (10 Atm), and the rebound in the tissue lasts somewhat longer. The wavefront in shock waves, where compression occurs, is a region in which sudden, enormous changes in tension, density, and temperature occur in the tissue, with pressure increases up to 100 MPa, almost 1000 Atm! Shock waves are generated either electromagnetically, electrohydraulically, or piezoelectrically; the technical details will not be discussed further here. It is important to distinguish between high-energy focused shock waves (also called fESWT or "hard shockwave") and low-energy radial pressure waves (often RSWT, rESWT, or "soft shockwave").

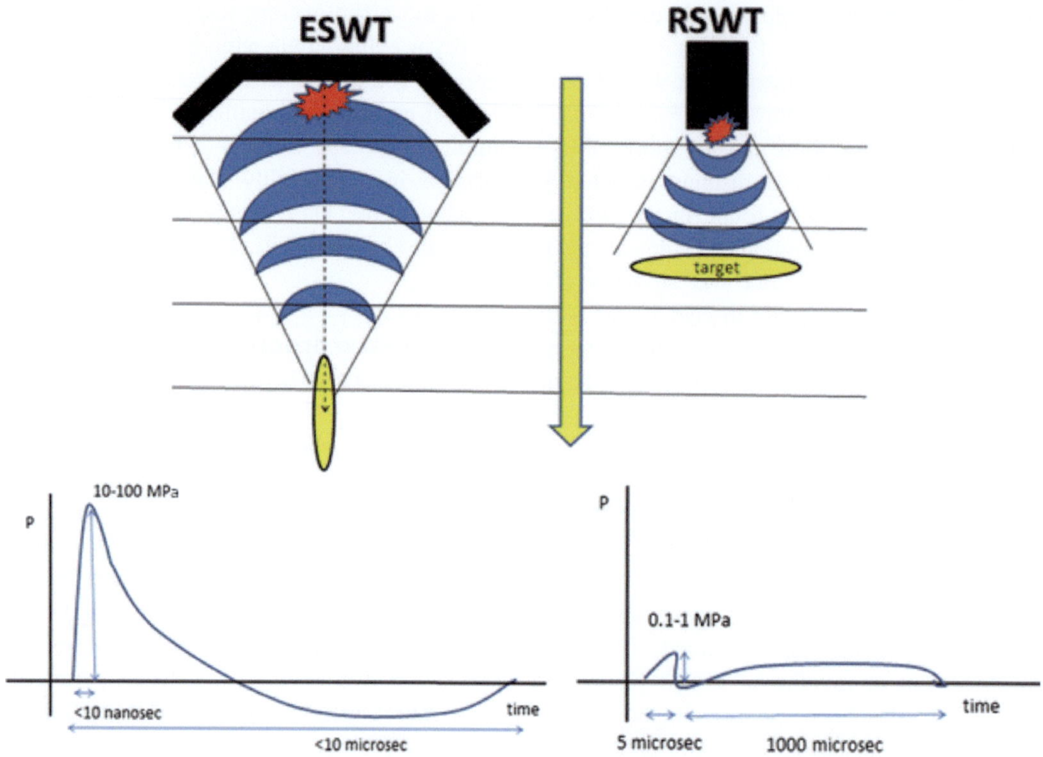

Fig. 5.12 Differences between extracorporeal shock waves (ESWT) and radial pressure waves (RSWT). Below: Course of the shock and pressure wave. MPa: Megapascal. From Notarnicola et al. 2012, with kind permission

For the sake of completeness, it should be mentioned that instead of RSWT, the term Extracorporeal Pulse Activation Therapy (EPAT) is also used. The difference between ESWT and RSWT is that the focused waves are concentrated, i.e., focused, on a specific point. Most of the energy is delivered at this point, and with this technique, depths of up to 20 cm can be reached, in contrast to the maximum 3.5–4 cm with the radial pressure wave device. It is mainly the spherically spreading pressure waves of radial pressure wave therapy that are used by therapists in the treatment of musculoskeletal pathologies, which is why only this method will be discussed below. Incidentally, the term "radial shock wave therapy" is incorrect; it would be correct to refer to pressure waves, as the pulse duration of pressure waves is significantly longer. Unfortunately, the term has become established, which often makes the interpretation of studies more difficult. In the following, the term "radial pressure wave therapy (rPWT)" will be used. Radial pressure waves are generated ballistically. For this purpose, a projectile is pneumatically or electromagnetically fired in a tube at a speed of about 5–25 m/s towards the treatment head, and the impact energy is transferred to the tissue. Comparisons with an air rifle are not far-fetched (Fig. 5.13).

5.12.1 Dosage of Radial Pressure Wave Therapy (rPWT)

Several parameters are important when dosing pressure wave therapy. In addition to the number of pulses delivered and their energy and frequency, there are the number of treatments per week, the total number of sessions, and the

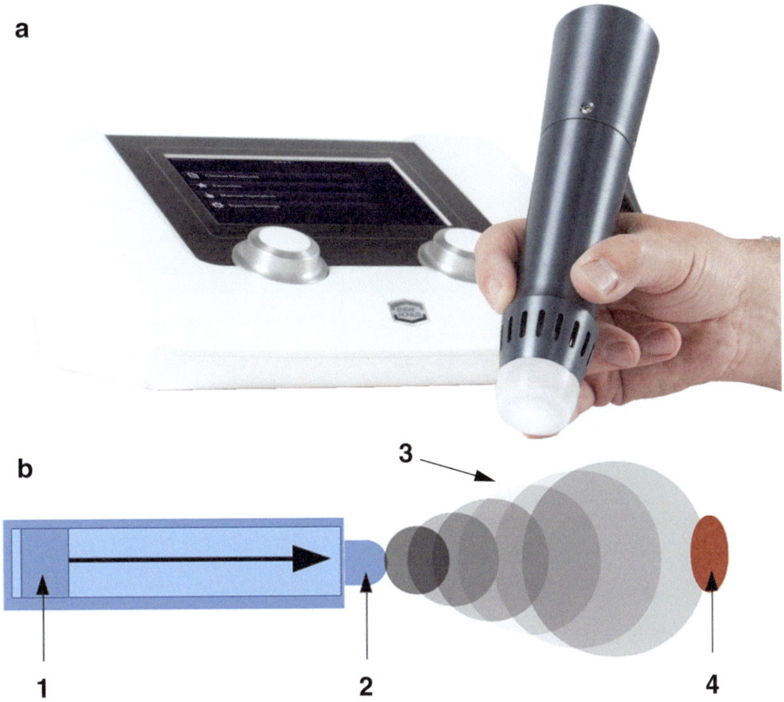

Fig. 5.13 **a** Pressure wave device. © Enraf-Nonius B.V. Delft, Netherlands, with kind permission. **b** Principle of a pressure wave device. 1: Projectile, 2: Applicator, 3: radial pressure wave, 4: Target

possible use of a local anesthetic, which is rather uncommon in rPWT. The energy or Energy Flux Density (EFD), i.e., the energy per area, is expressed in millijoules per mm^2 (mJ/mm^2) for the "true" focused ESWT devices. The energy delivered by the air pressure version of the rPWT device is given in bar, and for the electromagnetic version, in mJ. To annoy us clinicians (the author can see no other reason), many publications like to mix up the terminology. This is not helpful when trying to determine the dosages used. Here is a little help: When using a 15 mm^2 head on the rPWT device, 1 bar corresponds to 60 mJ, 2 bar to 90 mJ, 3 bar to 120 mJ, 4 bar to 150 mJ, and 5 bar to 180 mJ. The 3 bar correspond to 0.12 mJ/mm^2 on the fESWT device, and 5 bar correspond to 0.38 mJ/mm^2 on the fESWT device. Treatment with high-energy focused shock waves can be very painful, which is why a local anesthetic is often administered. However, this complicates the treatment, as the exact localization of the shocks often relies on the patient's feedback. It has also been found that a local anesthetic significantly reduces the effectiveness of the treatment (Klonschinski et al. 2011). The explanation seems plausible. The local anesthetic blocks the conduction of nociceptive C fibers. If these C fibers are stimulated, they express neuropeptides such as CGRP and substance P (SP), which play a key role in wound healing. These substances act on cells such as mast cells, immune cells, and muscle cells in the vessel wall and cause an inflammatory reaction. This reaction is called neurogenic inflammation because it is of neurogenic origin; it is characterized by redness and warmth (secondary to vasodilation), swelling (secondary to plasma extravasation), and increased sensitivity (secondary to changes in the excitability of certain nerve fibers): rubor, calor, tumor, and dolor (Herbert and Holzer 2002a, b). This neuropeptide release serves to maintain and protect

Table 5.7 Overview of possible mechanisms of action of pressure wave and shock wave therapy (list from Reilly et al. 2018)

Mechanism	Reference
Neovascularization at the tendon-bone junction	Wang et al. (2002)
Destruction of calcific deposits	Peters et al. (2004)
Increase in collagen synthesis, tissue remodeling	Bosch et al. (2007), Vetrano et al. (2011)
Leukocyte infiltration	Rompe et al. (1998)
Tenocyte proliferation	Chen et al. (2004)
Increase in glycosaminoglycan synthesis, protein synthesis	Bosch et al. (2007)
Increase in IL-6, IL-8, MMP-2, MMP-9, collagen synthesis	Waugh et al. (2015)
Increase in TGF-β1, IGF-1, collagen synthesis	Wang et al. (2002), Chen et al. (2004)
Mechanotransduction, increase in collagen synthesis	Bosch et al. (2007)
Enhanced osteoprogenitor cell differentiation	Wang et al. (2002)
Stimulation of C fibers with neuropeptide release	Klonschinski et al. 2011
Nociceptor hyperstimulation/gate control theory	Saggini et al. (2015a, b), Wess (2008), Vahdatpour et al. (2013), Zimmermann et al. (2009)
Increase in local pain-inhibiting substances	Saggini et al. (2015a, b), Wess (2008), Vahdatpour et al. (2013), Zimmermann et al. (2009)
Impairment of cell membrane receptor potential	Wess (2008)

IL = Interleukin; MMP = Matrix metalloproteinase; TGF-β1 = Transforming Growth Factor beta 1; IGF-1 = Insulin-like Growth Factor 1

the tissue. Substance P stimulates the proliferation of fibroblasts (in vitro), SP and CGRP have a promoting effect on angiogenesis and accelerate wound healing. Because the reaction is neurogenically induced, it does not occur or is less pronounced if the responsible nerve fibers are blocked by local anesthesia. Klonschinski et al. suggest that for very painful treatments, patients should be given conventional painkillers in advance, as these have a different mechanism of action and do not interfere with the effect of shock wave therapy. However, Reilly et al. advise against the use of NSAIDs, as this group of drugs could interfere with the inflammatory reaction responsible for the effect of fESWT and rPWT (Reilly et al. 2018).

5.12.2 Mechanism of Action of rPWT and fESWT

What exactly happens during rPWT and fESWT is still unclear. One thing is certain, however: the method is very low risk (Schmitz et al. 2015; Roerdink et al. 2017). Various mechanisms of action are discussed, but there is still no consensus among scientists. Table 5.7 provides an overview (after Reilly et al. 2018). A major problem is that the etiology of many conditions treated with these two methods remains a mystery to us. For example, if you have successfully treated plantar fasciitis but do not know exactly how this fasciitis developed, how can you then explain its recovery?

5.12.3 Application, Dosage

Many authors consider the use of ESWT justified in patients who do not respond to standard conservative therapeutic measures and for whom surgery is now being discussed. Since the results of the two methods are quite comparable, the current literature favors the use of the more cost-effective and less aggressive rPWT, although fESWT appears to be more effective in the treatment of so-called calcific shoulder, depending on the type of calcification. Both methods are used for many musculoskeletal conditions, albeit with mixed success (Reilly et al. 2018). This means,

Table 5.8 Pathologies for which reviews have provided assessments of effectiveness

Pathology	Dosage recommendation rPWT	Authors
Patellar tendon tendinopathy	Pulses > 2000 Energy > 2 bar Frequency 6–1 Hz Sessions 2–5	Leal et al. (2015)
Calcific tendinitis type I and II (according to Gärtner & Simons) fESWT is clearly superior	Pulses 2500 Energy 500 × 1.5 bar, 2000 × 2.5 bar Frequency 500 × 4.5 Hz, 2000 × 10 Hz Sessions 4, 1/week	Cacchio et al. (2011) Review by Huisstede et al. (2011)
Shoulder tendinitis without calcification	Pulses 2200 Energy 1.7 bar Frequency 5 Hz Sessions 7	Malliaropoulos et al. (2017) Review by Testa et al. (2020)
Carpal tunnel syndrome	Pulses 1000 and 5000 Energy 1.5 bar and 4 bar Frequency 5, 6 and 15 Hz Sessions 1 and 3 (1/week)	Testa et al. (2020). Three usable studies, but very heterogeneous
Achilles tendon tendinopathy	Pulses 500+2500, 2000, 3000 Energy 1.5 bar, 2.5 bar, 3 bar Frequency 8 Hz, 15 Hz Sessions 2 to 5, 1/week	Stania et al. (2019), several usable studies, but very heterogeneous
Plantar fasciitis	No usable dosage information for rPWT	Review by Wang et al. (2019) demonstrates effectiveness, but does not mention usable dosages
Trigger points		No reviews on rPWT

firstly, that not all conditions respond equally well to therapy, and secondly, that there are always different outcomes within patient groups with the same condition. The optimal treatment protocol must be determined anew for each condition and each patient, although fortunately, usable values from studies can be used as a basis. Table 5.8 lists pathologies for which reviews have provided assessments of effectiveness. It should be explicitly mentioned that these are dosage recommendations for radial pressure wave therapy. It is unclear whether the results of focused ESWT can be directly transferred to those of radial pressure wave therapy. Much more research is needed.

5.12.4 General Information on Radial Pressure Wave Therapy (rPWT)

The ultrasound heads used in rPWT come in various shapes. The most commonly used heads have a surface area of about 1.5–2 cm^2 and are either slightly convex or slightly concave. The concavity is intended to focus the pressure wave somewhat.

As mentioned above, the energy is given in bar for pneumatic devices. If the projectile strikes a head with a diameter of 15 mm and one with a diameter of 30 mm at the same pressure, the impact energy is delivered over a smaller area with the smaller head, and the application is logically more intense locally. Therefore, it would make sense to always specify the energy delivery in mJ/mm^2.

The total energy of a treatment is calculated by multiplying the pulse energy by the number of pulses, for example, $0.05\ mJ/mm^2 \times 2000 = 100\ mJ/mm^2$.

An important factor in treatment is the pulse frequency. Firstly, higher frequencies above 10 Hz are described by most patients as more pleasant—or, let's say, less unpleasant. Therefore, it is often recommended to start with a higher frequency in the first session and then gradually decrease it during the treatment until the desired frequency is reached. The frequency also influences the penetration depth, with higher frequencies penetrating somewhat less deeply than lower ones. Huber et al. (1999) were able to show that frequencies above 5 Hz cause more cavitation than frequencies between 0.5 and 5 Hz. It is unknown to what extent this affects the treatment outcome.

In 2015, Schmitz and colleagues compiled the following list in a Cochrane review. Unfortunately, the investigators lumped fESWT and rPWT together (Schmitz et al. 2015):

- ESWT is effective.
- ESWT is safe.
- For certain orthopedic conditions, the RCTs on ESWT are the most frequent RCTs in the PEDro database and/or achieved the highest scores among the therapeutic applications studied.
- There is no quality difference between RCTs with negative and positive results.
- The administration of a local anesthetic negatively affects the outcome of ESWT.
- Too low energy negatively affects the outcome of ESWT.
- There is no scientific evidence regarding treatment outcomes that favors the use of either rPWT or fESWT.
- The designation of radial ESWT as "low-energy ESWT" and focused ESWT as "high-energy ESWT" is incorrect and should not be used.
- There is no scientific evidence that any particular fESWT technology is superior to another.
- It appears that an optimal treatment protocol for ESWT consists of treatments with 2000 impulses at the highest possible intensity, administered in three sessions at one-week intervals.

5.13 Low Intensity Pulsed Ultrasound (LIPUS)

Fracture treatment is not exactly part of everyday physiotherapy practice, but the procedure will nevertheless be briefly discussed. Low Intensity Pulsed Ultrasound (LIPUS) is an ultrasound application used to stimulate fracture healing. LIPUS is also used for conditions that are traditionally treated with "conventional" ultrasound, since the same biological effects have been observed in the laboratory. The question of whether LIPUS is more effective than conventional ultrasound has not yet been answered. The following parameters are most commonly used for fracture treatment: 1–1.5 MHz carrier frequency, pulse frequency 1 kHz, 0.1–0.3 W/cm^2 (SATA), treatment duration 20 min per day. In the laboratory, it can be demonstrated that LIPUS stimulates cyclooxygenase-2 (Wadhwa et al. 2002; Reher et al. 2002), which in turn stimulates prostaglandin production (Saini et al. 2011). This, in turn, stimulates the expression of genes such as c-fos and aggrecan, which support bone formation (Warden et al. 2001; Yang et al. 1996). In principle, these are reactions that have already been demonstrated with conventional therapeutic ultrasound. Reviews from 2007 (Leighton 2007), 2016 (Aleem and Bhandari 2016, Rutten et al. 2016), 2017 (Poolman et al. 2017, Schandelmeier et al. 2017), and 2019 (Arand 2019; Lou et al. 2018) found no reason to use LIPUS in fracture treatment. Although healing is stimulated, this does not lead to a faster functional improvement, apart from a nicer X-ray image. Leighton et al. and Arand see its use primarily as an alternative for poorly healing fractures in high-risk cases where surgery is to be avoided.

5.14 Summary: Ultrasound

- Ultrasound is primarily a mechanical application. The rapid movements in the tissue cause friction, which leads to an increase in temperature in the tissue, especially at the interfaces.
- This heating leads to improved extensibility of collagen tissue (scars, tendons, ligaments) when the tissue is heated to 40–45 °C and this elevated temperature is maintained for at least 5 min.
- In addition, there is improved blood flow, pain relief, and stimulation of metabolic processes.
- The mechanical stimulus can be applied continuously or in pulses. Pulsing is intended to

give the circulatory system the opportunity to compensate for a temperature increase in the tissue. The thermal effect is more pronounced with continuously administered ultrasound.

- The concept of half-value depth must be questioned.
- 3 MHz ultrasound heats tissue at greater depths than previously assumed and is more efficient than 1 MHz ultrasound.
- Due to pressure changes in the tissue, stable acoustic cavitation occurs.
- Cavitation causes vortex flows in the intercellular fluid around the gas bubbles formed, which have mechanical effects on the surrounding cells. Cell membranes are temporarily mechanically destabilized, resulting in improved permeability.
- At higher dosages, unstable cavitation may occur, with potentially tissue-damaging effects.

5.15 Indications and Contraindications

- Indications are diseases and injuries of the musculoskeletal system, whether inflammatory or degenerative, acute or chronic.
- Because of the effective heating of dense tissue such as scars, ligaments, joint capsules, and tendons, problems in these structures are the most likely indications.
- The treatment area should not be larger than two to three times the ERA of the ultrasound head, and the structure to be treated should not be deeper than about 5 cm.

For the vast majority of contraindications, there are no studies that demonstrate the risks, and the few that do exist were conducted in rodents. Therefore, common sense should be used. Contraindications are thus as follows:

- Use of a device that is not regularly checked.
- Use of an ultrasound head that shows damage, such as scratches or dents.
- All conditions in which local heat is contraindicated, such as acute infections, thrombophlebitis, deep vein thrombosis, severe advanced circulatory disorders.
- Tumors are an absolute contraindication for local treatment (Maxwell 1995; Sicard-Rosenbaum et al. 1995).
- Of course, patients with unclear pathologies should not be treated, nor should patients with impaired thermal sensitivity.
- The presence of cognitive disorders is a relative contraindication. This also includes patients who believe that more is better and do not report pain.
- Local ultrasound treatment is also contraindicated over the testicles, ovaries, pregnant uterus, and the eye. Whatever one might wish to treat there.
- There is no consensus regarding ultrasound over active epiphyseal plates. Lyon et al. found that ultrasound applied to rabbit knees, 1 MHz, 2.2 W/cm^2, pulsed, ERA 2 cm^2, 20 min static, daily for 6 weeks, not unexpectedly led to burns of the skin and significant changes in the bone and epiphyseal plates (Lyon et al. 2003). The sonicated lateral side was higher than the medial side. The authors describe the dosage as high and "not therapeutic." Ogurtan et al. (2002) sonicated rabbit forelimbs with 0.2 and 0.5 W/cm^2, ERA 5 cm^2, 1 MHz, pulse 2:8, 5 min for 10, 15, and 20 days. The investigators found no significant difference between the treated and untreated sides and concluded that ultrasound with the parameters used in the study is not harmful to growth plates. They failed to mention that this recommendation applies to the treatment of rabbits.

Epiphyseal Plates, Author's Opinion

It is interesting that low-dose pulsed ultrasound has been shown in vitro to stimulate the growth of cells such as fibroblasts and osteoblasts; see also LIPUS. Okay, a poorly healing diaphysis is not a normally growing epiphysis, and the cells may respond differently. However, the evidence is very thin, and the author therefore advises against the use of ultrasound, both pulsed and continuous, in active epiphyseal plates until there is clear evidence of safety.

- The presence of (deep) metal implants and endoprostheses in the treatment area is not an absolute contraindication, as these reflect the ultrasound completely (Brunner et al. 1958; Skoubo-Kristensen and Sommer 1982; Arnold 1983; Kocaoğlu et al. 2011; Andrades et al. 2014). The metal reflects the ultrasound by almost 100%. In addition, only convex metal parts are practically used in orthopedics, so the ultrasound is scattered in all directions. The recommendation to reduce the intensity over metal is unfounded and also impractical. If, for example, a patient with a superficially located plate on the radius reports an unpleasant sensation every time, simply avoid that spot.

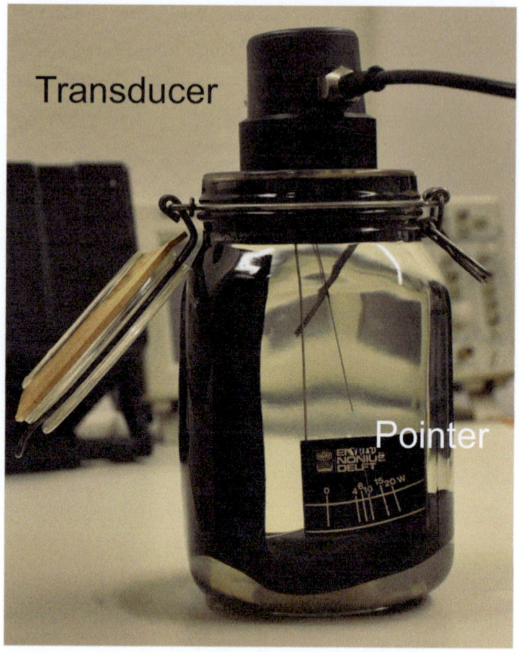

Fig. 5.14 Ultrasound scale

The International Society for Medical Shockwave Treatment mentions the following contraindications for radial pressure waves in its "Consensus Statement" from 2016:

- Malignant tumors in the treatment area
- Fetus in the treatment area

The author believes that the above-mentioned contraindications may be added without hesitation.

5.16 Precautions

There are two things that should be given special attention when using ultrasound: the mandatory regular calibration of the device and hygiene.

It has already been mentioned that the devices must be calibrated. We are legally obliged to do so. There are very good and expensive devices for this purpose. So expensive that usually only the manufacturers and officially recognized calibration centers have such a device. When the author inquired at the official calibration authority in Switzerland—the Federal Institute of Metrology in Bern—about the cost of calibrating an ultrasound head, the answer was that it would be more sensible, in the event of a dropped ultrasound head, to simply replace the head. That would be cheaper. However, there are very simple so-called ultrasound scales (Fig. 5.14) that measure the sound pressure. For this, the ultrasound head is placed on top of a water-filled preserving jar. Inside the jar is a construction with a thin metal plate and levers. The ultrasound hits the plate, which sets the levers in motion. This causes a pointer on a scale to indicate the sound energy. The method is suitable for quickly and inexpensively checking whether any sound is coming out of the head at all. But that's all. You do not know what the sound beam looks like, whether the sound energy is distributed reasonably evenly, or whether perhaps half of the element is not producing any sound. So if an ultrasound head has been dropped, do yourself and your patients a favor and replace the head. You don't want to be seen as a fraud.

Hygiene is a tiresome topic. Physiotherapists in hospitals are extremely mobile and thus confirmed vectors for the spread of nosocomial infections (Crowcroft et al. 1996). Many factors play a role here, one of which is the handling of electrotherapy devices (Lambert et al. 2000; Schabrun et al. 2006; Schabrun and Chipchase 2006). It is not uncommon for these devices to be placed in a convenient location where everyone (including patients) walks by, as no one wants to walk to the equipment room every time. In addition, the devices are rarely covered, anyone can fiddle with them (and then the key is even left in the laser device). The myth that ultrasound heads should not be cleaned with alcohol persists stubbornly. That. Is. Not. True. This only applies to ultrasound heads for sonography. These have a kind of filter at the front, which really should not be cleaned with alcohol. There are special wipes for this. Older heads are particularly tricky (Fig. 5.15a). A lot can accumulate in the rim at the front (Fig. 5.16). Fortunately, modern ultrasound heads are constructed differently (Fig. 5.15b). Incidentally, the culture in the image comes from a small "practice bottle" of ultrasound gel, which was conveniently refilled from a large container in the hospital pharmacy. Everywhere in the hospital where this gel was used, it was drawn from the same contaminated container: in orthopedics, rheumatology, gynecology … It goes without saying that after this result, they immediately switched to individual small gel bottles. A bit more expensive, but less expensive than a nosocomial infection in the hospital, which can quickly cost €3,000 (Pittet et al.

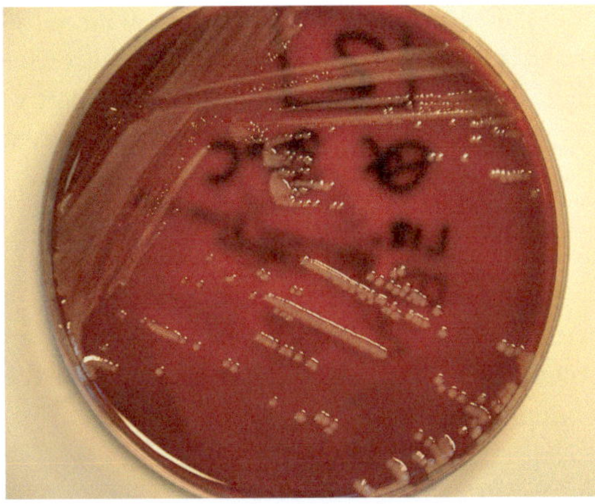

Fig. 5.16 Burkholderia cepacia. Already shown before, but always impressive

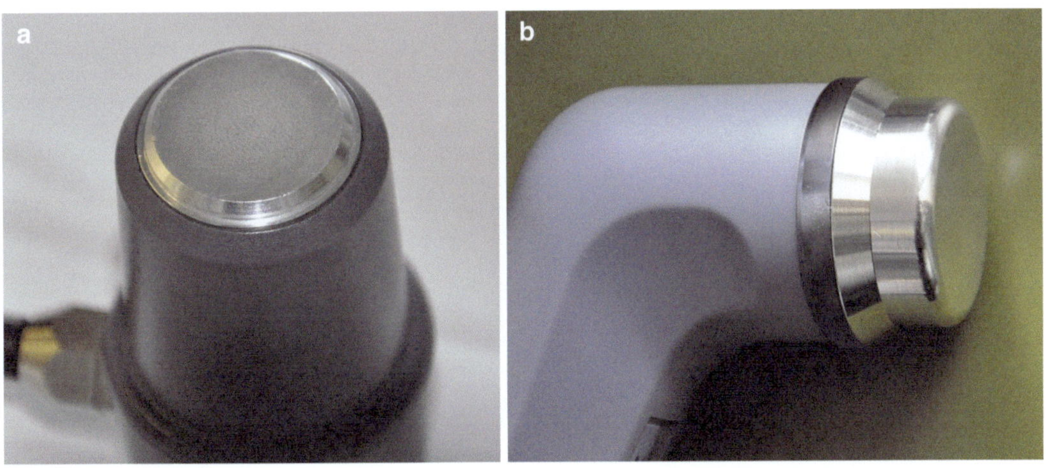

Fig. 5.15 **a** Older ultrasound head, note the rim, quite difficult to clean. **b** Newer model ultrasound head, easy to clean with 70% alcohol

2000). Unfortunately, the problem with ultrasound gel is quite widespread (Oleszkowicz et al. 2012). It is really worthwhile, as part of quality or risk management, to carry out regular checks.

5.17 A Few Numbers

Acoustic Impedance Z_F for Some Media, Unit: Ns/m^3

1. Air: 413
2. Water (at 10 °C): 1,440,000
3. Steel: 45,000,000

Overview of Reflection at Some Interfaces

1. Aluminum-air: 100%
2. Aluminum-contact medium: 60%
3. Ultrasound head-contact medium: 0%
4. Contact medium-skin: 0.1%
5. Skin-adipose tissue: 0.9%
6. Adipose tissue-muscle: 0.8%
7. Muscle-bone: 34.5%

Absorption Coefficient In Vitro at 1 MHz and 3 MHz

1. Bone: 3.22 and 0 mm
2. Skin: 0.62 and 1.86
3. Cartilage: 1.16 and 3.48
4. Tendon: 1.12 and 3.36
5. Muscle (ultrasound perpendicular to tissue): 0.76 and 2.28
6. Muscle (ultrasound parallel to tissue): 0.28 and 0.84
7. Fat: 0.14 and 0.42
8. Nerve: 0.2 and 0.6

Theoretical Half-Value Depth (HVD = D 1/2) for Various Media at 1 MHz and 3 MHz

1. Bone: 2.1 mm and 0 mm
2. Skin: 11.1 mm and 4 mm
3. Cartilage: 6 mm and 2 mm
4. Tendon: 6.2 mm and 2 mm
5. Muscle (ultrasound perpendicular): 9 mm and 3 mm
6. Muscle (ultrasound parallel): 24.6 mm and 8 mm
7. Fat: 50 mm and 16.5 mm
8. Water: 11,500 mm and 3,833 mm

Theoretical Penetration Depth for Various Media at 1 MHz and 3 MHz

1. Bone: 7 mm and 0 mm
2. Skin: 37 mm and 12 mm
3. Cartilage: 20 mm and 7 mm
4. Tendon: 21 mm and 7 mm
5. Muscle (ultrasound perpendicular): 30 mm and 10 mm
6. Muscle (ultrasound parallel): 82 mm and 27 mm
7. Fat: 165 mm and 55 mm
8. Water: 38,330 mm and 12,770 mm

References

Abd El Baky A, Waked IS (2011) Non-steroidal anti-inflammatory phonophoresis versus topical application in improvement of hand grip strength in psoriatic arthritic patients. J Am Sci 7(6):110–114

Abramson DI, Kahn A, Tuck S Jr, Turman GA, Rejal H, Fleischer C (1958) Relationship between a range of tissue temperature and local oxygen uptake in the human forearm. I. Changes observed under resting conditions. J Clin Invest 37:1031–1038

Adair HS, Levine D (2019) Effects of 1-MHz ultrasound on epaxial muscle temperature in horses. Front Vet Sci 6(6):177

Akinbo SR, Aiyejusunle CB, Akinyemi OA, Adesegun SA, Danesi MA (2007) Comparison of the therapeutic efficacy of phonophoresis and iontophoresis using dexamethasone sodium phosphate in the management of patients with knee osteoarthritis. Niger Postgrad Med J 14(3):190–194

Aleem IS, Bhandari M (2016) Cochrane in CORR: ultrasound and shockwave therapy for acute fractures in adults (review). Clin Orthop Relat Res 474:1553–1559

Alvarez-Román R, Merino G, Kalia YN, Naik A, Guy RH (2003) Skin permeability enhancement by low frequency sonophoresis: lipid extraction and transport pathways. J Pharm Sci 92(6):1138–1146

Andrades AO, Mazzanti A, Beckmann DV, Aiello G, Chaves RO, Santos RP (2014) Heating produced by therapeutic ultrasound in the presence of a metal plate in the femur of canine cadavers. Arq Bras Med Vet Zootec 66(5):1343–1350

Arand M (2019) Physikalische Verfahren mit Einfluss auf die Knochenheilung. Unfallchirurg 12:526–533

Arnold W (1983) Temperatureffekte an chirurgischen Metallimplantaten unter Elektrotherapie – Ultraschall. Z Physiother 35:253–258

Asano J, Suisha F, Takada M, Kawasaki N, Miyazaki S (1997) Effect of pulsed ultrasound on the transdermal absorption of indomethacin from an ointment in rats. Biol Pharm Bull 20(3):288–291

Ashton DF, Draper DO, Myrer JW (1998) Temperature rise in human muscle during ultrasound treatments using flex-all as a coupling agent. J Athl Train 33(2):136–140

Askin A, Savas S, Koyuncuoglu HR, Baloglu HH, Inci MF (2014) Low dose high frequency ultrasound therapy for stellate ganglion blockade in complex regional pain syndrome type I: a randomised placebo-controlled trial. Int J Exp Med 7(12):5603–5611

Bahadir C, Majlesi J, Unalan H (2009) The effect of high-power pain threshold ultrasound therapy on the electrical activity of trigger points and local twitch response on electromyography: a preliminary study. J Musculoskelet Pain 17(2):162–172

Baker RJ, Bell GW (1991) The effect of therapeutic modalities on blood flow in the human calf. J Orthop Sports Phys Ther 13(1):23–27

Bakhtiary AH, Fatemi E, Emami M, Malek M (2013) Phonophoresis of dexamethasone sodium phosphate may manage pain and symptoms of patients with carpal tunnel syndrome. Clin J Pain 29:348–353

Ballerini R, Casini A, Chinol M, Mannucci C, Giaccai L, Salvi M (1986) Study on the absorption of ketoprofen topically administered in man: comparison between tissue and plasma levels. Int J Pharmacol Res 6(1):69–72

Beetge E, du Plessis J, Müller DG, Goosen C, van Rensburg FJ (2000) The influence of the physicochemical characteristics and pharmacokinetic properties of selected NSAID's on their transdermal absorption. Int J Pharm 193(2):261–264

Benlidayi IC, Gokcen N, Basaran S (2018) Comparative short-term effectiveness of Ibuprofen gel and cream phonophoresis in patients with knee osteoarthritis. Rheumatol Int. https://doi.org/10.1007/s00296-018-4099-9

Bishop S, Draper DO, Knight KL, Feland JB, Eggett D (2004) Human tissue-temperature rise during ultrasound treatments with the Aquaflex gel pad. J Athl Train 39(2):126–131

Bosch G, Lin YL, van Schie HT, van De Lest CH, Barneveld A, van Weeren PR (2007) Effect of extracorporeal shock wave therapy on the biochemical composition and metabolic activity of tenocytes in normal tendinous structures in ponies. Equine Vet J 39(3):226–231

Boyaci A, Tutoglu A, Boyaci N, Aridici R, Koca I (2013) Comparison of the efficacy of ketoprofen phonophoresis, ultrasound, and short-wave diathermy in knee osteoarthritis. Rheumatol Int 33(11):2811–8013

Brunner GD, Lehmann JF, McMillan JA, Lane KE, Bell JW (1958) Can ultrasound be used in the presence of surgical metal implants: an experimental approach. Phys Ther Rev 38(12):823–824

Burr PO, Demchak TJ, Cordova ML, Ingersoll CD, Stone MB (2004) Effects of altering intensity during 1-MHz ultrasound treatment on increasing triceps surae temperature. J Sport Rehabil 13(4):275–286

Byl NN, McKenzie AL, West JM, Whitney JD, Hunt TK, Scheuenstuhl HA (1992) Low-dose ultrasound effects on wound healing: a controlled study with Yucatan pigs. Arch Phys Med Rehabil 73:656–664

Cacchio A, Rompe JD, Furia JP, Susi P, Santilli V, De Paulis F (2011) Shockwave therapy for the treatment of chronic proximal hamstring tendinopathy in professional athletes. Am J Sports Med 39(1):146–153

Cage SA, Rupp KA, Castel JC, Saliba EN, Hertel J, Saliba SA (2013) Relative acoustic transmission of topical preparations used with therapeutic ultrasound. Arch Phys Med Rehabil 94:2126–2130

Cagnie B, Vinck E, Rimbaut S, Vanderstraeten G (2003) Phonophoresis versus topical application of Ketoprofen: comparison between tissue and plasma levels. Phys Ther 83(8):707–712

Cameron MH, Monroe LG (1992) Relative transmission of ultrasound by media customarily used for phonophoresis. Phys Ther 72(2):142–148

Casarotto RA, Adamowski JC, Fallopa F, Bacanelli F (2004) Coupling agents in therapeutic ultrasound: acoustic and thermal behaviour. Arch Phys Med Rehabil 85:162165

Chan AK, Myrer JW, Measom GJ, Draper DO (1998) Temperature changes in human patellar tendon in response to therapeutic ultrasound. J Athl Train 3(2):130–135

Chen YJ, Wang CJ, Yang KD, Kuo YR, Huang HC, Huang YT, Sun YC, Wang FS (2004) Extracorporeal shock waves promote healing of collagenase-induced Achilles tendinitis and increase TGF-beta1 and IGF-I expression. J Orthop Res 22(4):854–861

Crowcroft N, Maguire H, Fleming M, Peacock J, Thomas J (1996) Methicillin-resistant Staphylococcus aureus: investigation of a hospital outbreak using a case-control study. J Hosp Infect 34(4):301–309

Cruz JM, Hauck M, Cardoso Pereira AP, Borges Moraes M, Noronha Martins C, da Silva PF, Della Mea Plentz R, Peres W, Vargas da Silva AM, Signori LU (2016) Effects of different ultrasound waveforms on endothelial function in healthy volunteers: a randomized clinical trial. Ultrasound Med Biol 42(2):471–480

Cullum N, Liu Z (2017) Therapeutic ultrasound for venous leg ulcers. Cochrane Database Syst Rev 5(5):CD001180

Curie J, Curie P (1880) Développement par compression de l'électricité polaire dans les cristaux hémièdres à faces inclinées. Bull Soc minér Fr 3(4):90–93

Dalecki D (2004) Mechanical bioeffects of ultrasound. Annu Rev Biomed Eng 6:229–248

Demmink JH, Helders PJM, Hobæk H, Enwemeka C (2003) The variation of heating depth with therapeutic ultrasound frequency in physiotherapy. Ultrasound Med Biol 29(1):113–118

Deniz S, Topuz O, Atalay NS, Sarsan A, Yildiz N, Findikoglu G, Karaca O, Ardic F (2009) Comparison of the effectiveness of pulsed and continuous diclofenac phonophoresis in treatment of knee osteoarthritis. J Phys Sci 21:331–336

Doan N, Reher P, Meghji S, Harris M (1999) In vitro effects of therapeutic ultrasound on cell proliferation, protein synthesis and cytokine production by human fibroblasts, osteoblasts and monocytes. J Oral Maxillofac Surg 57:409–419

Draper DO (2010) Ultrasound and joint mobilizations for achieving normal wrist range of motion after injury or surgery: a case series. J Athl Train 45(5):486–491

Draper DO (2014) Facts and misfits in ultrasound therapy: steps to improve your treatment results. Eur J Phys Rehabil Med 50:209–216

Draper DO, Ricard MD (1995) Rate of temperature decay in human muscle following 3 MHz ultrasound: the stretching window revealed. J Athl Train 30(4):304–307

Draper DO, Sunderland S (1993) Examination of the law of Grotthus-Draper: does ultrasound penetrate subcutaneous fat in humans? J Athl Train 28(3):246, 248–250

Draper DO, Sunderland S, Kirkendall DT, Ricard M (1993) A comparison of temperature rise in human calf muscles following applications of underwater and topical gel ultrasound. J Orthop Sports Phys Ther 17(5):247–251

Draper DO, Castel JC, Castel D (1995) Rate of temperature increase in human muscle during 1 MHz and 3 MHz continuous ultrasound. J Orthop Sports Phys Ther 22(4):142–150

Draper DO, Harris ST, Schulthies S, Durrant E, Knight KL, Ricard M (1998a) Hot-pack and 1 MHz ultrasound treatments have an additive effect on muscle temperature increase. J Athl Train 33(1):21–24

Draper DO, Anderson C, Schulthies S, Ricard MD (1998b) Immediate and residual changes in dorsiflexion range of motion using an ultrasound heat and stretch routine. J Athl Train 33(2):141–144

Draper DO, Mahaffey C, Kaiser D, Eggett D, Jarmin J (2010) Thermal ultrasound decreases tissue stiffness of trigger points in upper trapezius muscles. Physiother Theor Pract 26(3):167–172

Dular M, Požar T, Zevnik J, Petkovšek R (2019) High speed observation of damage created by a collapse of a single cavitation bubble. Wear 418–419:13–23

Dyson M, Luke DA (1986) Induction of mast cell degranulation in skin by ultrasound. IEEE Trans Ultrason Ferroelectr Freq Control 33(2):194–201

Ebrahimi S, Abbasnia K, Motealleh A, Kooroshfard N, Kamali F, Ghaffarinezhad F (2012) Effect of lidocaine phonophoresis on sensory blockade: pulsed or continuous mode of therapeutic ultrasound? Physiotherapy 98:57–63

Elder SA (1959) Cavitation microstreaming. J Acoust Soc Am 31(1):54–64

Emsen IM (2007) The effect of ultrasound on flap survival: an experimental study in rats. Burns 33:369–371

Ennis WJ, Lee C, Gellada K, Corbiere TF, Koh TJ (2016) Advanced technologies to improve wound healing: electrical stimulation, vibration therapy, and ultrasound-what is the evidence? Plast Reconstr Surg 138(3 Suppl):94S–104S

Everbach EC, Francis CW (2000) Cavitational mechanisms in ultrasound-accelerated thrombolysis at 1 MHz. Ultrasound Med Biol 26(7):1153–1160

Faisal Mohamed CK, Sumila M, Mathias L, Ajith S (2013) Comparative study on the effect of low-level laser therapy versus phonophoresis in the management of lateral epicondylitis. NUJHS 3(1):35–44

Francis C, Onundarson PT, Carstensen EL, Blinc A, Meltzer RS, Schwarz K, Marder VJ (1992) Enhancement of fibrinolysis in vitro by ultrasound. J Clin Invest 90(5):2063–2068

Franson J, Draper DO, Rigby JH, Johnson AW, Mitchell UH (2014) Tissues at a 3-cm depth vigorously heat using 3-MHz ultrasound. Athl Train Sports Health Care 6(6):267–272

Frenkel V, Kimmel E, Iger Y (1999) Ultrasound-induced cavitation damage to external epithelia of fish skin. Ultrasound Med Biol 25(8):1295–1303

Frye JL, Johns LD, Tom JA, Ingersoll CD (2007) Blisters on the anterior shin in 3 research subjects after a 1-MHz, 1,5 W/cm^2, continuous ultrasound treatment: a case series. J Athl Train 42(3):425–430

Fyfe MC, Chahl LA (1984) Mastcell degranulation and increased vascular permeability induced by „therapeutic" ultrasound in the rat ankle joint. Br Exp Path 65:671–676

Gallo JA, Draper DO, Thein Brody L, Fellingham GW (2004) A comparison of human muscle temperature increases during 3-MHz continuous and pulsed ultrasound with equivalent temporal average intensities. J Orthop Sports Phys Ther 34:395–401

Gan BS, Huys S, Sherebrin MH, Scilley CG (1995) The effects of ultrasound treatment on flexor tendon healing in the chicken limb. J Hand Surg (Br) 20:809–814

Gange KN, Kjellerson MC, Berdan CJ (2018) The Dynatron Solaris® ultrasound machine: slower heating than textbook recommendations at 3 MHz, 1.0 W/cm^2. J Sport Rehabil 27(1):22–29

Gann N (2003) Relationship between applied pressure and temperature change in a simulated model during therapeutic ultrasound. Physiotherapy 89(12):708–713

Garrett CL, Draper DO, Knight KL (2000) Heat distribution in the lower leg from pulsed short-wave diathermy and ultrasound treatments. J Athl Train 35(1):50–55

Grey K (2003) Distribution of treatment time in physiotherapeutic application of ultrasound. Physiotherapy 89(12):696–707

Gurcay E, Unlu E, Gurhan Gurcay A, Tuncay R, Cakci A (2012) Assessment of phonophoresis and iontophoresis in the treatment of carpal tunnel syndrome: a randomized controlled trial. Rheumatol Int 32:717–722

ter Haar G (1999) Therapeutic ultrasound. Eur J Ultrasound 9(1):3–9

ter Haar G (2007) Therapeutic applications of ultrasound. Prog Biophys Mol Biol 93(1–3):111–129

ter Haar G, Daniels S, Eastaugh KC, Hill CR (1982) Ultrasonically induced cavitation in vivo. Br J Cancer Suppl 5:151–155

Halle JS, Scoville CR, Greathouse DG (1981) Ultrasound's effect on the conduction latency of the superficial radial nerve in man. Phys Ther 61(3):345–350

Hardy M, Woodall W (1998) Therapeutic effects of heat, cold, and stretch on connective tissue. J Hand Ther 11(2):148–156

Harvey W, Dyson M, Pond JB, Grahame R (1975) The stimulation of protein synthesis in human fibroblasts by therapeutic ultrasound. Rheumatol Rehabil 14:237

Hauck M, Noronha Martins C, Borges Moraes M, Aikawa P, da Silva PF, Della Mea Plentz R, Teixeira da Costa S, Vargas da Silva AM, Signori LU (2019) Comparison of the effects of 1 MHz and 3 MHz therapeutic ultrasound on endothelium-dependent vasodilation of humans: a randomised clinical trial. Physiotherapy 105(1):120–125

Hayes BT, Merrick MA, Sandrey MA, Cordova ML (2004) Three-MHz ultrasound heats deeper into the tissues than originally theorized. J Athl Train 39(3):230–234

Herbert MK, Holzer P (2002a) Die neurogene Entzündung I. Grundlegende Mechanismen. Anaesth Intensivmed Notfallmed Schmerzther 37:314–325

Herbert MK, Holzer P (2002b) Die neurogene Entzündung II. Pathophysiologie und klinische Implikationen. Anaesth Intensivmed Notfallmed Schmerzther 37:386–394

Huang JJ, Shi YQ, Li RL, Hu A, Zhou HS, Cheng Q, Xu Z, Yang ZM, Hao CN, Duan JL (2014) Angiogenesis effect of therapeutic ultrasound on ischemic hind limb in mice. Am J Transl Res 6(6):703–713

Huber P, Debus J, Jöchle K, Simiantonakis I, Jenne J, Rastert R, Spoo J, Lorenz WJ, Wannenmacher M (1999) Control of cavitation activity by different shockwave pulsing regimes. Phys Med Biol 44(6):1427–1437

Huisstede BM, Gebremariam L, van der Sande R, Hay EM, Koes BW (2011) Evidence for effectiveness of Extracorporal Shock-Wave Therapy (ESWT) to treat calcific and non-calcific rotator cuff tendinosis – a systematic review. Man Ther 16(5):419–433

Hynynen K, Shimm D, Anhalt D, Stea B, Sykes H, Cassady JR, Roemer RB (1990) Temperature distributions during clinical scanned, focused ultrasound hyperthermia treatments. Int J Hyperth 6(5):891–908

Johns LD (2002) Nonthermal effects of therapeutic ultrasound: the frequency resonance hypothesis. J Athl Train 37(3):293–299

Johns LD, Straub SJ, Howard SM (2007a) Analysis of effective radiating area, power, intensity, and field characteristics of ultrasound transducers. Arch Phys Med Rehabil 88:124–129

Johns LD, Straub SJ, Howard SM (2007b) Variability in effective radiating area and output power of new ultrasound transducers at 3 MHz. J Athl Train 42(1):22–28

Joshi A, Raje J (2002) Sonicated transdermal drug transport. J Control Release 83(1):13–22

Kavros SJ, Coronado R (2018) Diagnostic and therapeutic ultrasound on venous and arterial ulcers: a focused review. Adv Skin Wound Care 31(2):55–65

van Kerkhof PH (2011) Ultraschall systematisch anwenden und dosieren – geht das? Auf einer Literaturrecherche basierender Vorschlag einer Dosierungsmatrix für therapeutischen kontinuierlichen Ultraschall. Physioscience 7(3):112–119

Kim Y, Kim J, Kwak K, Yoon BC (2014a) A preliminary study on the effect of high-power pain threshold ultrasound to desensitize latent trigger points: a double-blinded randomized study. J Musculoskelet Pain 22(2):175–181

Kim Y, Yang HR, Lee JW, Yoon BC (2014b) Effects of the high-power pain threshold ultrasound technique in the elderly with latent myofascial trigger points: a double-blind randomized study. J Back Musculoskelet Rehabil 7:17–23

Klonschinski T, Ament SJ, Schlereth T, Rompe JD, Birklein F (2011) Application of local anesthesia inhibits effects of low-energy extracorporeal shock wave treatment (ESWT) on nociceptors. Pain Med 12(10):1532–1537

Kocaoğlu B, Çabukoglu C, Özeras N, Seyhan M, Karahan M, Yalcin S (2011) The effect of therapeutic ultrasound on metallic implants: a study in rats. Arch Phys Med Rehabil 92:1858–1862

Kolb J, Nyborg WL (1956) Small-scale acoustic streaming in liquids. J Acoustic Soc Am 28(6):1237–1242

Kramer JF (1985) Effect of therapeutic ultrasound intensity on subcutaneous tissue temperature and ulnar nerve conduction velocity. Am J Phys Med 64(1):1–9

Kramer JF (1987) Sensory and Motor Nerve Conduction Velocities Following Therapeutic Ultrasound. Aus J Phys 33(4):235–243

Krasinski D, Thrasher AB, Miller MG, Holcomb WR (2013) Effects of transducer mass on intramuscular temperature during ultrasound treatments. J Sport Rehabil Nov 22(4):296–300

Lambert I, Tebbs SE, Hill D, Moss HA, Davies AJ, Elliott TS (2000) Interferential therapy machines as possible vehicles for cross-infection. J Hosp Infect 44(1):59–64

Leal C, Ramon S, Furia J, Fernandez A, Romero L, Hernandez-Sierra L (2015) Current concepts of shockwave therapy in chronic patellar tendinopathy. Int J Surg 24(Pt B):160–164

Lehmann J (1990) Therapeutic heat and cold, 4. Aufl. Williams & Wilkins, Baltimore, ISBN 0-683-04908-9

Lehmann JF, Masock AJ, Warren CG, Koblanski JN (1970) Effect of therapeutic temperatures on tendon extensibility. Arch Phys Med Rehabil 51(8):481–487

Leighton TG (2007) What is ultrasound? Prog Biophys Mol Biol 93(1–3):3–83

Levine D, Millis DL, Mynatt T (2001) Effects of 3.3-MHz ultrasound on caudal thigh muscle temperature in dogs. Vet Surg 30:170–174

Li J, Waugh LJ, Hui SL, Burr DB, Warden SJ (2007) Low-intensity pulsed ultrasound and nonsteroidal anti-inflammatory drugs have opposing effects during stress fracture repair. J Orthop Res 25:1559–1567

Lima LS, Oliveira DP, Costa-Junior JFS, Pinto PA, Omena TP, Costa RM, von Krüger MA, Pereira WCA (2017) Evaluation of gloves as a water bag coupling agent for therapeutic ultrasound. Res Biomed Eng 33(1):42–49

Lippmann G (1881) Principe de la conservation de l'électricité, ou second principe de la théorie des phénomènes électriques. J Phys Theor Appl 10(1):381–394

Lou S, Lv H, Li Z, Tang P, Wang Y (2018) Effect of low-intensity pulsed ultrasound on distraction osteogenesis: a systematic review and meta-analysis of randomized controlled trials. J Orthop Surg Res 12:205–215

Lyon R, Liu XC, Meier J (2003) The effects of therapeutic vs. high-intensity ultrasound on the rabbit growth plate. J Orthop Res 21:865–871

Majlesi J, Ünalan H (2004) High-power pain threshold ultrasound technique in the treatment of active myofascial trigger points: a randomized, double-blind, case-control study. Arch Phys Med Rehabil 85:833–836

Malliaropoulos N, Thompson D, Meke M, Pyne D, Alaseirlis D, Atkinson H, Korakakis V, Lohrer H (2017) Individualised radial extracorporeal shock wave therapy (rESWT) for symptomatic calcific shoulder tendinopathy: a retrospective clinical study. BMC Musculoskelet Disord 18:513–520

Mardiman S, Wessel J, Fisher B (1995) The effect of ultrasound on the mechanical pain threshold of healthy subjects. Physiotherapy 81(12):718–723

Maxwell L (1995) Therapeutic ultrasound and tumour metastasis. Physiotherapy 81:272–275

Meidan VM, Walmsley AD, Irwin WJ (1995) Phonophoresis – is it a reality? Int J Pharm 118:129–149

Mense S (1978) Effects of temperature on the discharges of muscle spindles and tendon organs. Pflugers Arch 374:15–166

Merino G, Kalia YN, Delgado-Charro MB, Potts RO, Guy RH (2003) Frequency and thermal effects on the enhancement of transdermal transport by sonophoresis. J Control Release 88(1):85–94

Merrick MA, Mihalyov MR, Roethemeier JL, Cordova ML, Ingersoll CD (2002) A comparison of intramuscular temperatures during ultrasound treatments with coupling gel or gel pads. J Orthop Sports Phys Ther 32:216–220

Miller MG, Longoria JR, Cheatham CC, Baker RJ, Michael TJ (2008) Intramuscular temperature differences between the mid-point and peripheral effective radiating area with ultrasound. J Sports Sci Med 7:286–291

Mitragotri S, Edwards DA, Blankschtein D, Langer R (1995a) A mechanistical study of ultrasonically enhanced transdermal drug delivery. J Pharm Sci 84(6):697–706

Mitragotri S, Blankschtein D, Langer R (1995b) Ultrasound-mediated transdermal protein delivery. Science 269(5225):850–853

Montgomery L, Elliott SB, Adair HS (2013) Muscle and tendon heating rate with therapeutic ultrasound in horses. Vet Surg 42:243–249

Moraska AF, Hickner RC, Kohrt WM, Brewer A (2013) Changes in blood flow and cellular metabolism at a myofascial trigger point with trigger point release (ischemic compression): a proof-of-principle pilot study. Arch Phys Med Rehabil 94(1):196–200

Mortimer AJ, Dyson M (1988) The effect of therapeutic ultrasound on calcium uptake in fibroblasts. Ultrasound Med Biol 14(6):499–506

Myrer JW, Measom GJ, Fellingham GW (2001) Intramuscular temperature rises with topical analgesics used as coupling agents during therapeutic ultrasound. J Athl Train 36(1):20–25

Nazer B, Ghahghaie F, Kashima R, Khoklova T, Perez C, Crum L, Matula T, Hata A (2015) Therapeutic ultrasound promotes reperfusion and angiogenesis in a rat model of peripheral arterial disease. Circ J 79:2042–2049

Notarnicola A, Tamma R, Moretti L, Fiore A, Vicenti G, Zallone A, Moretti B (2012) Effects of radial shock waves therapy on osteoblasts activities. Musculoskelet Surg 96(3):183–189

Nyborg WL (1982) Ultrasonic microstreaming and related phenomena. Br J Cancer Suppl 5:156–160

O'Brien W Jr (2007) Ultrasound-biophysics mechanisms. Prog Biophys Mol Biol 93(1–3):212–255

Ogurtan Z, Celik I, Izci C, Boydak M, Alkan F, Yilmaz K (2002) Effect of experimental therapeutic ultrasound on the distal antebrachial growth plates in one-month-old rabbits. Vet J 164:280–287

Oleszkowicz SC, Chittick P, Russo V, Keller P, Sims M, Band J (2012) Infections associated with use of ultrasound transmission gel: proposed guidelines to minimize risk. Infect Control Hosp Epidemiol 33(12):1235–1237

Oshikoya CA, Shultz SJ, Mistry D, Perrin DH, Arnold BL, Gansneder BM (2000) Effect of coupling medium temperature on rate of intramuscular temperature rise using continuous ultrasound. J Athl Train 35(4):417–421

Pan H, Zhou Y, Izadnegahdar O, Cui J, Deng CX (2005) Study of sonoporation dynamics affected by ultrasound duty cycle. Ultrasound Med Biol 31(6):849–856

Panus PC, Ferslew KE, Tober-Meyer B, Kao RL (1999) Ketoprofen tissue permeation in swine following cathodic iontophoresis. Phys Ther 79(1):40–49

Peters J, Luboldt W, Schwarz W, Jacobi V, Herzog C, Vogl TJ (2004) Extracorporeal shock wave therapy in calcific tendinitis of the shoulder. Skeletal Radiol 33(12):712–718

Pittet D, Hugonnet S, Harbarth S, Mourouga P, Sauvan V, Touveneau S, Perneger TV (2000) Effectiveness of a hospital-wide programme to improve compliance with hand hygiene. Infection control programme. Lancet 356(9238):1307–1312

Polak A, Franek A, Taradaj J (2014) High-voltage pulsed current electrical stimulation in wound treatment. Adv Wound Care (New Rochelle) 3(2):104–117

Polat BE, Hart D, Langer R, Blankschtein D (2011) Ultrasound-mediated transdermal drug delivery: mechanisms, scope, and emerging trends. J Control Release 152(3):330–348

Poltawski L, Watson T (2007) Transmission of therapeutic ultrasound by wound dressings. Wounds 19(1):1–12

Poolman RW, Agoritsas T, Siuemieniuk RAC, Harris IA, Schipper IB, Mollon B, Smith M, Albin A, Nador S, Sasges W, Schandelmeier S, Lytvyn L, Kuijpers T, van Beers LWAH, Verhofstad MHJ, Vandvik PO (2017) Low intensity pulsed ultrasound (LIPUS) for bone healing: a clinical practice guideline. BMJ 356:j576

Pye SD, Milford C (1994) The performance of ultrasound physiotherapy machines in Lothian Region, Scotland 1994. Ultrasound Med Biol 20(4):347–359

Quan KM, Shiran M, Watmough DJ (1989) Applicators for generating ultrasound-induced hyperthermia in neoplastic tumours and for use in ultrasound physiotherapy. Phys Med Biol 34(11):1719–1731

Qureshi F, Larrabee Z, Roth C, Hananel A, Eames M, Moore D, Snell J, Kassell N, Aubry J-F (2015) Thermochromic phantom for therapeutic ultrasound daily quality assurance. J Therapeutic Ultrasound 3(suppl 1):72–73

Reher P, Doan N, Bradnock B, Meghji S, Harris M (1999) Effect of ultrasound on the production of IL-8, basic FGF and VEGF. Cytokine 11:416–423

Reher P, Harris M, Whiteman M, Hai HK, Meghji S (2002) Ultrasound stimulates nitric oxide and prostaglandin E2 production by human osteoblasts. Bone 31:236–241

Reilly JM, Bluman E, Tenforde AS (2018) Effect of shockwave treatment for management of upper and lower extremity musculoskeletal conditions: a narrative review. PM&R 10(12):1385–1403

Rich KT, Hoerig CL, Rao MB, Mast TD (2014) Relations between acoustic cavitation and skin resistance during intermediate- and high-frequency sonophoresis. J Control Release 194:266–277

Robertson VJ, Ward AR (1995a) Subaqueous ultrasound: the depth efficiency of heating of 1 MHz and 45 kHz ultrasound machines compared. Arch Phys Med Rehabil 76:569–575

Robertson VJ, Ward AR (1995b) Subaqueous ultrasound: 45 kHz and 1 MHz machines compared. Arch Phys Med Rehabil 76(6):569–575

Roerdink RL, Dietvorst M, van der Zwaard B, van der Worp H, Zwerver J (2017) Complications of extracorporeal shockwave therapy in plantar fasciitis: systematic review. Int J Surg 46:133–145

Roman N (2017) Physiotherapy devices able to generate ethical dilemmas. MATEC Web Conf IManE E 112:1–7

Rompe JD, Kirkpatrick CJ, Küllmer K, Schwitalle M, Krischek O (1998) Dose-related effects of shock waves on rabbit tendo Achillis. A sonographic and histological study. J Bone Joint Surg (Br) 80(3):546–552

Rose S, Draper DO, Schulthies SS, Durrant E (1996) The stretching window part two: rate of thermal decay in deep muscle following 1-MHz ultrasound. J Athl Train 31(2):139–143

Rosim GC, Barbieri CH, Lanças FM, Mazzer N (2005) Diclofenac phonophoresis in human volunteers. Ultrasound Med Biol 31(3):337–343

Royer BC, de Fátima AC, da Silva CF, Walker Zancanaro G, Nakayama GK, Bertolini GRF (2018) Comparison of combined therapy with ultrasound-associated interferential current in healthy subjects. Br J Pain 1(1):51–54

Rutten S, van den Bekerom MPJ, Sierevelt IN, Nolte PA (2016) Enhancement of bone-healing by low-intensity pulsed ultrasound. A systematic review. JBJS Rev 4(3):e6

Saggini R, Di Stefano A, Saggini A, Bellomo RG (2015a) Clinical application of shock wave therapy in musculoskeletal disorders: part I. J Biol Regul Homeost Agents 29(3):533–545

Saggini R, Di Stefano A, Saggini A, Bellomo RG (2015b) Clinical application of shock wave therapy in musculoskeletal disorders: part II related to myofascial and nerve apparatus. J Biol Regul Homeost Agents 29(4):771–785

Said Ahmed MA, Saweeres ES, Abdelkader NA, Abdelmajeed SF, Fares AR (2019) Improved pain and function in knee osteoarthritis with dexamethasone phonophoresis: a randomized controlled trial. Indian J Orthop 53:700–707

Saini V, Yadav S, McCormick S (2011) Low-intensity pulsed ultrasound modulates shear stress induced PGHS-2 expression and PGE2 synthesis in MLO-Y4 osteocyte-like cells. Ann Biomed Eng 39:378–393

Sakharov DV, Hekkenberg RT, Rijken DC (2000) Acceleration of fibrinolysis by high-frequency ultrasound: the combination of acoustic streaming and temperature rise. Thromb Res 100:333–340

Sangtong K, Chupinijrobkob C, Putthakumnerd W, Kuptniratsaikul V (2019) Does adding transcutaneous electrical nerve stimulation to therapeutic ultrasound affect pain or function in people with osteoarthritis of the knee? A randomized controlled trial. Clin Rehab 33(7):1197–1205

Schabrun S, Chipchase L (2006) Healthcare equipment as a source of nosocomial infection: a systematic review. J Hosp Infect 63:239–245

Schabrun S, Chipchase L, Rickard H (2006 Jun) Are therapeutic ultrasound units a potential vector for nosocomial infection? Physiother Res Int 11(2):61–71

Schandelmeier S, Kaushal A, Lytvyn L, Heels-Ansdell D, Siemieniuk RAC, Agoritsas T, Guyat GH, Vandvik PO, Couban R, Mollon B, Busse JW (2017) Low intensity pulsed ultrasound for bone healing: systematic review of randomized controlled trials. BMJ 356:j656

Schmidt RF, Lang F, Heckmann M (2011) Physiologie des Menschen, mit Pathophysiologie. Springer, Berlin/Heidelberg, Print ISBN 978-3-642-01650-9

Schmitz C, Császár NBM, Milz S, Schieker M, Maffulli N, Rompe JD, Furia JP (2015) Efficacy and safety of extracorporeal shock wave therapy for orthopedic conditions: a systematic review on studies listed in the PEDro database. Br Med Bull 116:115–138

Shin SM, Choi JK (1997) Effect of indomethacin phonophoresis on the relief of temporomandibular joint pain. Cranio 15(4):345–348

Sicard-Rosenbaum L, Lord D, Danoff JV, Thom AK, Eckhaus MA (1995) Effects of continuous therapeutic ultrasound on growth and metastasis of subcutaneous murine tumors. Phys Ther 75:3–13

Simons DG, Travell JG (1999) Myofascial pain and dysfunction. The trigger point manual. Volume 1: upper half of body, 2. Lippincott Williams & Wilkins, Baltimore, ISBN 0-683-08363-5

Skoubo-Kristensen E, Sommer J (1982) Ultrasound influence on internal fixation with a rigid plate in dogs. Arch Phys Med Rehabil 63(8):371–373

Smith NB (2007) Perspectives on transdermal ultrasound mediated drug delivery. Int J Nanomedicine 2(4):585–594

Soyupek F, Kutluhan S, Uslusoy G, Ilgun E, Eris S, Askin A (2012) The efficacy of phonophoresis on electrophysiological studies of the patients with carpal tunnel syndrome. Rheumatol Int 32:3235–3242

Sprat HG, Levine D, Tillman L (2014) Physical therapy clinic therapeutic ultrasound equipment as a source for bacterial contamination. Physiother Theory Pract 30(7):507–511

Stania M, Juras G, Chmielewska D, Polak A, Kucio C, Król P (2019) Extracorporeal shock wave therapy for Achilles tendinopathy. Bio Med Res Int 26:3086910

Steiss JE, Adams CC (1999) Effect of coat on rate of temperature increase in muscle during ultrasound treatment of dogs. Am J Vet Res 60(1):76–80

Stewart HF, Harris GR, Herman BA, Robinson RA, Haran ME, McRall GR, Carless G, Rees D (1974) Survey of use and performance of ultrasonic therapy equipment in Pinellas County, Florida. Phys Ther 54(7):707–715

Straub SJ, Johns LD, Howard SM (2008) Variability in effective radiating area at 1 MHz affects ultrasound treatment intensity. Phys Ther 88:50–57

Sundaram J, Mellein BR, Mitragotri S (2003) An experimental and theoretical analysis of ultrasound-induced permeabilization of cell membranes. Biophys J 84(5):3087–3010

Taradaj J, Franek A, Brzezinska-Wcislo L, Cierpka L, Dolibog P, Chmielewska D, Blaszczak E, Kusz D (2008) The use of therapeutic ultrasound in venous leg ulcers: a randomized, controlled clinical trial. Phlebology 23(4):178–183

Testa G, Vescio A, Sessa G, Pavone V, Perez S, Consoli A, Costarella L (2020) Extracorporeal shockwave therapy treatment in upper limb diseases: a systematic review. J Clin Med 9:453–466

Tezel A, Mitragotri S (2003) Interactions of inertial cavitation bubbles with stratum corneum lipid bilayers during low frequency sonophoresis. Biophys J 85:3502–3512

Travell J, Simons D (1999) Myofascial pain and dysfunction. The trigger point manual. 1. Williams and Wilkins, Baltimore, ISBN 0-683-08366-X

Turner SM, Powell ES, Ng CSS (1989) The effect of ultrasound on the healing of repaired cockerel tendon: is collagen cross-linkage a factor? J Hand Surg (Br) 14B:428–433

Ueda H, Mutoh M, Seki T, Kobayashi D, Morimoto Y (2009) Acoustic cavitation as an enhancing mechanism of low-frequency sonophoresis for transdermal drug delivery. Biol Pharm Bull 32(5):916–920

Vahdatpour B, Alizadeh F, Moayednia A, Emadi M, Khorami MH, Haghdani S (2013) Efficacy of extracorporeal shock wave therapy for the treatment of chronic pelvic pain syndrome: a randomized, controlled trial. ISRN Urol 2013:972601

Vetrano M, D'Alessandro F, Torrisi MR, Ferretti A, Vulpiani MC, Visco V (2011) Extracorporeal shock wave therapy promotes cell proliferation and collagen synthesis of primary cultured human tenocytes. Knee Surg Sports Traumatol Arthrosc 19(12):2159–2168

Wadhwa S, Godwin SL, Peterson DR, Epstein MA, Raisz LG, Pilbeam CC (2002) Fluid flow induction of cyclo-oxygenase 2 gene expression in osteoblasts is dependent on an extracellular signal-regulated kinase signaling pathway. J Bone Miner Res 17:266–274

Wang CJ, Huang HY, Pai CH (2002) Shock wave-enhanced neovascularization at the tendon-bone junction: an experiment in dogs. J Foot Ankle Surg 41(1):16–22

Wang YC, Chen SJ, Huang PJ, Huang HT, Cheng YM, Shih CL (2019) Efficacy of different energy levels used in focused and radial extracorporeal shockwave therapy in the treatment of plantar fasciitis: a meta-analysis of randomized placebo-controlled trials. J Clin Med 8(9):1497

Ward AR, Robertson VJ (1996a) Dosage factors for the subaqueous application of 1 MHz ultrasound. Arch Phys Med Rehabil 77:1167–1172

Ward AR, Robertson VJ (1996b) Comparison of heating of nonliving soft tissue produced by 45 kHz and 1

MHz frequency ultrasound machines. J Orthop Sports Phys Ther 23(4):258–266

Warden SJ, Favaloro JM, Bennell KL, McMeeken JM, Ng KW, Zajac JD, Wark JD (2001) Low-intensity pulsed ultrasound stimulates a bone-forming response in UMR-106 Cells. Biochem Biophys Res Commun 286:443–450

van Warmel A, Kooiman K, Harteveld M, Emmer M, ten Cate FJ, Versluis M, de Jong N (2006) Vibrating microbubbles poking individual cells: drug transfer into cells via sonoporation. J Control Release 112(2):149–155

Warren CG, Lehmann JF, Koblanski JN (1971) Elongation of rat tail tendon: effect of load and temperature. Arch Phys Med Rehabil 52(10):465–474

Waugh CM, Morrissey D, Jones E, Riley GP, Langberg H, Screen HR (2015) In vivo biological response to extracorporeal shockwave therapy in human tendinopathy. Eur Cell Mater 29:268–280. discussion 280

Weaver SL, Demchak TJ, Stone MB, Bruckner JB, Burr PO (2006) Effect of transducer velocity on intramuscular temperature during a 1-MHz ultrasound treatment. J Orthop Sports Phys Ther 36(5):320–325

Webster DF, Harvey W, Dyson M, Pond JB (1980) The role of ultrasound-induced cavitation in the „in vitro" stimulation of collagen synthesis in human fibroblasts. Ultrasonics 18(1):33–37

Wess OJ (2008) A neural model for chronic pain and pain relief by extracorporeal shock wave treatment. Urol Res 36(6):327–334

Williams AR, McHale J, Bowditch M, Miller DL, Reed B (1987) Effects of MHz ultrasound on electrical pain threshold perception in humans. Ultrasound Med Biol 13(5):249–258

Wolloch L, Kost J (2010) The importance of microjet vs shock wave formation in sonophoresis. J Control Release 148(2):204–211

Yang KH, Parvizi J, Wang SJ, Lewallen DG, Kinnick RR, Greenleaf JF, Bolander ME (1996) Exposure to low-intensity ultrasound increases aggrecan gene expression in a rat femur fracture model. J Orthop Res 14(5):802–809

Yildiz N, Atalay NS, Gungen GO, Sanal E, Akkaya N, Topuz O (2011) Comparison of ultrasound and ketoprofen phonophoresis in the treatment of carpal tunnel syndrome. J Back Musculoskelet Rehabil 24:39–47

Young SR, Dyson M (1990) The effect of therapeutic ultrasound on angiogenesis. Ultrasound Med Biol 16(3):261–269

Žauhar G, Radojčić ĐS, Kaliman Z, Schnurrer-Luke-Vrbanić T, Jurković S (2019) Determination of physiotherapy ultrasound beam quality parameter from images derived using thermochromic material. Ultrasonics 99:1–6

Zimmermann R, Cumpanas A, Miclea F, Janetschek G (2009) Extracorporeal shock wave therapy for the treatment of chronic pelvic pain syndrome in males: a randomised, double-blind, placebo-controlled study. Eur Urol 56(3):418–424

6 Low-Level Laser Therapy (LLLT), Photobiomodulation (PBM)

First, a few explanatory words about the term "photobiomodulation."

What is that supposed to mean now? Photobiomodulation? Isn't that still called low-level laser therapy (LLLT)?

No, not really. A group of prominent figures from the "light scene" met in 2014 to discuss the designation for what they had been researching for many years: the therapeutic application of light (Anders et al. 2015). Since Endre Mester rather accidentally discovered the stimulating effect of weak laser radiation in the 1960s, this laser light has been used as a therapeutic agent in medicine. It was firmly believed that the biological effects could only be explained by the unique properties of the laser. That was until the first studies appeared showing that monochromatic light from other sources, such as LEDs (Light-Emitting Diodes), could trigger exactly the same biological effects. And with comparable intensities and dosages, and as a bonus, much more cost-effective than lasers. The therapy began to be called by different names, which was impractical, not least because PubMed used LLLT as a MeSH term. As a result, studies on photostimulation, light stimulation, and the like were overlooked. The majority of those present favored the term "photobiomodulation (PBM)" because this name better describes the application than LLLT. There was great joy when PubMed also included the new name in the MeSH database. Therefore, the term LLLT will no longer be used in the following, but rather PBM. Not that the debate between laser fans and LED enthusiasts has become any less heated! But more on that later.

6.1 Laser

When a metal is heated until white-hot, it emits light of different colors as it gets hotter. First dark red, then increasingly brighter and brighter, until white-hot. In the same way, the filament in a light bulb becomes hotter as the current increases, and the emitted light becomes whiter. Conversely, when incandescent light is dimmed, it becomes redder, or "warmer," as people say.

In 1900, Max Planck presented the explanation for why the colors of a material change at different temperatures when heated (Planck 1900). He postulated that radiation is emitted in small quantities (quanta), meaning not only as waves but also as particles. These particles are called photons.

The more energy such a quantum possesses, the shorter its wavelength and the brighter the emitted light. Dark red light—for example, from glowing iron with a wavelength of about 700 nm (1 nanometer = 1 billionth of a meter = $10–^{9}$ m) and a color temperature of 1000 K—is less energetic than blue light with a wavelength of 500

P. van Kerkhof, *Evidence-Based Electrotherapy*, https://doi.org/10.1007/978-3-662-73019-5_6

nm and a color temperature of 10,000 K. From a physical perspective, red light is therefore colder than blue light. We'll leave psychology aside here.

In 1917, Einstein explained the principles behind the generation of laser radiation with the theory of quantum mechanics. It took until 1960 for Theodore Maiman to construct the first laser.

The Hungarian researcher Endre Mester then tried in the early 1960s to induce cancer in mice using a laser (Mester et al. 1968). He shaved the backs of his mice, divided them into two groups, and irradiated one group with a HeNe laser with a wavelength of 694 nm. The experiment failed because his laser was far too weak. However, he noticed that hair growth was accelerated in the treated rodents. He called it "laser biostimulation." This was the birth of low-level laser therapy, a classic case of serendipity. Incidentally, the therapy would go on to receive many other names, such as soft laser, low intensity laser therapy, low level light therapy, and many more. Since it was found that many (perhaps even all...) effects of this laser therapy can also be triggered with LEDs, and because the term "low level" is somewhat ambiguous, the field eventually shifted from LLLT to photobiomodulation (PBM) (Hamblin 2016).

Laser is an acronym for "Light Amplification by Stimulated Emission of Radiation." Strictly speaking, it should be written "LASER," but "laser" has become established, as has the verb "to laser." We'll see what verb will be constructed from "LED."

6.2 Properties of Laser

If you were to look at normal light with a (nonexistent) super microscope, it would look as if you were looking down from a great height at a huge crowd of tourists on the Place de la Concorde in Paris: everyone is dressed differently, everyone moves at their own pace with their own stride length in their own direction—pretty chaotic, in other words. Laser light, on the other hand, would look like a column of soldiers on July 14th: everyone is dressed the same color and marches in step down the Avenue des Champs-Élysées.

Laser light differs from normal light for the following reasons:

- Because of its monochromaticity or single color: laser light has a specific fixed wavelength and therefore a specific fixed frequency.
- Because of its coherence: the radiation is in phase, meaning the maxima and minima of the waves always occur at the same time. This is called "temporal coherence." In addition, the waves travel in the same direction, which is called "spatial coherence." The distance over which the wave remains in phase is called the "coherence length." This varies from less than a millimeter to several hundred meters.
- Because of its collimation or parallelism: this term refers to the parallel direction of light rays. Because the radiation does not diverge significantly but is bundled, the energy is transmitted over very great distances. As an example, it is often mentioned that reflectors on the moon can reflect a laser pulse from Earth, allowing, among other things, the Earth-moon distance to be measured to within a centimeter. Since the moon is quite far away, the extremely low divergence of laser light still comes into play. The diameter of the "spotlight" on the moon is about 6 km. By the way, the pulse takes about 3 s for a round trip.

When laser light hits an object, it behaves just like normal light: it is reflected, absorbed, refracted, and scattered, and depending on the nature of the material, collimation and coherence are lost. As soon as a laser hits an object, a phenomenon typical of lasers can be observed, so-called speckles. These are flickering small spots that arise due to interference in the laser beam (Fig. 6.1).

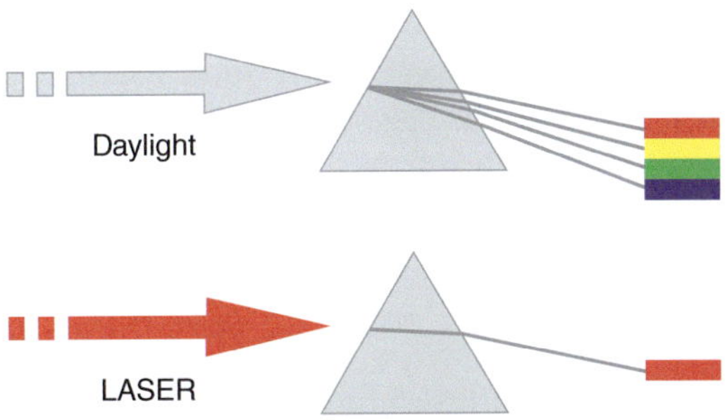

Fig. 6.1 Daylight consists of many different wavelengths, laser light is monochromatic

6.3 How is Laser Light Generated?

6.3.1 The Quantum Leap

Electrons are located in a kind of cloud around an atomic nucleus. In a greatly simplified way, this cloud was previously imagined as shells around the nucleus (Fig. 6.2). These shells correspond to different energy levels of the electrons. The further the electron is from the nucleus, the higher its energy level (for those interested: Bill Bryson (2004) explains such topics in his book A Short History of Nearly Everything in a very understandable and humorous way!).

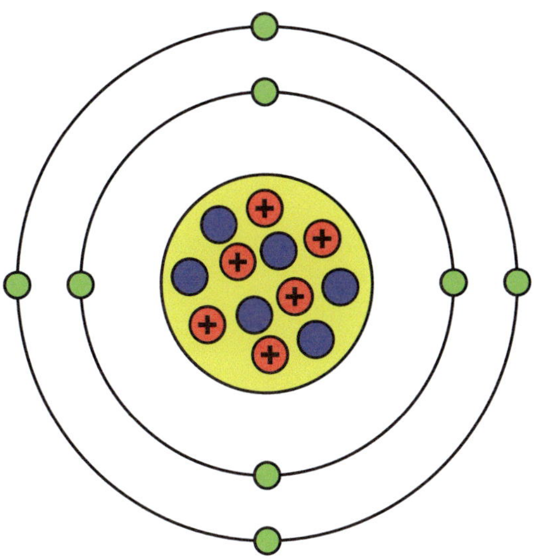

Fig. 6.2 The atomic model according to Niels Bohr

The electrons in the outer "shells" can be influenced by external forces. When energy is supplied to an atom, for example by heating or by intense flashes of light, these outer electrons can be made to move to a higher energy level. The step from one level to the next higher is the famous quantum leap: the abrupt transition of a system from one quantum state to another (Fig. 6.3a, b). However, these more energetic electrons will want to return to the previous, more stable level, and in this case, the electron must release the previously absorbed energy. This happens in the form of a quantum of energy: a photon (= light quantum). The wavelength and thus the frequency of such a photon depends on the difference between the two energy levels: the greater the difference, the shorter the wavelength, the higher the frequency, and the greater the energy of such a photon. If the electron falls

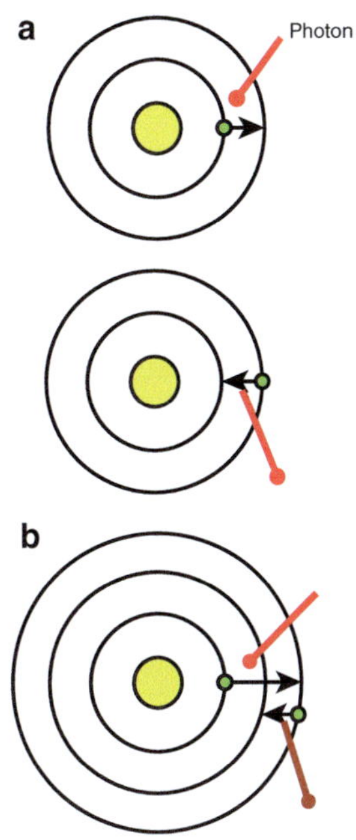

Fig. 6.3 (**a**) Quantum leap. A photon (red) excites an electron (green), which emits a photon when it falls back. (**b**) The electron was raised by two levels and falls back by one level

back to its old level, it releases the same amount of energy it had absorbed. If it is raised higher and does not fall all the way back, it releases less energy than it absorbed; in this case, the light has a different wavelength.

Red light has a longer wavelength than violet light: 750 nm vs. 370 nm. In physics, infrared radiation (short: IR radiation) refers to electromagnetic waves in the spectral range between visible light and the longer-wavelength microwave radiation. This corresponds to a wavelength range of about 780 nm to 1 mm. The frequencies for infrared light are between 0.3 THz and 380 THz (terahertz = 10^{12} Hz). A distinction is made between near, mid, and far infrared. Near infrared is the shortest wavelength in the infrared family. It comes in the spectrum immediately after visible light. Far infrared, on the other hand, is much longer in wavelength and extends up to the microwave region. There is no sharp division by wavelength (Fig. 6.4).

Ultraviolet radiation consists of electromagnetic waves with a wavelength of about 1–380 nm and a frequency of approx. 790 THz to 30 PHz (petahertz = 10^{15} Hz). A distinction is made between UV-A (wavelength λ = 315–400 nm), UV-B (λ = 280–315 nm), and UV-C (λ = 100–280 nm). Due to its shorter wavelength, UV light has higher energy, so with laser light from the blue and near-UV range, it would be possible to achieve some of the same effects as with red and IR laser light, but with an energy density lower by a factor of 10. However, short-wavelength UV light has a much lower penetration depth, because hemoglobin and melanin absorb most of it. In addition, it is extremely aggressive. For these reasons, PBM uses the longer-wavelength red light or IR laser or LED.

6.3.2 Stimulated Emission

When an electron is in a higher energy state, the atom is referred to as *excited*. This state usually lasts only about 10^{-8} s before the electron falls back to its ground state and emits a photon. For example, when the filament in a normal lamp is heated, the many different energy jumps result in just as many different wavelengths being emitted in all directions: in this so-called spontaneous emission, the familiar continuous spectrum from infrared to visible light (rainbow) is produced.

If this emission is forced in a single "pure" element, only defined jumps are possible: only photons with specific properties are emitted. Therefore, the spectrum in this case is narrowly limited and line-shaped. Photons, when absorbed, can excite an atom. For this to happen, the energy of such a photon must exactly correspond to the energy difference between the ground state and the excited state of an electron. If an electron is already in a higher energy state and the atom collides with a photon of the corresponding energy, the electron can fall back,

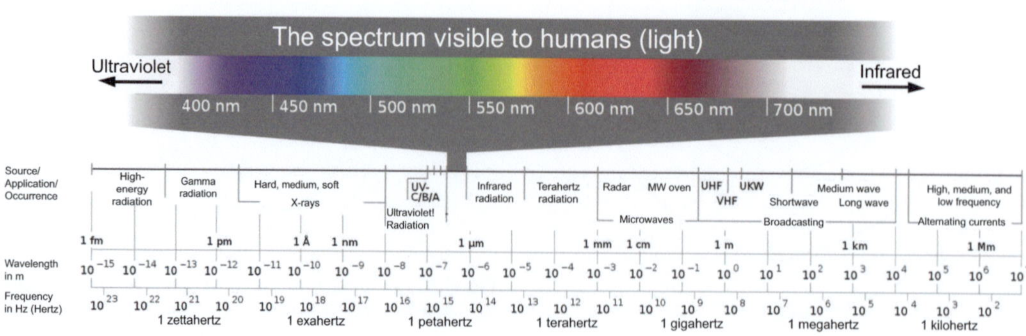

Fig. 6.4 The electromagnetic spectrum. Wikimedia Commons, licensed under Creative Commons License by-sa-2.0-de, http://creativecommons.org/licenses/by-sa/2.0/de/legalcode

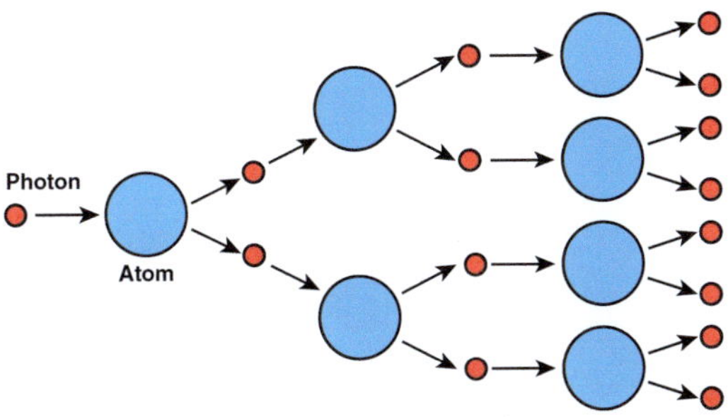

Fig. 6.5 Chain reaction. A photon excites an atom, which emits 2 photons that excite 2 atoms, and so on

emitting a photon that is completely identical to the colliding photon. This process is called "stimulated emission."

The presence of a large number of excited atoms can lead to amplification, because one photon "releases" a second photon, and these two photons then release another two, and so on: a snowball effect (Fig. 6.5).

However, this process only works if more electrons are in a higher energy state than in the ground state. This state does not normally occur in nature and is therefore called population inversion. Such a state can be achieved for a short time by using a large energy input—this is called pumping—to bring many atoms into a so-called metastable state. This is a relatively stable excited state in which the electrons have a higher energy level. This higher level can then only be given up by collision with other atoms or photons. The atoms remain in this state for a relatively long time (0.001 s), so that for a certain period, more electrons enter a metastable state than leave it. When they fall back to the ground state, the absorbed energy is released again.

6.4 Structure of a Laser

A laser fundamentally consists of three components:

- an active medium (laser material), in which the laser radiation is generated by stimulated emission,
- a pumping mechanism that supplies energy to the active medium,
- a resonator to amplify the laser radiation.

The excitation (pumping) of the atoms can occur through different pumping mechanisms depending on the type of laser:

- collision excitation of atoms, molecules, or plasmas (gas lasers, for example, helium-neon lasers),
- excitation by electromagnetic radiation (optical pumping), for example with intense flash lamps, continuously emitting high-pressure lamps, and pump lasers,
- excitation by chemical reactions (chemical lasers),
- excitation by electric current (laser diodes).

Any substance in which a population inversion can be achieved can serve as a laser medium. These can include the following materials:

- gaseous atoms or molecules in ionized or neutral form (gas lasers),
- dye molecules in solutions (dye lasers),
- atoms or ions in solids (solid-state lasers),
- doped semiconductors (diode lasers),
- free electrons (free electron lasers).

6.4.1 Functionality of a Ruby Laser

The ruby laser was constructed by Theodore Maiman in 1960 as the very first laser and consists of an artificially manufactured ruby rod made of chromium-doped aluminum oxide. Wrapped around the rod is a xenon flash tube. Both ends of the ruby rod are reflective, with one end being partially transparent so that some light can exit. A short (0.5 ms) flash excites the ruby molecules and raises many electrons to a higher energy level. However, atoms do not have just two potential excitation states, but several. As a result of the flash, the electrons are raised to the highest excitation state and almost immediately fall back to the second, the metastable state. Thus, a population inversion occurs. When relaxing from this level back to the ground state, photons with a wavelength of 694.3 nm are emitted.

These photons have exactly the right amount of energy to raise an electron in the ground state to a higher level. However, since more electrons are now in a higher level than in the ground state (the aforementioned population inversion), the emitted photons are more likely to collide with these metastable electrons. As a result, these electrons fall back to their lower energy level and release their portion of "extra energy" in the form of a photon. This process is rapidly amplified as more and more photons are emitted. This is now *stimulated emission of radiation*.

The photons are reflected between the two mirrored surfaces and repeatedly pass through the region where population inversion exists. Such an arrangement is called an *optical resonator*; in principle, this is an amplifier of oscillations in which standing waves are formed. Here, the light is increasingly amplified as it is reflected back and forth between the two mirrors, resulting in more and more collisions and emissions. The energy stored in the ruby molecules is released in a very short time in the form of a red light pulse. Completely identical photons with the same wavelength, frequency, and polarity exit from the transparent side of the ruby rod: laser light with a wavelength of 694.3 nm. Gas lasers such as HeNe lasers operate on the same principle, except that the "lasing" material here is a gas mixture in a tube (Fig. 6.6).

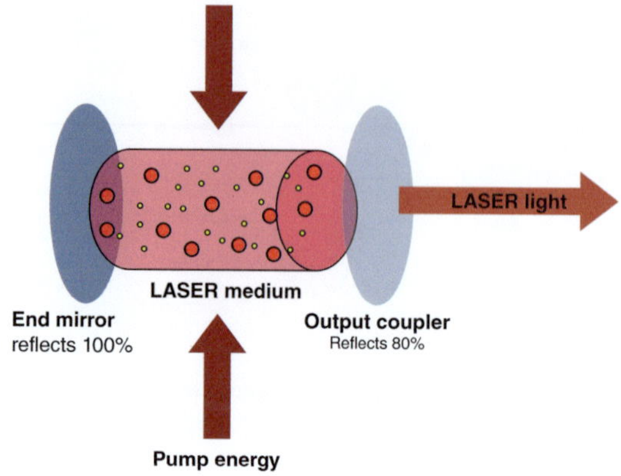

Fig. 6.6 Functionality of a ruby laser

6.4.2 Functionality of a Semiconductor Laser

This type of laser uses semiconductor diodes that emit light from the depletion layer when a voltage is applied. Semiconductors are solids whose electrical conductivity lies between that of conductors and insulators. These diodes are made of semiconductor compounds, with III/V semiconductors being the most commonly used. These are elements from the 3rd and 5th groups of the periodic table (the group between metals and insulators). The reason for this is that the energy relationships in these semiconductors are such that, during the so-called recombination of an electron with a hole, light is produced. The wavelength of the light is determined by the type of semiconductor materials and their ratio to each other. Important in this context are the so-called dopings: certain foreign atoms that are added to the semiconductor material to specifically influence the conductivity of these semiconductors. These are usually substances such as gallium phosphide (GaP), aluminum gallium arsenide (AlGaAs), or indium gallium nitride (InGaN).

In semiconductor lasers, transitions in the semiconductor are used to achieve population inversion. This works as follows: An n-type semiconductor is doped with an electron donor. This means that a foreign atom is added to an element, for example tetravalent silicon, to specifically change its conductivity. A foreign atom with more valence electrons than the semiconductor material is used, for example pentavalent arsenic (the red "As" in Fig. 6.7a). The semiconductor material silicon has 4 valence electrons in its outer shell, and these 4 outer electrons are needed to be incorporated into the semiconductor crystal (electron pair bonding). The doping atom arsenic has 5 valence electrons, and the

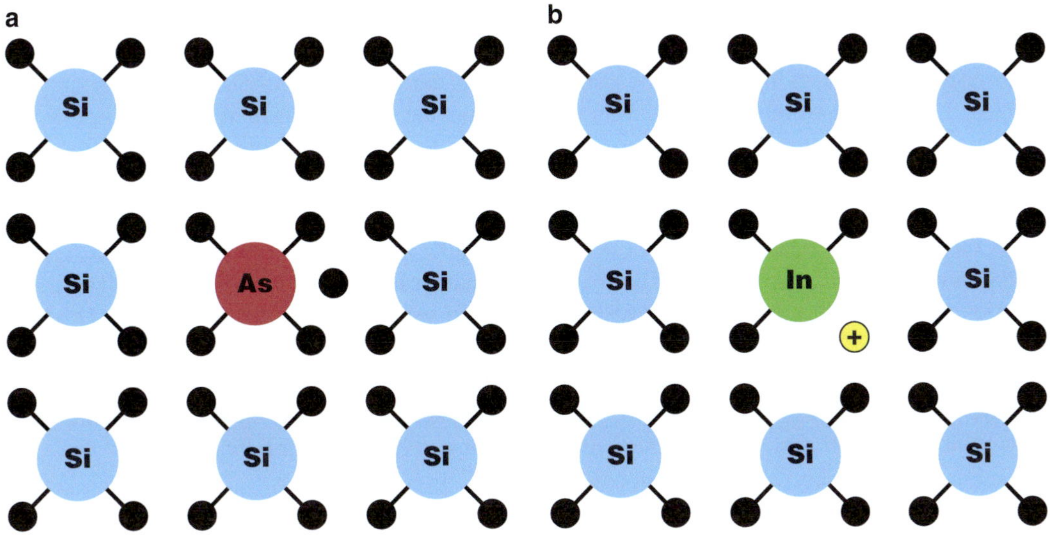

Fig. 6.7 (**a**) n-doped silicon, (**b**) p-doped silicon

5th outer electron is only very weakly bound to the positive atomic core of the arsenic atom, since only 4 are needed. The 5th electron can be detached from the arsenic atom with minimal energy input. Such an n-type semiconductor conducts current, similar to how it would normally flow through a power line, via the electrons supplied by the donor (the arsenic). These semiconductors are called "n-type semiconductors" because their electrical conductivity is due to the negative donor electrons.

A p-type semiconductor conducts current via so-called holes. These are regions in the material where there is a deficiency of electrons because the material has been doped with a foreign atom with fewer valence electrons, for example trivalent indium (the green "In" in Fig. 6.7b).

The indium now takes an electron from its surroundings to stabilize the bond (i.e., from the arsenic), and this electron "stolen" by the indium is now missing elsewhere in the crystal lattice. The regions where the electron is missing are now relatively positively charged, because the indium has taken an electron from the semiconductor. Indium is therefore called an "acceptor." The holes are not always in the same place, but "move" around. Semiconductors with such mobile (positively charged) holes are therefore called p-type semiconductors.

If you combine an n-type semiconductor and a p-type semiconductor, you get a semiconductor diode. At the interface, the p/n junction, between the two materials, electrons from the n-side penetrate into the p-side of the semiconductor, and in the p-side, the electrons are attracted by the positively charged holes. As soon as an electron fills such a free spot, a hole, this electron and the hole are no longer available as mobile charge carriers. This process is called recombination.

Similarly, holes move into the n-side and recombine with the free electrons. Thus, near the interface, the holes disappear in the p-side and the free electrons in the n-side. On both sides of the interface, there are no more mobile charge carriers. A thin layer almost devoid of mobile charge carriers is formed. This layer is called the depletion zone. It is about 1 μm = 1/1000 mm wide.

The penetration of electrons into the p-side and of holes into the n-side has another consequence: In the depletion zone, the charge balance is no longer neutral. Since some electrons have migrated from the originally electrically neutral n-side, they leave behind a thin layer with an excess of positive charge. In the p-side, a corresponding excess of negative charge is created. The two oppositely charged layers now generate, as in a plate capacitor, an electric force and an electric field directed from the n-side to the p-side. This so-called space charge field prevents further electrons and holes from diffusing to the other side and recombining. The recombination process is thus stopped by the built-up electric field. This process prevents the depletion zone from spreading throughout the entire crystal, limiting it to the aforementioned thickness of about 1/1000 mm. The thickness of the depletion zone, however, depends strongly on the doping and somewhat on the temperature.

If the semiconductor material is now biased in the so-called forward direction (n-side negative, p-side positive), the holes in the p-side move away from the anode into the depletion zone. On the p-side, the depletion zone thus becomes thinner. Similarly, electrons on the n-side migrate from the cathode toward the depletion zone. Thus, the depletion zone becomes narrower on both sides and even disappears completely at sufficient voltage.

The donor electrons from the n-zone continuously cross the interface and recombine with holes from the p-zone. Naturally, the energy that was used to create an electron-hole pair is released in the process. This energy is supplied by a voltage source. Depending on the semiconductor, this released energy is emitted as light, as in the case of an LED. LED light is monochromatic but not coherent, as in a laser diode. The LED light is emitted "chaotically" in all directions (Figs. 6.8 and 6.9).

The end faces of a laser diode are reflective, just like in a ruby laser. In this way, an optical resonator is formed between these surfaces, similar to the ruby laser described above. The photons are reflected within it as in the ruby laser and exit from the partially transmissive end of the diode. Unlike the light from an LED, this light is coherent: laser light.

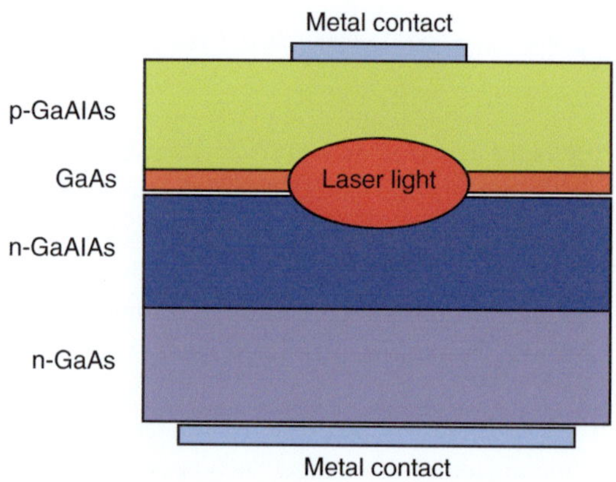

Fig. 6.8 Schematic representation of a laser diode. In reality, the chips are extremely thin

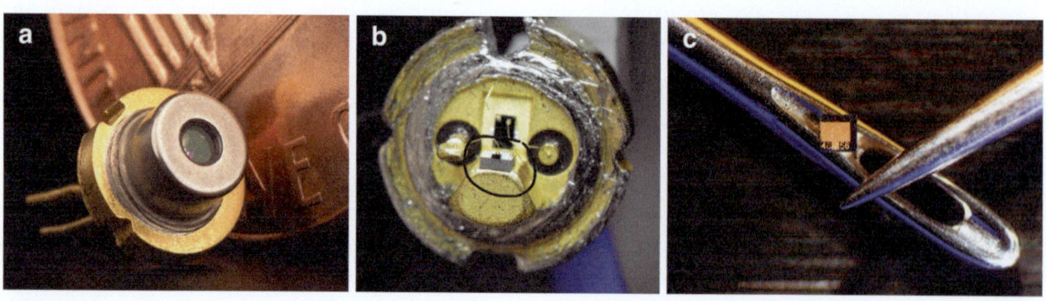

Fig. 6.9 (**a**) Laser diode. Jet Propulsion Laboratory, Wikimedia Commons, licensed under Creative Commons License by-sa-2.0-de, http://creativecommons.org/licenses/by-sa/2.0/de/legalcode. (**b**) The same diode, with the front removed. The laser chip is circled. John Maushammer, Wikimedia Commons, licensed under Creative Commons License by-sa-2.0-de, http://creativecommons.org/licenses/by-sa/2.0/de/legalcode. (**c**) The laser chip. Wikimedia Commons, licensed under Creative Commons License by-sa-2.0-de, http://creativecommons.org/licenses/by-sa/2.0/de/legalcode

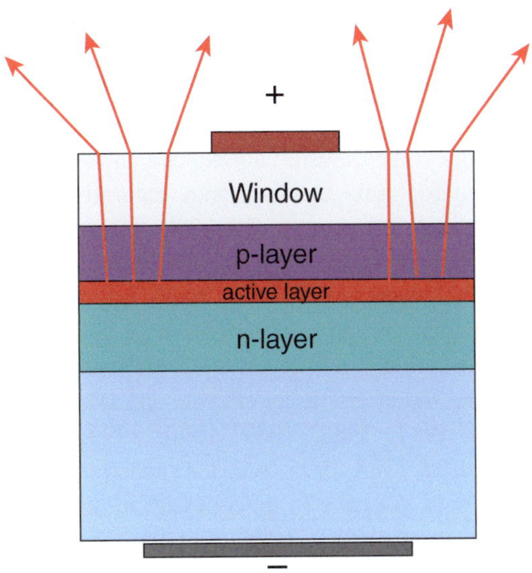

Fig. 6.10 Schematic representation of an LED

An LED works in a similar way. However, the light generated by recombination does not enter a resonator but is emitted directly. A lens (the window in Fig. 6.10) is placed above the luminous layer. This lens serves to protect the sensitive chip and distributes the generated light. The color of the emitted light is determined by the composition of the semiconductor material, with, for example, gallium arsenide (GaAs) or gallium arsenide phosphide (GaAsP) being used for red or infrared light, respectively. In therapy, gallium aluminum arsenide (GaAlAs) lasers are most commonly used. By varying the Ga/Al ratio, different wavelengths can be emitted, which can be delivered continuously or in pulses. Sometimes, several laser diodes or LEDs are combined in a so-called cluster, so that larger areas can be treated.

Laser diodes are by far the most commonly used lasers today. The advantages of these diodes are clear: they are compact, highly efficient, and the power supply is simple and highly modulatable. In addition, the devices are quite robust, which is a significant advantage in a physiotherapy practice. However, LEDs are increasingly being used in PBM, and for many years there has been a sometimes quite emotional debate between proponents of lasers and those of LEDs as to whether lasers possess certain unique properties that make laser therapy more effective (Heiskanen and Hamblin 2018). Time will tell. In any case, a major advantage of LEDs is that the cost per mW of output is a hundred times lower than for laser diodes, and that these devices can be used by patients at home with virtually no risk.

6.5 Effect of Laser Light on Tissue

There is an enormous variety of laser sources with a corresponding diversity in application methods, wavelengths, and power. Unfortunately, treatment parameters are not always mentioned in studies, and there is no clear consensus on how dosage should be described—more on this below. Patient groups are also often very heterogeneous in terms of their diagnoses. Therefore, many studies are unfortunately not comparable with each other.

This makes the assessment of the therapeutic effect of lasers very difficult. Nevertheless, the efficacy of laser treatment for a variety of pathologies is now undisputed (Bjordal et al. 2003, 2006; Huang et al. 2009, 2011). Today, it is no longer about proving *that* lasers work; we even have a very good understanding of *how* lasers work. This is primarily due to the significant contributions of researcher Tiina Karu and her team, who in the 1980s and 1990s laid the foundations for understanding the mechanisms of action of laser light.

The effect of light on specialized photoreceptors such as rhodopsin, the visual pigment in the retina of vertebrate eyes, and on chlorophyll, the pigment that gives plants their green color and enables them to convert light energy into a usable form during photosynthesis, is particularly well studied. In short: the light is absorbed and triggers a chemical reaction. However, irradiation of cells without such specific photoreceptors with light of certain wavelengths can also influence certain cellular biochemical reactions.

These reactions are mediated by so-called photoacceptors (Karu 1999, 2010) and form the basis for the effects observed in PBM. Photoacceptors are not specialized for the absorption and processing of light like photoreceptors, but their function can nevertheless be influenced by light energy. It should be noted, however, that the photochemical conversion by light-absorbing molecules is not a specific effect of laser light. The same reactions occur when irradiated with light sources such as LEDs, provided the appropriate wavelengths are used.

The laser is a very practical application tool because the devices today are usually not much larger than a very thick felt-tip pen and also no longer cost a fortune. It is quite conceivable that in the future, the significantly more cost-effective LEDs will be used instead of lasers. Whether LEDs can be used for the same conditions as lasers remains to be seen in research (Laakso et al. 1993; Chaves et al. 2014; Heiskanen and Hamblin 2018).

The photobiological reaction is based on the absorption of photons of a specific wavelength by a molecule that, due to its chemical composition, can be excited by irradiation with light—a so-called photoacceptor molecule.

The absorption of (laser) light in cells takes place in the cytochromes located in the mitochondrial membrane. Cytochromes are found in all living organisms and are enzymatically active, membrane-bound colored proteins (hence the name: cell pigment) that act as redox catalysts in cellular respiration and other biochemical processes. The iron ion in the active center of the cytochromes can switch between the divalent (ferro form, Fe^{2+}, Fe(II)) and trivalent (ferri form, Fe^{3+}, Fe(III)) states during an electron transfer reaction. The molecule changes from its Fe(III) form to the reduced Fe(II) state by accepting an electron. The same happens with the copper ion, which can switch between Cu(II) and Cu(I) by accepting and releasing an electron. In the reduced state of these ions, the electrons can be passed on to the next carrier, and so on—hence the term electron transport chain. The biological function of cytochromes is thus electron transfer, and they are also called "electron carriers."

Because cytochromes have excitable electrons, they can be stimulated by light, even though cytochromes do not depend on light irradiation for their function: they naturally function in the dark as well. Every cell in the human body contains such cytochromes and can therefore be stimulated by light. There is much evidence that certain wavelengths have a specific "all-or-nothing" effect on such photoacceptors and can therefore trigger enzyme-specific effects (Karu 1987, 1988, 1989, 1990, 1999, 2010; Karu et al. 1984, 1995, 2005). As mentioned, the light does not have to be coherent: in principle, any monochromatic light of a specific wavelength at adequate intensity has the same effect.

The main effect is the stimulation of cellular metabolism, with the light being absorbed by enzymes of the respiratory chain. It has been shown that there is a "dose window" for this stimulation: over- and underdosing have no effect or even an inhibitory (so-called biosuppressive) effect (Karu 1990; Huang et al. 2009, 2011). It has also been demonstrated that cells in which optimal metabolic conditions already exist cannot be further stimulated. This is probably also a reason why some studies have failed to demonstrate an effect: in a process that is already running optimally, there is probably nothing left to stimulate.

6.5.1 The Respiratory Chain

The cell converts glucose and oxygen into carbon dioxide and water. This process is exothermic, releasing energy. This energy is "stored" in ATP. The respiratory chain is the final stage of glucose breakdown, with the goal of this breakdown being the synthesis of ATP. The process is also called oxidative phosphorylation. In the final phase of this process, oxygen combines with hydrogen to form water, releasing energy. This reaction is known as the *oxyhydrogen reaction*. We know this reaction from chemistry class: the teacher produced H_2 and O_2 by electrolysis and introduced these gases into a test

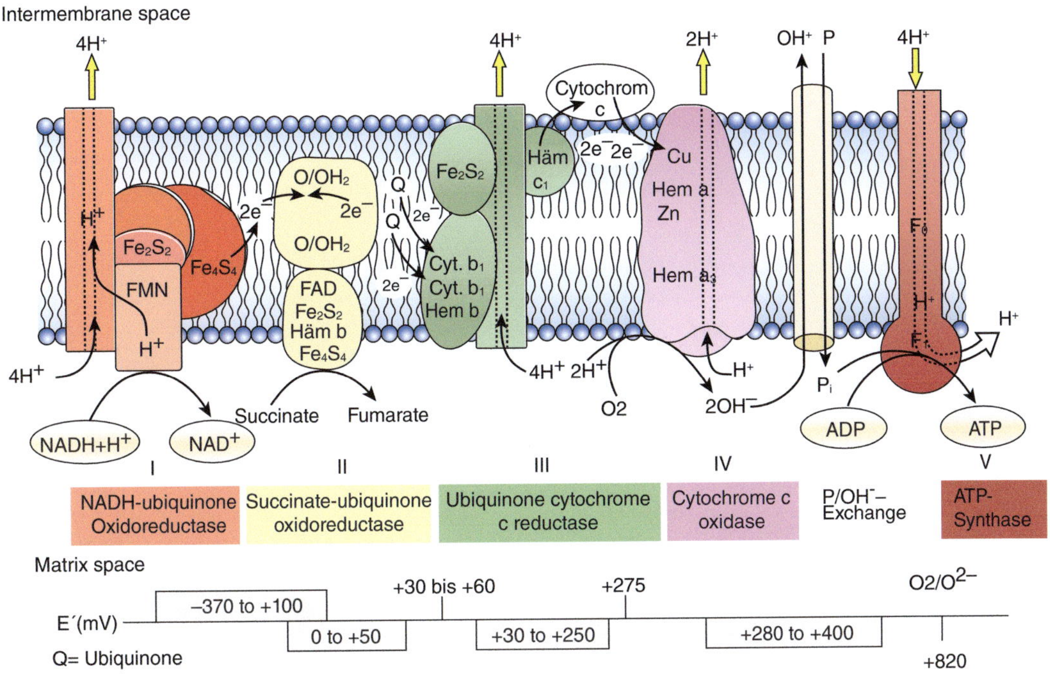

Fig. 6.11 The respiratory chain. PBM acts on the step involving cytochrome (IV). © Spektrum, Heidelberg, with kind permission

tube. Then he ignited the mixture, and there was a "pfüüüt" in the test tube, releasing energy in the form of heat, light, and some sound. And, of course, some water. The same thing happened to the Hindenburg in Lakehurst in 1937.

So that the cell is not destroyed by this reaction, Mother Nature allows it to proceed in a so-called electron transport chain in several harmless steps, with only a small amount of energy released at each stage. The net energy yield remains the same. This energy is used, among other things, to synthesize ATP from ADP and phosphate.

It is now fairly certain that lasers primarily accelerate electron transport. Electrons in the excited state are less tightly bound to the Fe and Cu ions than in the stable ground state. The energy of the absorbed photons is chemically transferred to the redox centers of the enzymes of the respiratory chain, making oxidation easier and increasing ATP synthesis. In addition, thermal activation of the enzymes is discussed, but this is negligibly small in vivo. In particular, cytochrome c oxidase, which is involved in the respiratory chain, responds to laser stimulation with increased activity (Fig. 6.11). Stimulation of this intracellular process triggers a variety of different secondary reactions, such as increased RNA and protein synthesis—processes that continue long after irradiation has ceased.

6.5.2 Laser Effects

Four main effects of lasers are described (Table 6.1):

- increased cell proliferation,
- an anti-inflammatory effect,
- an anti-edematous effect,
- an analgesic effect.

There is a great deal of evidence for the anti-inflammatory effect in particular: the production

Table 6.1 Laser effects

Effect	Authors
Decrease in PGE_2, inhibition of COX-2	Honmura et al. (1993a, b), Shimizu et al. (1995), de Jesus et al. (2015), Prianti et al. (2014), Freitas and Hamblin (2016)
Stimulation of angiogenesis	Ihsan (2005), Kipshidze et al. (2001), Agaiby et al. (2000)
Reduction of edema	Honmura et al. (1992), Medrado et al. (2003), Albertini et al. (2004)
Anti-inflammatory effect	Aimbire et al. (2005, 2006, 2007), Pessoa et al. (2004), Medrado et al. (2003)
Anti-inflammatory effect, comparable to NSAIDs	Honmura et al. (1993a, b), Campana et al. (1999), Aimbire et al. (2005), Albertini et al. (2004)
Release of β-endorphin, ACTH	Laakso et al. (1994)
Release of serotonin	Ceylan et al. (2004)

of PGE2, TNF-alpha, and IL1 is inhibited, as is cyclooxygenase-2 (COX2). The anti-inflammatory effect of PBM is even as pronounced as that of indomethacin, celecoxib, and diclofenac. The dosage used in these studies was around 7.5 J/cm^2 (0.7–19 J/cm^2). These effects influence edema formation in the first 72 h after an injury and thus affect blood flow as well as the formation of necroses and hematomas. Bjordal (2006) recommends, after this period, influencing wound healing with a dose of 2 J/cm^2 per point. By the way: In studies with negative results, underdosing was consistently observed: significantly less than 5 J/cm^2 total dose.

The analgesic effect is attributed to the release of β-endorphin (Laakso et al. 1994). Laser light causes mast cells and macrophages to release, among other things, interleukin-1. Interleukin activates the release of CRH from the hypothalamus and thus the hypothalamic-pituitary-adrenal axis (Sapolski et al. 1987). CRH causes the anterior pituitary to split proopiomelanocortin (POMC) into ACTH and β-endorphin. However, Laakso could not confirm the involvement of β-endorphins with certainty, as naloxone only slightly reduced pain relief. Bjordal (2006) therefore doubts the involvement of β-endorphins in pain relief.

Another explanation for pain relief involves the participation of serotonin (Ceylan et al. 2004). The investigators found that after treatment with a HeNe laser, the concentration of 5-hydroxyindoleacetic acid in the urine was significantly increased, several days before the onset of pain relief. 5HIAA is a metabolite of serotonin.

Laser is used in dermatology for the treatment of poorly healing wounds and ulcers. Laser is also successfully used in the treatment of problems in orthopedics and rheumatology, such as arthritis, bursitis, trigger point therapy, and stimulation of acupuncture points.

6.5.3 Types of Lasers

PBM devices are available in various designs. PBM refers to the therapeutic application of lasers with light of such low intensity that tissue damage never occurs. Laser light is intended to stimulate, not heat. In practice, this means that the power density must remain below 5 mW/mm^2 or below 500 mW/cm^2. This value is the lowest at which tissue heating has ever been detected.

Basically, there are lasers that emit their energy continuously and those that pulse. In addition, there are lasers that emit their energy in the invisible infrared range (IR) and those that produce visible red light. Lasers of other colors are not of interest for therapy because they have extremely low penetration depth. The wavelength ranges between 670 and 690 nm (red light) and between 760 and 900 nm (IR) positively influence the redox process of the respiratory chain (Chung et al. 2012; de Freitas and Hamblin 2016), so a therapeutic laser should cover at least one of these ranges. This positive effect was first discovered purely by chance; later, the effect was confirmed by creating so-called action spectra (also called effect spectra). Such an action spectrum shows the magnitude of a biological effect as a function of the wavelength used, for example, measured by O_2 production. An absorption spectrum is the graphical representation of the absorption capacity, for example, of enzymes as a function of the wavelength of light. This spectrum largely coincides with the action spectrum (Fig. 6.12). The action spectrum can be used to identify the enzyme responsible for a particular process. If the action spectrum of a particular enzyme is known, its function can be stimulated with the corresponding wavelength (Karu and Kolyakov 2005).

IR lasers with a wavelength of about 780 nm and above are also therapeutically effective, but with increasing wavelength, the therapeutic effects are reportedly weaker; in other words, the required power density increases. However, compared to red light, the longer-wavelength IR light has a greater penetration depth of about 3 mm, while for red light lasers this depth is about 1 mm. The penetration depth is the depth at which the energy is still 37% of the emitted intensity. Some authors (Laakso et al. 1993) claim, however, that the 830 nm IR laser penetrates up to 5 cm deep and stimulates endorphin production more strongly than a red light laser. Since the action spectra at 800 nm also show increased RNA synthesis (albeit somewhat less pronounced than at 600 nm), it certainly makes sense to use such a laser.

Whether the effect of a red light laser differs significantly from that of an IR laser is unclear. In addition to stimulation of the respiratory chain, an influence on membrane molecules is suspected, such as the transient receptor potential (TRP) Ca^{2+} ion channels, which are activated with 980 nm IR light (Wang et al. 2016). This could then influence the Ca^{2+} concentration in

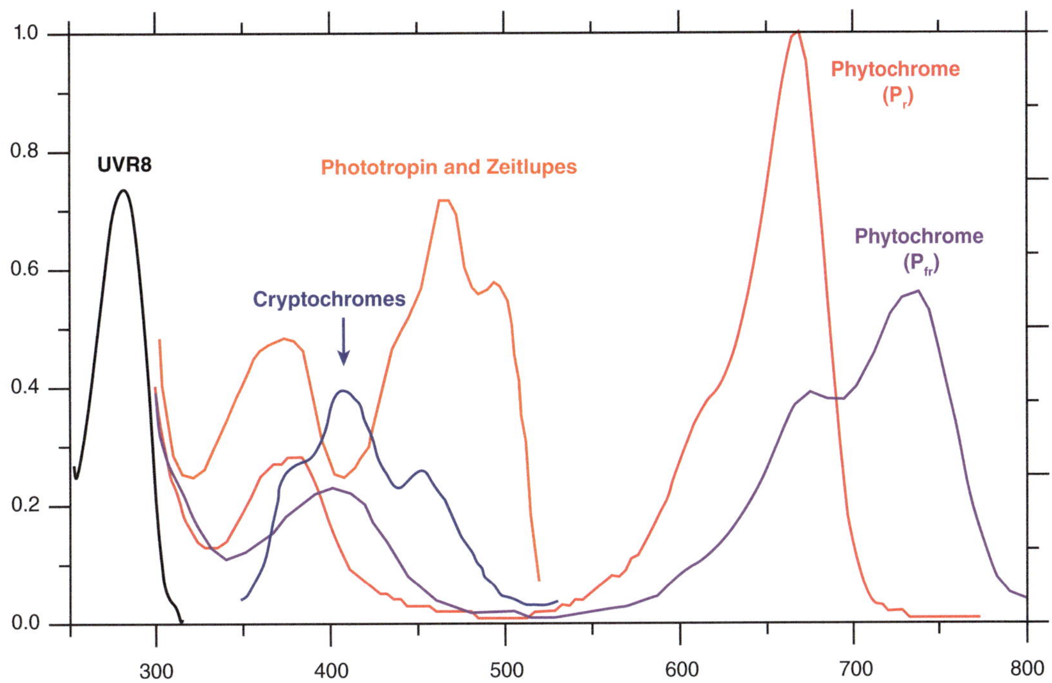

Fig. 6.12 Action spectrum. Abscissa: wavelength in nm, ordinate: relative absorption. The reactions of several photosynthetic pigments of plants observed in this example are stimulated with different wavelengths, for example, phytochromes (Pr) with 650 nm. With kind permission, Eichhorn Bilodeau et al. 2019, https://creativecommons.org/licenses/by/4.0/

the cytosol and mitochondria. However, it seems rather unlikely that there is a sharp boundary between the mechanisms of action in the visible and infrared range. It would, of course, be equally possible that such photophysical processes play a role with red light lasers as well.

Close to the laser source, the energy decreases exponentially. Studies have shown that the decrease in power further from the source (in tissue) is almost linear. In one study, the energy of a 200 mW GaAlAs laser was only 16 mW after 15 mm in tissue. Deeper in the tissue, the power decreased slowly, reaching 1.4 mW at 34 mm.

6.5.4 Laser Type and Wavelength

There is a so-called optical window in tissue that defines which wavelengths can penetrate optimally (Fig. 6.13). Wavelengths shorter than 650 nm are strongly absorbed by hemoglobin and melanin, while waves from the long-wavelength IR range from about 1200 nm are strongly absorbed by water in the tissue. This creates a window for wavelengths between 650 nm and 1200 nm, and that is why almost exclusively red light and near-infrared lasers are used for therapy (Huang et al. 2009).

The lasers used in therapy are usually indium lasers. Most commonly, this refers to the gallium-aluminum-indium-phosphide laser, abbreviated GaAlInP, with the order of the letters varying. This semiconductor laser emits (like the helium-neon = HeNe gas laser) visible red light in the wavelength range 630–670 nm and is most effective for problems of the skin and mucous membranes, including herpes and shingles, facial palsy, trigeminal neuralgia, leg ulcers, varicose leg ulcers, and pressure ulcers.

A second type of laser is the aluminium laser. The full name is gallium-aluminium -arsenide, abbreviated GaAlAs. The wavelength is between 780 and 890 nm, i.e., in the invisible near-infrared range. This semiconductor laser usually operates continuously but can be pulsed and has an in vitro penetration depth of up to 2 mm (Kolari and Airaksinen 1993). It is best suited for the treatment of tendons but can also

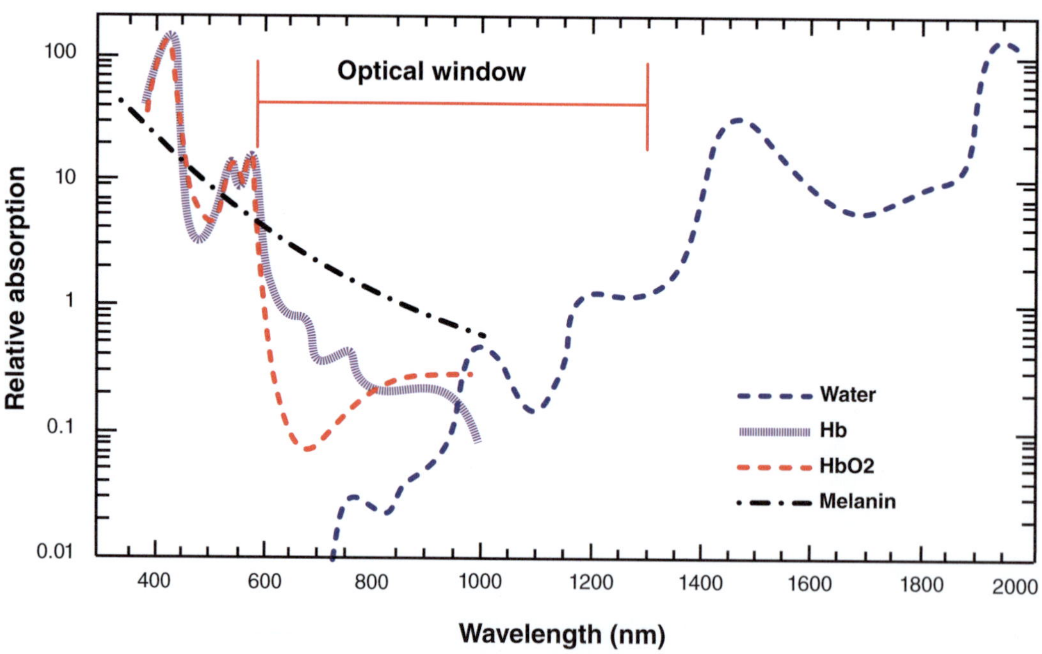

Fig. 6.13 Optical window. Wavelengths < 650 nm and > 1200 nm are absorbed too strongly. After Chung et al. 2012, with kind permission

be used in the treatment of skin diseases such as leg ulcers and herpes zoster.

The third type is the gallium laser. The full name is gallium-arsenide laser, abbreviated GaAs. This semiconductor laser emits invisible infrared radiation with a wavelength of 904 nm. It always operates in pulsed mode with extremely short pulses (superpulsed, 100–200 ns. 1 ns = 1 ns = 1 billionth of a second = 1×10^{-9} = 0.000000001 s) of high intensity (1–20, sometimes up to 50 W peak power), roughly like a flash lamp. The depth of effect is therefore significantly greater than with a laser of the same wavelength that is not superpulsed. Measurements show that, depending on the application technique and tissue, the penetration depth is 3–5 cm. This laser is best suited for deep-seated problems in the back, neck, shoulders, and knees, for tendonitis, osteoarthritis, and myofascial pain. The deeper penetration is explained by a kind of "photobleaching phenomenon": the first pulse bleaches the tissue (more precisely: the chromophores, i.e., the molecular components responsible for color), so that the second pulse can penetrate deeper, then comes the third pulse, and so on (Kusnetzow et al. 2001; Joensen et al. 2012).

6.6 Application of the Laser

The application of the laser is extremely simple. Of course, the instructions in the respective user manuals must be observed.

For pain point treatment (myofascial trigger points, tender points, Ah-Shi points, etc.), the laser is held vertically on the pain point with more or less pressure, depending on the symptoms. The pressure causes local hypoperfusion, resulting in less laser light being absorbed by hemoglobin and allowing more energy to penetrate deeper layers. The treatment time is set on the device or the probe.

For the treatment of arthritis, several points on the joint are treated depending on the size of the joint (see the list under "Dosage" 6.7.6).

In general, the dose should be increased if there is no response. As with other therapies, the method should be discontinued if there is no improvement after about 5–6 treatments. This, of course, taking the pathology into account. By the way: be careful with tattoos in the treatment area. First, the pigments used in tattoos absorb the light very strongly, which massively reduces the effect. Second, tattoos are too expensive for the patient to accept any possible color change.

6.7 Treatment Parameters

Parameters include wavelength, dose, pulse frequency, frequency of treatments, power density, pulse structure, polarization, coherence, and treatment method.

6.7.1 Wavelength

See above under "Laser Type and Wavelength" (Sect. 6.5.4).

6.7.2 Treatment Dose

The power ("strength") of a laser primarily determines the length of treatment per point. A certain dose is reached more quickly with a strong laser than with a weak one. However, power is not decisive for a good result. With a strong laser, one could even achieve less favorable results due to too short an irradiation time.

Power density indicates how much power (in watts) is delivered per cm^2. Some researchers prefer the term "irradiance" or illuminance (Huang et al. 2009, 2011). For example, if a laser has a power of 250 mW and delivers this over an area of 0.2 cm^2, the power density is 100 times greater than if the same energy is delivered over an area of 20 cm^2.

Light can be circularly or linearly polarized. Or not at all. It is unclear whether this has any effect on treatment. In any case, the polarization disappears as soon as the light penetrates the skin, and whether polarization has a specific effect on tissue is unclear.

The pulse structure refers to the maximum energy in watts, the pulse frequency (Hz), the pulse duration (s), and the duty cycle (%). For a pulsed laser, the average energy delivered should also be specified in addition to the maximum energy. This is calculated as follows:

$$\text{Average power (W)} = \text{maximum power (W)} \times \text{pulse duration (s)} \times \text{pulse frequency (Hz)}$$

$$\text{Maximum power (W)} = \text{pulse energy (Joule)} \times \text{pulse frequency (Hz)}$$

Please note: In the calculation, the energy is given in watts, not in mW (milliwatts).

If the power is 10 W with a pulse duration of 150 ns and a frequency of 100 Hz, the average power is 0.15 mW. A single pulse in this example has an energy of 1.5 μJ. At a frequency of 1000 Hz, the average power is 1.5 mW. If a dose of 4 J/point is to be achieved with such a laser, the treatment time at 1000 Hz is 2666 s (about 45 min); at 30,000 Hz (if possible on the device), the average power is 45 mW, and the treatment time per point is 88 s.

6.7.3 Pulse Frequency

With a gallium laser, the desired pulse frequency must always be set. Low frequencies (10–100 Hz) are said to have a stronger analgesic effect, while high frequencies (2500–5000 Hz) are reportedly most effective for inflammatory processes. Medium frequencies (500–1000 Hz) appear to be best suited for the treatment of edema and swelling, as well as, for example, bone regeneration. However, much more research is needed on this topic (Hashmi et al. 2010).

6.7.4 Dose Calculation

The energy absorbed by the tissue during a treatment, also called the dose, is expressed in joules (J) and is usually calculated using the formula:

$$\text{Dose (J)} = \text{laser power(W)} \times \text{treatment time(s)}$$

$$\text{Or : dose (J)/power (W)} = \text{treatment time (s)}$$

However, if the dose is given only in joules, this leads to problems. Example: One wants to treat a trigger point with 5 J. This dose is reached with a 1000 mW laser after 5 s. With a 250 mW laser, the same dose is reached after 20 s. But this does not mean that the therapeutic effect is the same (van Breugel and Bär 1992). Laser users are familiar with this phenomenon in practice; there seems to be a certain soft spot for treatment. In fact, there are a variety of processes in which a nonlinear dose-response relationship (biphasic dose response) can be observed (Huang et al. 2009, 2011; Hamblin et al. 2019). Too low an energy density or too short an irradiation has no effect on the pathology, while too high an energy density or excessively long irradiation times can have an inhibitory effect or even be harmful. In their 2011 review, Huang et al. list a variety of studies supporting this observation; we omit their publication here for reasons of space. Huang et al. attribute this phenomenon to the intracellular production of ROS (Reactive Oxygen Species, formerly known as "oxygen radicals"). The investigators believe that two types of these compounds are involved in this phenomenon: one type is produced under the influence of rather low power densities and in connection with the stimulated function of the respiratory chain. These ROS stimulate many intracellular processes that are important for cell survival (Ristow 2014; Shadel and Horvath 2015). At higher power densities, i.e., when more energy is "pumped in," a second ROS peak occurs, which causes mitochondrial damage and ultimately apoptosis. It is still unclear whether these are different chemical compounds or whether the "radicals" simply occur in greater quantities.

When specifying doses, one must therefore state the power and wavelength of the laser, the energy delivered per cm^2, the power density in J/cm^2, and the irradiation time in seconds.

The power of a laser is measured directly at the diode, and this power is usually indicated by the manufacturer on the device. However, there are lasers in which the laser light must travel through a more or less long optical path before it exits the probe. Depending on the properties of this optical system, power losses of up to 50% can occur before reaching the exit point. Not entirely insignificant.

6.7.5 Dosage Recommendations for Chronic Joint Problems

The dosage suggestions in Table 6.2 are based on a thorough literature review by Bjordal and colleagues from 2003.

Generally speaking: When referring to "dose per point," one point usually, but not always, corresponds to 1 cm^2. In well-designed studies, the area is precisely defined. For myofascial trigger points, a dose of 1–4 J/point is recommended depending on depth; for the treatment of acupuncture points, 0.5–2 J/point is recommended.

For the treatment of inflammatory processes, doses between 0.4 and 19 J at a power density of 5–21 mW/cm^2 are recommended. For such treatment, the depth of the problem and the size of the area to be treated must be taken into account.

The authors assume that enormous energy losses occur when passing through the skin: with a HeNe laser, 90%; with a GaAlAs laser, 80%; and with a pulsed GaAs laser, 50% energy loss. Thereafter, the energy for infrared lasers decreases by a further (estimated) 5% per mm. The energy decrease for HeNe lasers is 10% per mm of tissue.

In PBM studies on anti-inflammatory effects that yielded positive results, dosages as in Table 6.2 were generally used. In studies with negative results, underdosing (often significantly) was usually the case. At doses significantly higher than those mentioned above (5 to 10 times), a weaker biological effect is observed (for example, in wound healing and inflammation). At even higher doses, the so-called biosuppressive range is reached, and inhibitory effects must be expected. However, the dosages mentioned above show that such inhibition obviously requires a considerable amount of energy.

Table 6.2 Dosage recommendations according to Bjordal et al. (2003)

	Dose per point
Finger, toe joints, temporomandibular joint, depth about 1.5–5 mm (skin to synovial membrane), treat 1 point	
GaAlAs and Nd:YAG (infrared, continuous), wavelength 820, 830, 1060 nm, power density (PD) 15–105 mW/cm^2	0.5–15 J
GaAs (infrared, pulsed), wavelength 904 nm, PD 6–42 mW/cm^2	0.2–1.4 J
HeNe (red, continuous), wavelength 632 nm, PD 30–210 mW/cm^2	6–30 J
Knee joint, anteromedial and anterolateral, depth about 1.5–5 mm, treat 3 points	
GaAlAs and Nd:YAG (infrared, continuous), wavelength 820, 830, 1060 nm, power density (PD) 30–210 mW/cm^2	6–180 J
GaAs (infrared, pulsed), wavelength 904 nm, PD 12–60 mW/cm^2	1.2–84 J
HeNe (red, continuous), wavelength 632 nm, PD 90–500 mW/cm^2	9–2700 J
Cervical spine, depth of zygapophyseal joints about 12 mm (8–20 mm), treat 3 points	
GaAlAs and Nd:YAG (infrared, continuous), wavelength 820, 830, 1060 nm, power density (PD) 50–350 mW/cm^2	11–360 J
GaAs (infrared, pulsed), wavelength 904 nm, PD 24–60 mW/cm^2	0.8–56 J
HeNe (red, continuous), wavelength 632 nm, PD 150–500 mW/cm^2	5–150 J
Lumbar spine, depth of zygapophyseal joints about 30 mm (25–35 mm), treat 3 points	
GaAlAs and Nd:YAG (infrared, continuous), wavelength 820, 830, 1060 nm, power density (PD) 180–500 mW/cm^2	48–480 J
GaAs (infrared, pulsed), wavelength 904 nm, PD 30–210 mW/cm^2	15–105 J
HeNe	Impossible

6.7.6 Dosage Recommendations of the World Association of Photobiomodulation Therapy (WALT)

For 780–860 nm Lasers

The WALT (World Association for Photobiomodulation Therapy, formerly the World Association for Laser Therapy) recommends treatment either daily for 2 weeks or every other day for 3–4 weeks. Treatment should begin with the proposed dose. If improvement occurs, the dose should be reduced by 30% (Tables 6.3, 6.4, 6.5, and 6.6). The recommendations can be downloaded from the WALT website (WALT Dosage Recommendations 2020). WALT regularly reviews the information and adjusts it as necessary based on new findings. The recommendations listed below were reviewed by the author in October 2024; it is advisable to visit the WALT website regularly. These are minimum recommendations based on clinical studies. The number of points and the dose may need to be increased. The studies were conducted with individuals with light skin. For

Table 6.3 Dosage recommendations for 780–860 nm GaAlAs lasers, class 3B. Continuous or pulsed. Treatment time should be 20–300 s

Tendinitis	Points or cm^2	Joules (780–860 nm)	Note
Carpal tunnel syndrome	2–3	8	Minimum 4 J/point
Epicondylitis lat/med	1–2	4	Maximum 100 mW/cm^2
Long head of biceps brachii	1–2	6	–
Supraspinatus	2–3	8	Minimum 4 J/point
Infraspinatus	2–3	8	Minimum 4 J/point
Greater trochanter	2–4	8	–
Patellar tendon	2–3	8	–
Iliotibial tract	1–2	4	Maximum 100 mW/cm^2
Achillodynia	2–3	8	Maximum 100 mW/cm^2
Plantar fasciitis	2–3	8	Minimum 4 J/point
Trigger points	–	1–4	= Dose per point
Acupuncture points	–	0.5–2	= Dose per point
Wound treatment	–	0.1–1	= Dose per cm^2

Table 6.4 Dosage recommendations for 780–860 nm GaAlAs lasers, class 3B. Continuous or pulsed. Treatment time should be 20–300 s

Arthritis	Points or cm^2	Joules (780–860 nm)	Note
MCP, PIP, DIP	1–2	4	Foot same
Wrist	2–4	8	–
Radiohumeral	1–2	4	–
Ulnohumeral	2–4	8	–
Glenohumeral	2–4	8	Minimum 4 J/point
Acromioclavicular	1–2	4	–
Temporomandibular	1–2	4	–
Cervical spine	4–12	16	Minimum 4 J/point
Thoracic spine	No recommendation from WALT available		
Lumbar spine	4–8	16	Minimum 4 J/point
Hip	2–4	12	Minimum 6 J/point
Knee per side	3–6	12	Minimum 4 J/point
Ankle joint	2–4	8	–

Table 6.5 Dosage recommendations for 904 nm GaAs lasers, class 3B. Maximum pulse energy > 1 W, average power > 5 mW, 5 mW/cm^2. Treatment duration 30–600 s

Tendinitis	Points or cm^2	Joules (904 nm)	Note
Carpal tunnel syndrome	2–3	4	Minimum 2 J/point
Epicondylitis lat/med	2–3	2	Maximum 100 mW/cm^2
Long head of biceps brachii	2–3	2	–
Supraspinatus	2–3	4	Minimum 2 J/point
Infraspinatus	2–3	4	Minimum 2 J/point
Greater trochanter	2–3	2	–
Patellar tendon	2–3	2	–
Iliotibial tract	2–3	2	Maximum 100 mW/cm^2
Achillodynia	2–3	2	Maximum 100 mW/cm^2
Plantar fasciitis	2–3	4	Minimum 2 J/point
Trigger points	–	1–4	= Dose per point
Acupuncture points	–	0.5–2	= Dose per point
Wound treatment	–	0.01–0.1	= Dose per cm^2

Table 6.6 Dosage recommendations for 904 nm GaAs lasers, class 3B. Maximum pulse energy > 1 W, average power > 5 mW, energy density 5 mW/cm^2. Treatment duration 30–600 s

Arthritis	Points or cm^2	Joules (904 nm)	Note
MCP, PIP, DIP	1–2	1	Foot same
Wrist	2–3	2	–
Radiohumeral	2–3	2	–
Ulnohumeral	2–3	2	–
Glenohumeral	2–3	2	Minimum 1 J/point
Acromioclavicular	2–3	2	–
Temporomandibular	2–3	2	–
Cervical spine	4	4	Minimum 1 J/point
Thoracic spine	No recommendation from WALT available		
Lumbar spine	4	4	Minimum 1 J/point
Hip	2	4	Minimum 2 J/point
Knee per side	4–6	4	Minimum 1 J/point
Ankle joint	2–4	2	–

patients with darker skin, the dosages must be adjusted upward. The author assumes no responsibility for the accuracy of the recommendations.

For GaAs Lasers 904 nm

Due to the photobleaching effect, pulsed infrared GaAs laser light is said to penetrate deeper. Therefore, according to some authors, different dosage recommendations apply here. In addition, the pulse frequency should be taken into account (see Sect. 6.7.3).

6.7.7 Wound Treatment

Laser not only stimulates postoperative wound healing (Woodruff et al. 2004; Gál et al. 2018) and poorly healing wounds (Machado et al. 2017), but is also effective in the treatment of extremely painful aphthae (Suter et al. 2017), especially as they frequently occur during chemotherapy (He et al. 2018).

The following procedure is used for wound treatment:

The 632.8 nm (Enwemeka et al. 2004) and the 658 nm laser (Machado et al. 2017) appear to be the most effective for wound treatment. The area to be treated is divided into a one-centimeter grid, and each cm^2 is irradiated separately without contact with the wound. This is the best method because it allows the dose to be controlled most accurately. The probe is held as close as possible to the wound without direct contact (0.5 cm distance). A kind of grid made of fine wires would be very helpful here. An idea for device manufacturers?

A second, less precise method is so-called scanning: The probe is moved "hovering" over the wound area at a small distance (0.5 cm) and the irradiation is performed as evenly as possible. To do this, the size of the wound area must first be determined and the appropriate treatment time set. Special care must be taken not to "tilt" the probe, otherwise an unknown amount of laser radiation will be reflected and the dosage will be incorrect. The tissue directly adjacent to the wound is treated using the same method as described under "Application of the Laser Sect. 6.6." It goes without saying that utmost hygiene must be observed!

Aphthae

For the treatment of painful oral inflammations, as often occur during chemotherapy, the following treatment protocol is recommended (Zecha et al. 2016): Wavelength 633–685 or 780–830 nm, power between 10 and 150 mW, energy density 2–3 J/cm^2, but not more than 6 J/cm^2, 2 to 3 times per week up to daily. Treating individual points on the mucosa is more effective than scanning the entire mucosal surface. Application can be continuous or pulsed (< 100 Hz). Low-frequency pulsed light appears to be more effective for wound healing in this case. Extraoral PBM can be effective for treating the buccal mucosa, vestibule, and inner epithelial surfaces of the lips, in combination with intraoral treatment.

At this point, reference should be made to the work of Birger Kaada (Chap. 5, TENS). It certainly makes sense to combine local laser therapy with Kaada stimulation. Of course, the course of treatment should be documented. See also the discussion of wound healing under "TENS" Sect. 3.5.

6.7.8 Effective Depth, Penetration Depth

There is no exact penetration limit for laser light. Laser light spreads in all directions and is absorbed in the tissue. The light intensity becomes weaker the further one moves from the point of incidence on the surface. There is a threshold at which the light intensity becomes so low that the light no longer produces a biological effect. This threshold is referred to as the effective depth. The effective depth depends on various factors: wavelength of the light, type of tissue (skin and adipose tissue are "more transparent" than well-perfused muscle), and pigmentation. Laser light even penetrates bone (approximately as it does muscle tissue).

An important factor is the displacement of blood in the tissue. When a laser probe is pressed lightly against the skin, the blood is pushed aside. The tissue in front of the probe becomes bloodless, and since hemoglobin in the blood is the light-absorbing factor, this significantly improves penetration.

Other important factors are power density and treatment technique (treatment with skin contact or at a distance). So-called scanners have only very low power and, depending on the size of the treatment area, sometimes require extremely long treatment times.

6.7.9 Treatment Technique

A distinction is made between local treatment and systemic treatment. Normally, treatment is local, i.e., directly in the problem area. Systemic treatment means treating sites that are remote from the actual problem area. An example of systemic treatment is the treatment of so-called trigger points: Not the entire painful area is treated, but only the point responsible for the pain symptoms. Another example is laserpuncture, in which one or more acupuncture points are stimulated with laser light instead of needles.

Laserpuncture

Laserpuncture (laser acupuncture) is enjoying great popularity (Law et al. 2015). The method is sterile and painless and is therefore gladly accepted by patients who are "needle-phobic." In particular, painful needling in the face can be very well replaced by laserpuncture. Both laserpuncture and conventional acupuncture have been proven to have effects via AP points, although the effects are not always identical. However, they can complement each other, comparable to AP point treatment with TENS.

6.7.10 Treatment Intervals

Bjordal et al. (2003) mention that appropriate time intervals between treatments are more effective than treatments that are too closely spaced. It has also been shown that the effect of laser treatment is cumulative (i.e., the dose of one treatment adds to the dose of the previous one). Therefore, it is important that treatments are not performed too close together. Usually, treatment is given every second or third day for two weeks, then at longer intervals. Acute problems generally respond more quickly to treatment. Chronic complaints are usually treated at longer intervals. Skin diseases are mostly treated daily.

6.8 Risks and Side Effects

According to their potential danger to humans, lasers are classified into device classes (Table 6.7). Classification according to DIN EN 60825-1 is carried out by the manufacturer.

To avoid potential problems, both the patient and the therapist should always wear protective goggles. Never allow a patient to stare directly into a laser probe aimed at the eyes. However, if this accidentally happens for a brief moment, it usually does not result in any serious consequences.

Table 6.7 Classification of lasers according to DIN EN 60825-1 (2004)

Laser class	Description
1	The accessible laser radiation is harmless (for example, CD player)
1M	The accessible laser radiation is harmless as long as no optical instruments such as magnifying glasses or binoculars are used
2	The accessible laser radiation is only in the visible spectral range (400–700 nm). It is harmless to the eye for short exposure durations (up to 0.25 s). Longer exposure is prevented by the natural blink reflex (*)
2M	Like class 2, as long as no optical instruments such as magnifying glasses or binoculars are used (*)
3R	The accessible laser radiation is dangerous to the eye
3B	The accessible laser radiation is dangerous to the eye and, in certain cases, also to the skin
4	The accessible laser radiation is very dangerous to the eye and dangerous to the skin. Even diffusely scattered radiation can be hazardous. The laser radiation can cause fire or explosions

*Note on laser class 2 and 2M: Scientific studies (FH Cologne) have shown that the blink reflex (which, incidentally, occurs within 0.25 s; longer exposure damages the eye) was present in less than 20% of test subjects. Therefore, one should not generally assume that the blink reflex will protect the eyes. Thus, if laser radiation of class 2 or 2M enters the eye, one should consciously close the eyes or immediately turn away. Furthermore, it should be noted that the blink reflex only occurs with visible light. Laser radiation, for example in the infrared range, does not trigger a blink reflex, as the radiation is not perceived by the eye. Therefore, particularly careful handling of invisible laser radiation is important

6.8.1 Please pay special attention to the following

- Special laser safety goggles, which are tuned to a specific laser wavelength range, are completely useless for other wavelengths. Ordinary sunglasses provide no protection whatsoever and may even increase the risk of eye damage, as the wearer may mistakenly believe that nothing can happen.
- In most treatment rooms, in addition to mirrors, there are many other reflective surfaces: Please do not beam into them.
- A laser warning sign must be placed on the entrance door of the treatment room (Fig. 6.14).
- Many laser devices are secured with a lock to prevent unauthorized use. As part of good risk management, the key must always be removed after treatment and stored in a safe place.

Fig. 6.14 Laser warning sign

- Laser devices (like all devices used in therapy) must be regularly checked for safety and performance. The inspection must be documented in writing and should take place annually. If a laser probe has ever been dropped, it is very likely no longer delivering the desired performance and should not be used again without inspection by a qualified professional.

6.8.2 Reactions to Treatment

It can happen that pain disappears almost immediately after a laser treatment. In such cases, it is important that the affected area is not overused. It is very important that the patient is informed that such states of "apparent recovery" can occur and that the patient must absolutely avoid overexertion.

Patients often report feeling very tired during or after a laser treatment. This could be due to endorphin release.

It is quite common, especially when treating chronic problems, for a patient to experience more pain the day after treatment. This is because the problem enters an "acute stage" as healing begins. This phenomenon is comparable to the reaction to other treatments, such as TENS or acupuncture, and is usually not due to overdose. The reaction should be interpreted as a positive response to the treatment, and patients must be informed about this possible pain reaction. Uninformed patients might interpret this reaction as "laser damage."

6.9 Indications

PBM sometimes appears to be a kind of universal remedy for all sorts of complaints without risks or side effects. Laser has a primarily local effect, which triggers a number of secondary effects that can also act at a distance from the stimulation site. For this reason, treatment can have local and systemic stimulating, anti-inflammatory, and analgesic effects. Therefore, a wide variety of pathologies can be treated with laser.

If a patient does not respond to treatment, the various treatment parameters should be checked. A lack of effect may be due to an unsuitable type of laser, too low or too high a dose, incorrect diagnosis, too few treatments, incorrect pulse frequency, incorrect power density, a defective device, etc. Patients also vary in their sensitivity to a given dose and respond very differently to laser treatment. Some can "feel the laser all the way to their toes," while others seem completely unaffected, similar to the "responders" and "non-responders" in acupuncture. The more experience the therapist has with laser treatment, the more successful they will be. It must also be emphasized that laser therapy is only one of many therapies.

6.10 Contraindications

There are not many absolute contraindications for treatment with PBM.

- Tumors, the eyes, the testes, and active epiphyseal plates are, of course, not treated.
- In addition, as is generally the case in physiotherapy, all unclear pathologies, patients in poor general condition, or with fever.
- Older laser literature often mentions, for example, pacemakers, pregnancy, epilepsy, and the like as contraindications for laser treatment.
  - Pacemakers are encased in metal and are completely unaffected by light, and therefore do not constitute a contraindication.
  - With regard to pregnancy, the usual medical assessment of the mother's condition applies. Laser light itself does not affect the fetus, as very little light penetrates. However, when treating acupuncture points in pregnant women, the relevant contraindications must be observed (see EAP/trigger point treatment Sect. 3.7.3.3).
  - It is known that pulsed visible light, especially with pulse frequencies in the range of 5–10 Hz, can trigger epileptic seizures. Therefore, one must of course be careful with instruments that produce flashing visible light. However, it is rare for PBM laser devices to emit pulsed visible light. There is no information in the literature that pulsed invisible light could trigger epileptic seizures.

References

Agaiby AD, Ghali LR, Wilson R, Dyson M (2000) Laser modulation of angiogenic factor production by T-Lymphocytes. Lasers Surg Med 26(4):357–363

Aimbire F, Albertine R, de Magalhães RG, Lopes-Martins RAB, Castro-Faria-Neto HC, Zângaro RA, Chavantes MC, Pacheco MTT (2005) Effect of LLLT Ga–Al–As (685 nm) on LPS-induced inflammation of the airway and lung in the Rat. Lasers Med Sci 20:11–20

Aimbire F, Albertini R, Pacheco MTT, Castro-Faria-Neto HC, Leonardo PSLM, Iversen VV, Lopes-Martins RAB, Bjordal JM (2006) Low-level laser therapy induces dose-dependent reduction of TNFα levels in acute inflammation. Photomed Laser Surg 24(1):33–37

Aimbire F, Lopes-Martins RAB, Albertini R, Pacheco MTT, Castro-Faria-Neto HC, Martins PSLL, Bjordal JM (2007) Effect of low-level laser therapy on hemorrhagic lesions induced by immune complex in rat lungs. Photomed Laser Surg 25(2):112–117

Albertini R, Aimbire FSC, Correa FI, Ribeiro W, Cogo JC, Antunes E, Teixeira SA, De Nucci G, Castro-Faria-Neto HC, Zângaro RA, Lopes-Martins RAB (2004) Effects of different protocol doses of low power Gallium–Aluminum–Arsenate (Ga–Al–As) laser radiation (650 nm) on Carrageenan Induced Rat Paw Oedema. J Photochem Photobiol 74(2–3):101–107

Anders JJ, Lanzafame RJ, Arany PR (2015) Low-level light/laser therapy versus photobiomodulation. Photomed Laser Surg 33(4):183–184

Bjordal J, Couppé C, Chow R, Tuner J, Ljunggren EA (2003) A systematic review of low laser therapy with location-specific doses for pain and chronic joint disorders. Aust J Physiother 49:107–116

Bjordal JM, Johnson MI, Iversen V, Aimbre F, Lopes-Martins RAB (2006) Low-level laser therapy in acute pain: a systematic review of possible mechanisms of action and clinical effects in randomized placebo-controlled trials. Photomed Laser Surg 24(2):158–168 van Breugel HHFI, Bär PRD (1992) Power density and exposure time of He-Ne laser irradiation are more important than total energy dose in photo-biomodulation of human fibroblasts in vitro. Lasers Surg Med 12:528–537

Bryson B (2004) A short history of nearly everything, 1. Aufl. (September 14). Broadway Books, Portland, ISBN-13: 978-0767908184

Campana VR, Moya M, Gavotto A, Soriano F, Juri HO, Spitale LS, Simes JC, Palma JA (1999) The realtive effects of He-Ne laser and Meloxicam on experimentally induced inflammation. Laser Ther 11:36–41

Ceylan Y, Hizmetli S, Siliğ Y (2004) The effects of infrared laser and medical treatments on pain and serotonin degradation products in patients with myofascial pain syndrome. A controlled trial. Rheumatol Int 24(5):260–263

Chaves MEA, Araújo AR, Costa Cruz Piancastelli A, Pinotti M (2014) Effects of low-power light therapy on wound healing: LASER x LED. An Bras Dermatol 89(4):616–623

Chung H, Dai T, Sharma SK, Huang Y, Carroll JD, Hamblin MR (2012) The nuts and bolts of low-level laser (light) therapy. Ann Biomed Eng 40:516–533

Eichhorn Bilodeau S, Wu BS, Rufyikiri AS, MacPherson S, Lefsrud M (2019) An update on plant photobiology and implications for cannabis production. Front Plant Sci 10:296

Enwemeka CS, Parker JC, Dowdy DS, Harkness EE, Sanford LE, Woodruff LD (2004) The efficacy of low-power lasers in tissue repair and pain control: a meta-analysis study. Photomed Laser Surg 22(4):323–329

Ferreira DM, Zângaro RA, Balbin Villaverde A, Cury Y, Frigo L, Picolo G, Longo I, Barbosa DG (2005) Analgesic effect of He-Ne (632.8 nm) low-level laser therapy on acute inflammatory pain. Photomed Laser Surg 23(2):177–181

Freitas de Freitas L, Hamblin MR (2016) Proposed mechanisms of photobiomodulation or low-level light therapy. IEEE J Sel Top Quantum Electron 22(3):7000417

Gál P, Stausholm MB, Kováč I, Erik Dosedla E, Luczy J, Sabol F, Bjordal JM (2018) Should open excisions and sutured incisions be treated differently? A review and meta-analysis of animal wound models following low-level laser therapy. Lasers Med Sci 33(6):1351–1362

Hamblin MR (2016) Photobiomodulation or low-level laser therapy. Biophotonics 9(11–12):1122–1124

Hamblin MR, Huang YY, Heiskanen V (2019) Non-mamalian hosts and photobiomodulation: do all life-forms respond to light? Photochem Photobiol 95(1):126–139

Hashmi JT, Huang YY, Osmani BZ, Sharma SK, Naeser MA, Hamblin MR (2010) Role of low-level laser therapy in neurorehabilitation. PM R Dec 2(12 Suppl 2):S292–S305

He M, Zhang B, Shen N, Wu N, Sun JA (2018) Systematic review and meta-analysis of the effect of Low-Level Laser Therapy (LLLT) on chemotherapy-induced oral mucositis in pediatric and young patients. Eur J Pediatr 177(1):7–17

Heiskanen V, Hamblin MR (2018) Photobiomodulation: lasers vs. light emitting diodes? Photochem Photobiol Sci 17(8):1003–1017

Honmura A, Yanase M, Obata J, Haruki E (1992) Therapeutic effect of Ga-Al-As diode laser irradiation on experimentally induced inflammation in rats. Lasers Surg Med 12(4):441–449

Honmura A, Akemi Ishii A, Yanase M, Obata J, Haruki E (1993a) Analgesic effect of Ga-Al-As diode laser irradiation on hyperalgesia in carrageen induced inflammation. Lasers Surg Med 13(4):463–469

Honmura A, Ishii A, Yanase M, Obata J, Haruki E (1993b) Therapeutic effect of GaAlAs diode laser on experimentally induced inflammation in rats. Lasers Surg Med 13:463–469

Huang YY, Chen ACH, Carroll JD, Hamblin MR (2009) Biphasic dose response in low level light therapy. Dose-Response 7:358–383

Huang YY, Sharma SK, Carroll J, Hamblin MR (2011) Biphasic dose response in low level light therapy – an update. Dose Response 9(4):602–618

Ihsan FRM (2005) Low-level laser therapy accelerates collateral circulation and enhances microcirculation. Photomed Laser Surg 23(3):289–294

de Jesus JF, Spadacci-Morena DD, dos Anjos Rabelo ND, Pinfildi CE, Fukuda TY, Plapler H (2015) Low-Level Laser Therapy in IL-1β, COX-2, and PGE2 modulation in partially injured Achilles Tendon. Lasers Med Sci 30(1):153–158

Joensen J, Ovsthus K, Reed RK, Hummelsund S, Iversen VV, Lopes-Martins RÁ, Bjordal JM (2012) Skin penetration time profiles for continuous 810 nm and Superpulsed 904 nm lasers in a rat model. Photomed Laser Surg 30(12):688–694

Karu T (1987) Photobiological fundamentals of low power laser therapy. IEEE J Quantum Electron 23(10):1703–1717

Karu T (1988) Molecular mechanisms of the therapeutic effect of low-level laser therapy. Lasers Life Sci 2(1):1245–1249

Karu T (1989) Photobiology of low-power laser effects. Health Phys 56(5):691–704

Karu T (1990) Effects of visible radiation on cultured cells. Photochem Photobiol 52(6):1089–1098

Karu T (1999) Primary and secondary mechanisms of action of visible to near-IR radiation on cells. J Photochem Photobiol 49:1–17

Karu T (2010) Multiple roles of cytochrome c oxidase in mamalian cells under action of red and IR-A radiation. IUBMB Life 62:607–610

Karu T, Kolyakov M (2005) Exact action spectra for cellular responses relevant to phototherapy. Photomed Laser Surg 23(4):355–361

Karu T, Tiphlova O, Fedoseyeva G (1984) Biostimulating action of low-intensity monochromatic visible light: is it possible? Laser Chem 5:19–25

Karu T, Pyatibrat L, Kalendo G (1995) Irradiation with He-Ne laser increases ATP-levels in cells cultivated in vitro. J Photochem Photobio 27:219–223

Karu T, Pyatibrat L, Kolyakov S, Afanasyeva N (2005) Absorption measurements of a cell monolayer relevant to phototherapy: reduction of cytochrome C oxidase under near IR radiation. J Photochem Photobiol 81:98–106

Kipshidze N, Nikolaychik V, Keelan MH, Shankar LR, Khanna A, Kornowski R, Leon M, Moses J (2001) Low-power helium:neon laser irradiation enhances production of vascular endothelial growth factor and promotes growth of endothelial cells in vitro. Lasers Surg Med 28(4):355–64N

Kolari PJ, Airaksinen O (1993) Poor penetration of infrared and helium neon low power laser light into the dermal tissue. Acupunct Electrother Res 18(1):17–21

Kusnetzow A, Dukkipati A, Babu KR, Singh D, Vought BW, Knox BE, Birge RR (2001) The photobleaching sequence of a short-wavelength visual pigment. Biochemistry 40(26):7832–7844

Laakso EL, Richardson C, Cramond T (1993) Quality of light – is laser necessary for effective photobiostimulation? Aust J Physiother 39:87–92

Laakso EL, Cramond T, Richardson C, Galligan JP (1994) Plasma ACTH and β-endorphin levels in response to Low Level Laser Therapy (LLLT) for myofascial trigger points. Laser Therapy 6:133–142

Law D, McDonough S, Bleakley C, Baxter GD, Tumilty S (2015) Laser acupuncture for treating musculoskeletal pain: a systematic review with meta-analysis. J Acupunct Meridian Stud 8(1):2–16

Machado RS, Viana S, Sbruzzi G (2017) Low-level laser therapy in the treatment of pressure ulcers: systematic review. Lasers Med Sci 32(4):937–944

Medrado ARAP, Pugliese LS, Reis SRA, Andrade ZA (2003) Influence of low level laser therapy on wound healing and its biological action upon myofibroblasts. Lasers Surg Med 32(3):239–244

Mester E, Szende B, Gärtner P (1968) The effect of laser beams on the growth of hair in mice. Radiobiol Radiother 9(5):621–626

Pessoa ES, Melhado RM, Theodoro LH, Garcia VGA (2004) Histologic assessment of the influence of low-intensity laser therapy on wound healing in steroid-treated animals. Photomed Laser Surg 22(3):199–204

Planck M (1900) On the theory of the energy distribution law of the normal spectrum. Verhandl Dtsch phys Ges 2: 237. http://www.ffn.ub.es/luisnavarro/nuevo_maletin/Planck%20(1900),%20Distribution%20Law.pdf. Zugegriffen im Januar 2008.

Prianti AC Jr, Silva JA Jr, Dos Santos RF, Rosseti IB, Costa MS (2014) Low-level laser therapy (LLLT) reduces the COX-2 mRNA expression in both subplantar and total brain tissues in the model of peripheral inflammation induced by administration of carrageenan. Lasers Med Sci Jul 29(4):1397–1403

Ristow M (2014) Unraveling the truth about antioxidants: mitohormesis explains ROS-induced health benefits. Nat Med 20:709–711

Sapolski R, Rivier C, Yamamoto G, Plotsky P, Vale W (1987) Interleukin-1 stimulates the secretion of hypothalamic corticotropin-releasing factor. Science 238(4826):522–524

Shadel GS, Horvath TL (2015) Mitochondrial ROS signaling in organismal homeostasis. Cell 163:560–569

Shimizu N, Yamaguchi M, Goseki T, Shibata Y, Takiguchi H, Iwasawa T, Abiko Y (1995) Inhibition of prostaglandin E2 and interleukin-1 beta production by low power laser irradiation in stretched human periodontal ligament cells. J Dent Res 74:1382–1388

Suter VGA, Sjölund S, Bornstein MM (2017) Effect of laser on pain relief and wound healing of recurrent aphthous stomatitis: a systematic review. Lasers Med Sci 32(4):953–963

Walt Dosierungsvorschläge. https://waltza.co.za/documentation-links/recommendations/dosage-recommendations/. Zugegriffen am 13.06.2020.

Wang Y, Huang YY, Wang Y, Lyu P, Hamblin MR (2016) Photobiomodulation of human adipose-derived stem cells using 810 nm and 980 nm lasers operates via different mechanisms of action. Biochim Biophys Acta 2:441–449

Woodruff LD, Bounkeo JM, Brannon WM, Dawes KS, Barham CD, Waddell DL, Enwemeka CS (2004) The efficacy of laser therapy in wound repair: a meta-analysis of the literature. Photomed Laser Surg 22(3):241–247

Zecha JAEM, Raber-Durlacher JE, Nair RG, Epstein JB, Elad S, Hamblin MR, Barasch A, Migliorati CA, Milstein DMJ, Genot MT, Lansaat L, van der Brink R, Arnabat-Dominguez J, van der Molen L, Jacobi I, van Diessen J, de Lange J, Smeele LE, Schubert MM, Bensadoun RJ (2016) Low-level laser therapy/photobiomodulation in the management of side effects of chemoradiation therapy in head and neck cancer: part 2: proposed applications and treatment protocols. Support Care Cancer 24(6):2793–2805

7 High-Frequency Therapy (HF)

7.1 Definition of High-Frequency Therapy

High-frequency therapy (HF) refers to the use of electromagnetic waves with a frequency higher than 300 kHz up to a maximum, depending on the author, of 100 GHz. The upper limit is chosen because this is approximately where the infrared range begins and the radio wave range ends, although the transition is gradual. Radio waves do not trigger action potentials in tissue, nor do they induce electrochemical processes such as those that occur, for example, with direct current. The waves generate heat, and it is likely that the electromagnetic energy also has an additional effect on certain physiological processes. Since the heat is generated rather deep within the tissue, the therapy is also called diathermy, which literally means “deep heating.” As we will see later, the name is somewhat unfortunately chosen. The method is not exactly new; it dates back to applications recommended by the French physicist and physician Jacques-Arsène d’Arsonval as early as 1892 (Kowarschik 1926). HF is not used only in physiotherapy. The method is also employed for coagulating blood vessels and for cutting in surgery, for warming people who have become severely hypothermic, for example, in an avalanche (Hébette 2012), or after thoracic surgery in which the patient has been significantly cooled (Schmicke 1984), as well as for the removal of warts. HF is also used in cancer therapy for hyperthermia, in which the whole body or a body part is heated to 40–43 °C.

At international conferences in 1947 in Atlantic City (USA) and 1959 in Geneva (Switzerland), certain frequencies were reserved exclusively for medical purposes. Had this not been done, it would have led to unimaginably chaotic situations, since the devices used for therapy are very powerful transmitters that could interfere with normal radio communication and radio and television reception over a wide area. For example: An amateur radio operator in Germany can use his small citizen band radio with a power output of 0.5–12 W, depending on the antenna, to communicate up to 80 km. A modern shortwave device for therapy has a peak output of 1000 W (pulsed). The claim that in the 1960s a shortwave device in a clinic in the Swiss Jura interfered with air traffic communications may be an “urban legend,” but it is certainly possible.

The frequencies used therapeutically are:

- 27.12 MHz, with a wavelength of 11.06 m, called shortwave (SW)
- 433.92 MHz, wavelength 69 cm, also called decimeter wave (DM) (has fallen out of use)
- 2450 MHz, wavelength 12.5 cm, also called radar, microwave (MW), or centimeter wave

P. van Kerkhof, *Evidence-Based Electrotherapy*, https://doi.org/10.1007/978-3-662-73019-5_7

In the following, continuous shortwave application will be referred to as "SW" and pulsed SW application as "pulsed-SW." The use of decimeter waves will not be discussed in detail. In terms of depth of penetration, its application is closer to MW than to inductive SW application.

If the frequency f is known, the wavelength λ can be calculated using the formula $c = \lambda \times f$, where c is the propagation speed in the respective medium. If the speed of light in a vacuum is assumed for c, the wavelength of SW in a vacuum is 11.06 m. In the human body, the wavelengths change depending on the type of tissue. The frequencies, however, remain the same. For this reason, some authors prefer to refer to the applications by their frequency rather than by their wavelength.

The three applications mentioned have comparable physiological effects, so they will be discussed together below. The physical properties, especially the penetration depths, differ, and this has consequences for their areas of application. This will be discussed in the relevant sections.

7.2 Pulsing

HF is, a priori, a heat therapy. The development of a pulse mechanism in 1935, in which the continuous energy output is regularly interrupted, made it possible to use HF even in pathologies where heat is contraindicated. For the first time, "athermal effects" were discussed (Ginsberg 1961). The pauses between pulses result in a slower rise in temperature and allow the circulatory system to dissipate the heat. The pulse intensity in watts can be freely selected, as can the pulse frequency. Some devices also allow the pulse duration to be set. A low frequency with short pulses and low intensity logically leads to a lower energy output and consequently to a reduced thermal effect. It is essential to note during application that there are no thermoreceptors where a large part of the energy is delivered. A patient therefore only feels warmth when, after some time, it reaches the skin by conduction and convection. It cannot be ruled out that the physiological effects observed in "athermal" pulsed mode occur due to weak thermal effects (Kitchen and Partridge 1992; Low 1995; Bricknell and Watson 1995; Draper et al. 1999; Al-Mandeel and Watson 2010). Incidentally, this shows that the term diathermy is somewhat unfortunate. An "athermal diathermy" is an oxymoron.

7.3 Heat Generation

Heat in tissue is generated by an electric field alternating at high frequency. This electric field is produced in three different ways: with a capacitor (capacitive) or with a coil (inductive) in SW, with a resonant circuit generator in DM, and with a magnetron in MW.

7.3.1 Capacitor Field Method

A plate capacitor consists of two parallel electrodes with an insulating material in between, the so-called dielectric. The plates are connected to a power source and can store charge. This results in an electric field forming between the plates. The polar molecules in the dielectric, such as water and proteins, align themselves according to their charge in this electric field; this is called orientation polarization. If the direction of the electric field is reversed, these molecules realign, which is called a relaxation process. In nonpolar molecules, the charge within the molecule shifts; this is called displacement polarization. Both processes together are referred to as electric polarization. In the SW capacitor field method, this alignment occurs 27,120,000 times per second, leading to heat production by friction in the dielectric. In a therapeutic application, the patient, or a part of them, is the dielectric. Heat production now depends on the physical properties of the different tissue types, as well as on the arrangement of the electrodes (the capacitor plates) and the tissue layers. The alternating electric field also sets ions in motion, both polar and nonpolar molecules, at the frequency of the alternating field.

This is called electrical conduction and also contributes to heat generation through friction.

Polar molecules are those in which the electric charge is not evenly distributed, such as the water molecule, which has a positively and a negatively charged side; it is a dipole. In nonpolar molecules, the electric charge is evenly distributed. Under the influence of the electric field, however, the charge distribution in such a nonpolar molecule is altered so that it behaves like a polar molecule; it acquires a so-called temporary dipole moment.

The relative permittivity, also called dielectric conductivity, indicates how permeable a material or tissue is to electric fields. Permittivity is the product of the permittivity of a vacuum ε_0 and the relative permittivity ε_r. The greater the number, the more the dipoles in the tissue can be aligned when exposed to an electric field. Muscle tissue has an ε_r of 108 at 27 MHz, while that of fat is 20. Ideally, this method could generate heat very effectively in tissue with a high proportion of dipoles (water), as is the case with muscle. However, electrode placement and anatomy come into play. In a transverse application, for example with one electrode medial and one lateral to the knee, the electric field is almost perpendicular to the course of the tissue layers. This is shown in a highly simplified manner in Fig. 7.1.

The electric field will deliver most of its energy where the electrical resistance is greatest: in the skin and subcutaneous fat. In addition, at the boundaries between different tissue types, charge accumulation occurs due to electric polarization. This ultimately leads to the deeper layers being practically shielded, and most of the energy is delivered very superficially, to the skin and subcutaneous fat tissue. The specific absorption rate (SAR, in W/kg) in this case is about 10 times lower for muscle tissue than for skin and fat tissue. The strong local superficial temperature increase can quickly lead to pain, which forces the use of rather low intensities. Therefore, with this application, significant deep heating with temperatures in the therapeutic range (40–44 °C) is not to be expected (Lehmann 1990). Any warming of the joint capsule of a somewhat deeper joint will only occur due to convection and conduction of the superficially generated heat. If the application were used as a "longitudinal application" (Fig. 7.2), the current generated by the electric field would take the path of least resistance through the muscle.

Theoretically, the SAR for muscle tissue in this case would be 20 to 30 times higher than for the superficial layers. Unfortunately, this does not work in practice, since the first layers that must be overcome are also perpendicular to the electrodes. In longitudinal application, there are even areas where no heat is generated at all. For example, in such an application to the lower leg (one electrode proximal at the knee, one under the foot), a temperature increase will occur mainly somewhere ventral at the distal lower

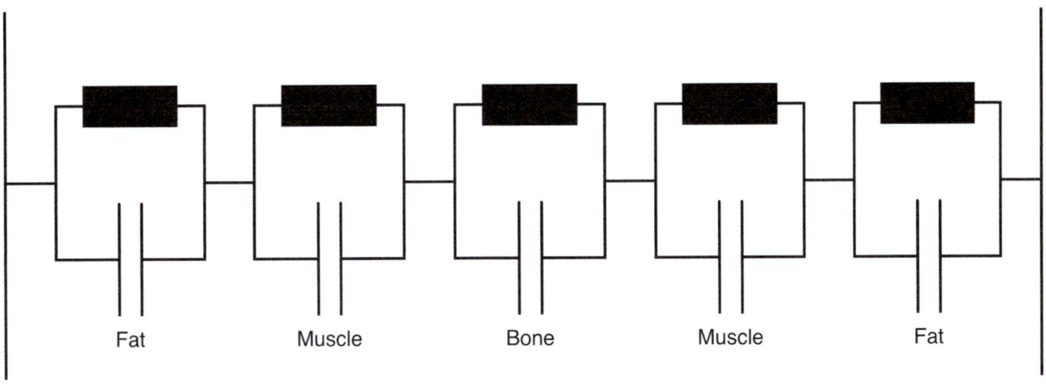

Fig. 7.1 Series circuit in tissue

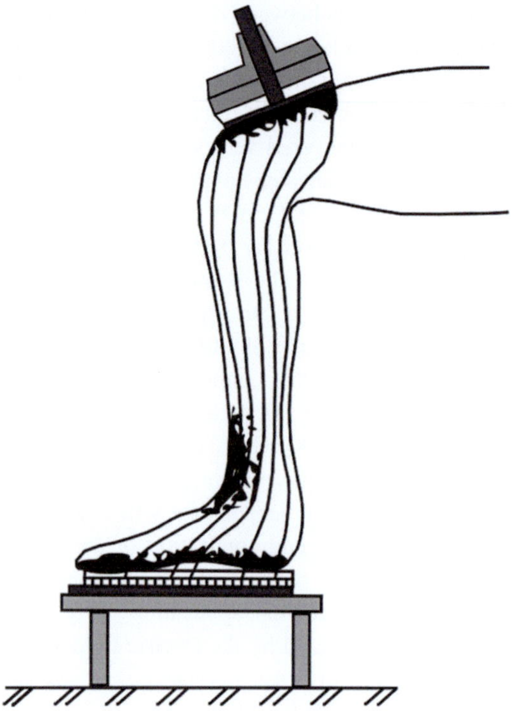

Fig. 7.2 Longitudinal application. A shell electrode at the knee, a rubber electrode under the foot. © Enraf-Nonius, Delft, Netherlands, with kind permission

leg, certainly not throughout the entire lower leg. The capacitor field method is therefore mainly suitable for rather superficially localized pathologies.

A small study of 10 subjects by Oosterveld et al. (1992) showed the following: After an SW application (continuous, 15 min, 180 W, Schliephake (disc) electrodes Ø 13 cm, medial and lateral to the knee, electrode-skin distance 3 cm), the skin temperature increased on average from 27.6 °C to 30 °C and the intra-articular temperature from 32.5 °C to 33.9 °C. This 1.4 °C increase is just enough to stimulate metabolic processes (Lehmann 1990). The 30 °C skin temperature is well below the threshold of about 44 °C for thermal nociceptors in the skin. However, a lignoparaffin pack (50 °C, 10 min) was able to raise the intra-articular temperature from 32.5 to 36 °C (ΔT 3.5 °C). So much for the depth effect of the SW capacitor field method.

7.3.2 Coil Field Method

When an electric current flows through a wire, this current generates a magnetic field around the wire. With direct current, this is called a static field or a static magnetic field. If alternating current flows, the magnetic field changes direction at the same frequency as the alternating current. Magnetic fields generated by alternating electric fields are called magnetic eddy fields. These alternating magnetic fields in turn generate alternating electric fields, and the process repeats itself, the wave propagates. In this context, we speak of electromagnetic waves. These waves have, depending on their parameters and method of generation, interesting properties. They can be used to transmit conversations or to heat food. The fact that alternating electric waves generated by capacitor plates can be used to heat human tissue and thus trigger therapeutic effects has already been mentioned. A coil can do this as well, but works somewhat differently.

Alternating current that changes direction less than 3000 times per second (frequency below 3000 Hz) is referred to by physicists as low-frequency current. Alternating current that does this more than 3000 times per second (frequency above 3000 Hz) is called high-frequency current. All radio applications fall into the high-frequency range. High-frequency current can be emitted as an electromagnetic wave via antennas. Therefore, it is also referred to as high-frequency electromagnetic radiation (sometimes the threshold for high frequency is given as 30,000 Hz [30 kHz] or 100,000 Hz [100 kHz]).

To generate alternating magnetic fields, alternating current is passed through a wire, since every current flow generates a magnetic field. If the wire is formed into a loop, a magnetic field is created inside the loop. If two or more such loops are used, it is called a coil. In a coil, the magnetic fields of the individual loops add up, creating a relatively strong magnetic field inside the coil, which then generates an electric field. In HF therapy, this is referred to as a radiator, for example a minode, monode, or diplode/flexiplode. In electrically conductive tissue, these alternating magnetic fields now induce eddy currents, and it is these electric currents that are responsible for heat generation in the tissue. Compared to the electric field, the influence of magnetic fields on polar molecules in tissue is negligibly small.

This is related to the so-called magnetic susceptibility, which in turn is related to magnetic permeability. The latter is the same for human tissue as for a vacuum and is zero. For the interested reader, the "Tipler" (Tipler et al. 2019) is recommended at this point.

A magnetic field, as described above, can, in contrast to the electric field, easily penetrate deeper tissue and induce an electric field there. If the coil is constructed so that the electric field generated by the alternating magnetic field is parallel to the deeper muscle tissue, significantly more heat will be generated here than with the capacitor field method, sparing the skin and superficial fat layer.

It is essential to note that the magnetic field is weakest in the center of the coil, and consequently, the generated electric field is also weakest there. Therefore, the strongest heating occurs *beside* the central axis of the coil. Consequence: The center of the applicator should not be aimed at the area to be treated, but slightly beside it. The user manual provides further information on this.

An electric field is also generated with a coil, which causes strong superficial heating. One method to reduce the effect of the electric field is the construction of a kind of Faraday cage on a monode, as is the case, for example, with the Circuplode®. This metal grid attached to the front of the applicator diverts part of the electric field and thus reduces the surface load of the capacitive effect, allowing greater energy delivery to deeper layers (Fig. 7.3).

The electric eddy field always exists, regardless of whether conductive tissue is present or

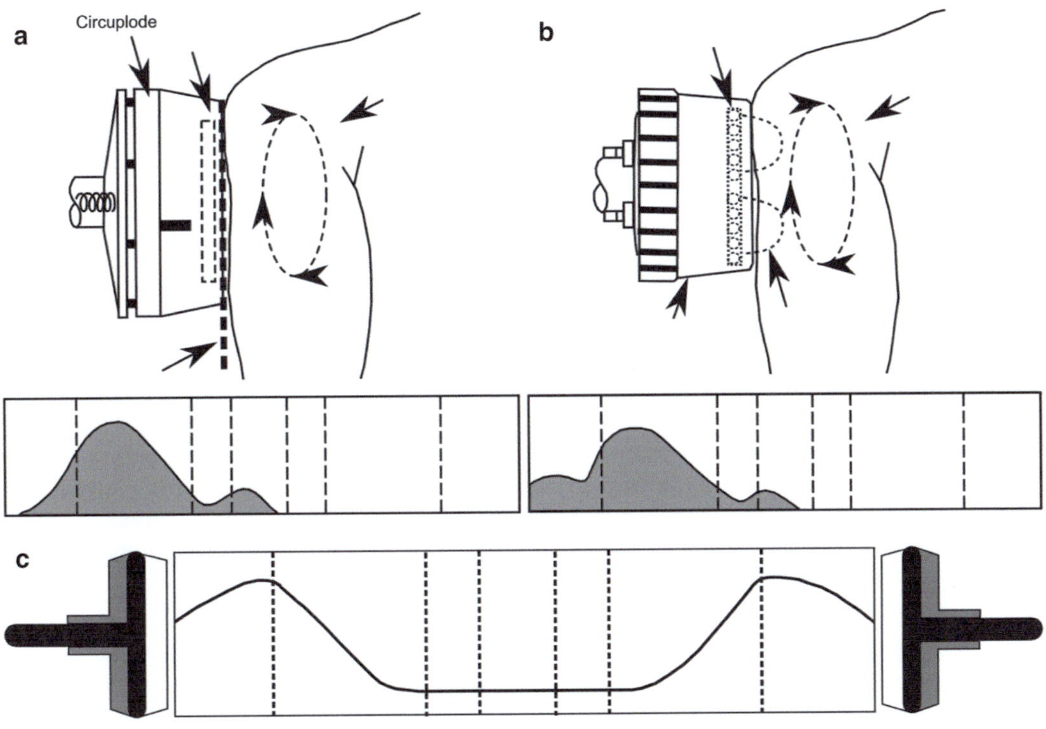

Fig. 7.3 (**a**) Energy distribution with a Circuplode® (inductive). Note the low fat load; (**b**) Energy distribution with a normal coil (monode, inductive); (**c**) Energy distribution when using 2 shell electrodes (capacitive method). Note the high fat load compared to the inductive method. © Enraf-Nonius, Delft, Netherlands, with kind permission

not. However, electric current is only generated in conductive tissue. If a tissue is not homogeneously conductive, but has areas of better and worse conductivity, as in muscle, the eddy current will take the path of least resistance and cause the strongest heating there. This leads to uneven and, above all, unpredictable heating.

7.4 Application of High-Frequency Therapy

Therapeutic effects of heat occur when the tissue to be treated reaches a temperature of 40–44 °C and this temperature is maintained for at least 5 min (Lehmann 1990). This applies to improving blood circulation, enhancing the viscoelastic properties of various tissue types, reducing muscle tension, and relieving pain.

7.4.1 Improvement of Blood Circulation

It is well known that an increase in temperature affects blood circulation (McMeeken 1994; Malanga et al. 2015). In this context, Lehmann et al. elegantly confirmed the cooling effect of increased blood flow (Lehmann 1990). In a healthy subject, an SW application was performed on the thigh using a coil, and the temperature was measured at various depths. The coil-skin distance was 3.5 cm. The intensity was set so that the person experienced "only mild pain" after 12 min, allegedly the highest setting on the device (400 W). The application lasted 22 min. During the first 12 min, the skin temperature rose from 32 to about 42 °C, at a depth of 0.7 cm from 34 to 44 °C, and at 1.6 cm depth from 35 to 43 °C. After 12 min, the temperature quickly dropped by about 2 °C at each depth. After circulation was interrupted with a tourniquet, the temperature quickly rose again to the highest value within about 2 min and remained there for several minutes after the device was turned off. Conclusion: After a critical temperature was reached, probably 44 °C, the increased blood flow efficiently transported the heat away. In another study with the same parameters, but using the direct contact method with a terry cloth as an intermediate layer, the temperature of 44 °C at a depth of 1.2 cm was reached after just 6 min, and the same phenomenon of the cooling effect of blood flow was observed. It was also shown that superficial heating with the contact method was clearly stronger in this case compared to the "distance method." Because some subjects experienced excessive pain, the study had to be discontinued for them. Al-Mandeel and Watson studied the effect of pulsed-SW (27.12 MHz) on blood flow in the lower leg and on skin temperature in healthy subjects and found that after an average energy delivery of 24 W over 10 min, blood flow had doubled (Al-Mandeel and Watson 2010). Skin temperature increased by just under 2 °C. Only 11 of 31 subjects perceived the temperature increase. More on this later.

7.4.2 Viscoelastic Properties

We know that collagen behaves elastically under tension at body temperature. If the temperature is increased above 50 °C, the tissue shrinks and then liquefies. At temperatures up to 44 °C, viscosity changes and, under tension, plastic adaptation occurs, with the structure experiencing a lasting elongation of a few percent. However, some authors assume that the effects occur when the temperature is increased by a certain value. For example, the extensibility of collagen is said to improve when the local temperature increases by about 4 °C. However, if the initial temperature, as in the case of a knee joint, is about 31 °C and the temperature is raised to 35 °C, this temperature is well below the required therapeutic range and can only stimulate local metabolism. However, there are studies showing that this 4 °C increase is sufficient as a pretreatment for mobilization (Draper et al. 2004a, b; Seiger and Draper 2006). Lehmann's values are therefore not set in stone.

Peres et al. (2002) showed in healthy subjects that after pretreatment with pulsed-SW (coil 200 cm^2, 15 min, 800 Hz, 400 µs pulse, max. 150 W, Ø 48 W, 43.2 kJ, 216 J/cm^2), passive mobility of the ankle joint was significantly improved. Draper et al. (2004a, b) showed in healthy subjects that pretreatment with pulsed-SW (coil 200 cm^2, 15 min, 800 Hz, 400 µs pulse, max. 150 W, Ø 48 W, 43.2 kJ, 216 J/cm^2) significantly improved the extensibility of the hamstrings. There are also publications from the Draper group describing how pulsed-SW can be successfully used as a pretreatment for mobilization of joints with restricted mobility, even in the presence of osteosynthesis material (Draper et al. 2004a, b; Seiger and Draper 2006). Robertson et al. (2005) showed in healthy subjects that an SW application to the lower leg (rubber electrodes 12 × 17 cm, on both sides of the lower leg, 15 min "pleasantly warm") improved extensibility significantly more than a hot pack (25 × 30 cm, 80 °C, 2 layers of terry cloth, 15 min). Wright and Johns had already objectively demonstrated in 1960 in patients with rheumatoid arthritis that their (hand and finger) joints were significantly less stiff after warming to 43 °C. Every patient can confirm this, but it simply had to be objectified. Bäcklund and Tiselius confirmed the correlation between subjective and objective findings (Bäcklund and Tiselius 1967). In this case, it is of course important to note that in active synovitis or arthritis, enzymatic processes that destroy cartilage are activated at temperatures around 35–36 °C (Harris and McCroskery 1974). Interestingly, in vitro, the activity of such destructive enzymes decreases markedly above 38 °C after an initial increase, probably because the proteins are denatured. That stronger heating of an inflamed joint leads to improvement seems counterintuitive, but the idea is not new (Weinberger et al. 1988; Jeziorski 2018) and the method has already been successfully used in patients with gonarthrosis (Takahashi et al. 2011). Although data from whole-body hyperthermia show successful treatments, for example in patients with ankylosing spondylitis, little is known about local treatment.

7.4.3 Muscle Tone

Mense demonstrated in 1978 that muscle spindle activity decreases with heating "in the therapeutic range," and this can lead to a reduction in muscle tone (Mense 1978). If a heat application relieves pain, this can also have a normalizing effect on muscle tone (Malanga et al. 2015).

7.4.4 Pain Relief

Heat relieves pain in various ways (Malanga et al. 2015): by improving blood circulation (Charkoudian 2010), by improving metabolism (Nadler et al. 2004), by improving mobility due to changes in the viscoelastic properties of collagen and synovial fluid (Bleakley and Costello 2013), and by stimulating skin receptors and consequently activating descending pain inhibition mechanisms (Palazzo et al. 2008).

7.4.5 Metabolism

For the stimulation of metabolic processes, van't Hoff's law applies, according to which every chemical reaction is stimulated by a factor of 2–3 when the temperature is increased by 10 °C (Abramson et al. 1961; Atkins and De Paula 2014). This means that each degree of temperature increase accelerates metabolic processes by about 13%, of course only within certain physiological limits. This can be exploited in the treatment of poorly healing wounds or in the stimulation of chronic "burned-out" pathologies.

7.5 Temperature Measurements

Unfortunately, there are very few studies in which the increase in temperature was measured in vivo in humans. The studies by Lehmann regarding the temperature increase in the thigh have already been mentioned; the various values are detailed in Tables 7.1 and 7.2. Lehmann describes these studies in his book (1990). The author notes that the intensity was maximal, which for the device used (Siemens Ultratherm® 608 at level 5) corresponds to a power output of 400 W. The size of the applicator is unknown, but illustrations in his book suggest a monode with an area of about 200 cm^2. This implies an energy delivery after 6 min of about 144 kJ (720 J/cm^2) and after 12 min of about 290 kJ (1450 J/cm^2). After a temperature of 44 °C was reached, the temperature decreased by 2 °C due to improved blood flow (Tables 7.1 and 7.2).

Draper et al. also conducted studies on in vivo temperature increase using pulsed shortwave. The choice of parameters seems rather arbitrary, presumably determined in preliminary experiments. His results (Draper et al. 1999) with the inductive method: "coil" (not further defined, probably Faraday-shielded) 200 cm^2, coil-skin distance 2.5 cm, plastic housing in contact with the skin without terry cloth or similar.

Measurement at 3 cm depth in the gastrocnemius, 800 Hz, 400 μs bursts, 850 μs burst interval, maximum intensity 150 W/burst, average energy output 48 W. After 5 min, this corresponds to an energy delivery of about 14.5 kJ = 72 J/cm^2, 10 times less than with Lehmann.

Temperature increases:

- Initial temperature 35.84 °C ± 0.93 °C
- after 5 min Δt 1.36 °C ± 0.9 °C
- after 10 min Δt 2.87 °C ± 1.44 °C
- after 15 min Δt 3.78 °C ± 1.19 °C
- after 20 min Δt 3.49 °C ± 1.13 °C
- maximum thus 39.80 °C

This is roughly equivalent to the result of an ultrasound application with 1 MHz, 1.5 W/cm^2, 10 min, 2 times ERA (10 cm^2), although with this coil a significantly larger area can be efficiently heated (Peres et al. 2002).

With Lehmann, the temperature at about 3 cm after 6 min (144 kJ, 720 J/cm^2) had increased by a good 5 °C, while with Draper at 3 cm depth after 5 min (14.5 kJ = 72 J/cm^2) it was just under 1.5 °C. These are at least data that can be used in clinical practice.

In a study comparing heating with pulsed shortwave and ultrasound of the gastrocnemius (Garrett et al. 2000), it was confirmed that ultrasound is completely unsuitable for heating large

Table 7.1 27.12 MHz, coil, thigh musculature. Intensity 400 W, coil-skin distance 3.5 cm, 0.6 cm fat layer, after 12 min "mild pain"

Measurement depth in cm	Temperature at start °C	Temperature after 12 min °C	Δt °C
Skin	32	41.8	9.8
1.07	34	44	10
1.60	34.8	43.4	8.6
2.54	35.8	43.3	7.5
3.47	36	38.2	2.2
4.14	36.2	39.2	3

Table 7.2 27.12 MHz, coil, thigh musculature. Intensity 400 W, coil-skin distance 0.3 cm, 1 cm fat layer, after 6 min in some subjects discontinued due to "severe pain"

Measurement depth in cm	Temperature at start °C	Temperature after 7 min °C	Δt °C
Skin	30.8	42.2	11.4
0.6	32.4	43.8	11.4
1.2	34	44.2	10.2
3.22	35.8	41	5.2
3.48	37	41.2	4.2
3.89	37.2	41	3.8

areas. Parameters: pulsed shortwave as above in Draper et al. (1999). Ultrasound: 1 MHz, 1.5 W/cm^2, ERA 5 cm^2, 20 min, continuous, area = 40 times the ERA (200 cm^2!). Measurements were taken at three different sites at 3 cm depth. Heating with pulsed shortwave after 20 min: between 3.02 °C ± 1.02 °C and 4.58 °C ± 0.87 °C (in the center of the treatment area). With ultrasound: 0.17 °C ± 0.40 °C to 0.43 °C ± 0.41 °C. Almost like laying on of hands.

Martin and Herrick conducted an in vivo study with MW (2450 MHz). The temperature in the quadriceps at 5 cm depth was measured after 20 min of MW application (Martin and Herrick 1955). Unfortunately, no technical details or information on intensity were provided. The authors only mention that the power was determined based on the maximum tolerated intensity of the subjects and corresponded to 50–100 % of the device's output, which is also unknown. They note that temperature increases of 3–5 °C occurred with varying thicknesses of the subcutaneous fat layer (4–25 mm). Nothing is known about the exact correlations between fat layer, intensity, and temperature increase. At least it was shown that muscle tissue at a depth of 5 cm can be adequately heated, but probably only with intensities that are unusually high by today's standards.

Al-Mandeel and Watson in 2010 investigated the effect of pulsed shortwave (27.12 MHz) on blood flow in the lower leg and skin temperature in 31 healthy subjects of different ages. The effects of "high" intensity (average energy output 24 W) and "low" intensity (Ø 3 W) were compared with a placebo group (Ø 0.05 W). Applicator: Faraday-shielded coil, 200 cm^2.

Parameters:

- 24 W: max. intensity 150 W, 200 μs pulse, 800 Hz, 10 min (14.4 kJ, 72 J/cm^2)
- 3 W: max. intensity 150 W, 100 μs, 200 Hz, 10 min (1.8 kJ, 9 J/cm^2)
- Placebo 0.05 W: 150 W, 20 μs, 50 Hz, 10 min (0.03 kJ, 0.15 J/cm^2)

Results:

- Blood flow in the 24 W group was more than doubled in the treated lower leg and on the contralateral side (only relative values were reported).
- Blood flow in the 3 W group increased very slightly, but only on the treated side.
- Skin temperature in the 24 W group increased by 1.96 °C on the treated side, and by 0.45 °C contralaterally.
- Skin temperature in the 3 W group increased by 0.34 °C on the treated side, and decreased by 0.13 °C contralaterally.
- The placebo group and the control group showed no significant changes in blood flow or temperature.

The inductive method with the mentioned special electrode (type Circuplode®) primarily generates heating in deeper, well-perfused layers; this heat only reaches the thermoreceptors in the skin after a certain time. Thus, if the skin temperature had increased by almost 2 °C, this implies a greater heating in deeper layers, possibly in the range of 3–4 °C or more.

It was particularly remarkable that in the 24 W group only 11 of the 31 subjects perceived the temperature increase, and in the 3 W group only one person out of 31. Note that these were healthy subjects whose sensitivity had been checked beforehand! Pulsed shortwave is preferably used in acute pathologies where heating is to be avoided. The results of this study highlight two problems in determining intensity: First, the investigators showed that even at very low intensities (Ø 3 W), thermal effects occur, and second, that when determining intensity in this so-called athermal application, one cannot rely on the patient's statements. Not exactly trivial.

Microwaves, 2450 MHz (MW)

After the Americans received the necessary technology from the British following World War II, the specialists allegedly took a long time to understand the underlying physics. The following is a highly simplified explanation of the effect for the interested colleague. For those who want the full details, Tipler (2019) is recommended.

Microwaves, whether in the kitchen or the military, are generated with a magnetron. A magnetron consists of a metal cavity with a so-called heated cathode in the center (Fig. 7.4). The outer wall of the cavity is the anode. When a current flows, the cathode begins to glow and emits electrons. These move toward the positively charged outer wall. Two magnets, one above and one below, generate a magnetic field in the cavity, forcing the electrons into a spiral circular motion around the cathode. Eventually, they circle past the cavities in the outer wall. This causes alternating charge displacements in the cavities, resulting in the generation of electromagnetic fields, with the size of the cavities determining their frequency. Some electrons are slowed down during their flight, others are accelerated. This creates groups of electrons, a kind of pattern that looks like a spoked wheel rotating around the cathode. This amplifies the generation of microwaves. The MW are conducted outward and radiated via an antenna.

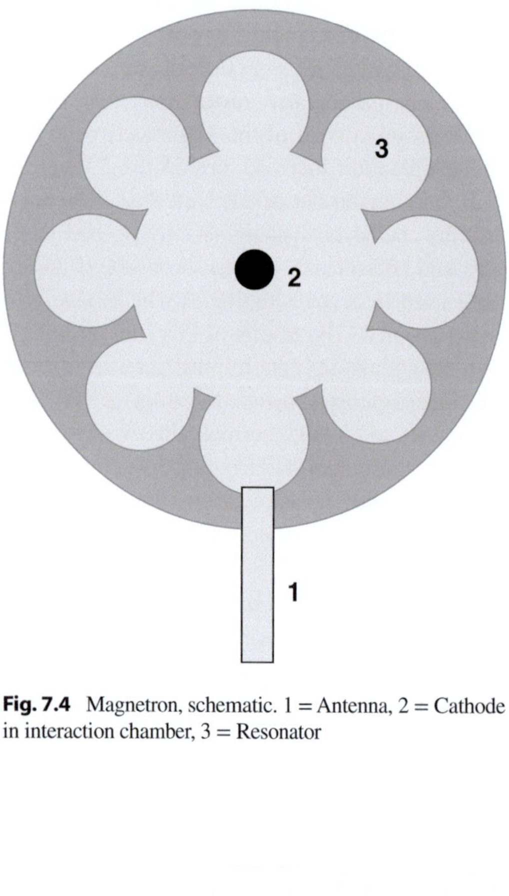

Fig. 7.4 Magnetron, schematic. 1 = Antenna, 2 = Cathode in interaction chamber, 3 = Resonator

As already mentioned, the penetration depth of electromagnetic waves is frequency-dependent: the higher the frequency, the lower the depth of penetration. MW energy, like SW, is preferentially delivered to well-conducting, water-rich tissue such as muscle and can penetrate fat tissue with relatively little loss. However, in vivo, an unknown proportion of the energy is reflected at the fat-muscle interface, which, due to the formation of standing waves, can lead to relatively strong heating in the fat tissue, with correspondingly large energy losses. The remaining energy does not penetrate very deeply into the muscle tissue; some authors mention a half-value depth of at most about 1 cm for MW, with SW being theoretically somewhat better. Compared to inductive SW application, MW therapy has several disadvantages. First, as mentioned, standing waves can occur due to reflections at tissue boundaries, leading to hotspots with local temperature peaks. When and where these hotspots occur is unpredictable. It is also unpredictable how much energy actually penetrates the tissue and how much is lost as stray energy and released to the environment. From today's perspective, this is somewhat problematic in terms of radiation hygiene and can also cause interference with devices in the immediate vicinity. The debate as to whether the energy of these radio frequencies is harmful to health in the long term continues. The fact is that all authors advise against prolonged exposure to the radiation (Delpizzo and Joyner 1987; Shields et al. 2004; Andrikopoulos et al. 2017).

7.6 Indications

HF therapy has been (and continues to be) used for a wide variety of pathologies that are not typically part of everyday physiotherapy practice. These include, for example, pathologies from dermatology, internal medicine, ENT, and gynecology. Much of the literature on these treatments comes from the early years of SW therapy, and as with any new therapy, it is understandable that its introduction at the time triggered a real hype—naturally also because the pharmaceutical options were very different from today. Accordingly, there is little that was not treated, and some indications have survived on indication lists more for traditional than rational reasons. Nevertheless, there is some more recent literature on "unusual" indications that, despite the usual methodological shortcomings, justifies the use of HF therapy, namely:

- Maxillary sinusitis (Shinde and Jayawant 2012; Heggannavar et al. 2017)
- Dysmenorrhea (Jo and Lee 2018; Machado et al. 2019)
- Chronic pelvic conditions (Lamina et al. 2011)

HF is now used primarily for pathologies of the musculoskeletal system, including post-traumatic, postoperative, degenerative, and inflammatory conditions. In addition, successes have been reported in the treatment of skin defects (McGaughey et al. 2009) and neurological conditions such as carpal tunnel syndrome (Fu et al. 2019).

HF application in continuous mode is clearly a thermotherapy, and it is understandably impossible to distinguish thermal from non-thermal effects.

For the following pathologies, clinical studies have shown a positive effect of HF therapy. The studies may be of good to very good methodological quality according to Cochrane, Consort, or PEDro criteria, but unfortunately, they almost all share the same serious flaw: the dosage is very rarely traceable (Table 7.3):

- Knee osteoarthritis pain (MW and SW, continuous and pulsed) (Takahashi et al. 2011; Atamaz et al. 2012; Laufer and Dar 2012; Rabini et al. 2012; Wang et al. 2017; Ozen et al. 2019)
  - For the treatment of knee osteoarthritis pain, the results of using pulsed SW or SW are controversial. Ozen et al. and Wang

Table 7.3 Critique of studies on high-frequency therapy

The intensity in pulsed applications is almost always described as "athermal," and in continuous applications mostly as "pleasantly warm" or "according to tolerance," without more precise power specifications	Al-Mandeel and Watson showed in 2010 how unreliable this information is
Some authors mention that the device they used has a certain maximum output, but the intensity used is rarely specified; often, information such as "according to manufacturer's instructions" is provided	The information is worthless If the manufacturer is mentioned, it is possible to determine the intensity
Very few authors mention the applicator, let alone its area in cm^2	If you know the intensity and the area, you can calculate the energy per cm^2, which makes the study results comparable. 50 kJ on 12 cm^2 is quite different from 50 kJ on 200 cm^2
The electrode-skin distance and the distance from the coil to the skin are rarely mentioned	Lehmann showed with in vivo measurements how strongly energy delivery in deeper layers depends on the coil-skin distance
The local anatomical conditions (fat layer) are not mentioned	A thick fat layer "absorbs" more energy than a thin one
Treatment duration varies from 10 to 60 min	This makes it difficult to compare treatments or their results
The inductive method is mainly used	If you are lucky, somewhere in the publication "drum" (German: "barrel," here: coil) or "capacitive" (capacitive, condenser field) is mentioned. Sometimes you can guess, because certain devices always use coils or because the publication contains images

et al. found a positive effect of pulsed SW, while Laufer et al. (2005) found no effect.
- Knee osteoarthritis synovitis (pulsed SW) (Jan et al. 2006)
- Wound healing, pressure ulcers (pulsed SW) (Goldin et al. 1981; Masayoshi et al. 1991; McGaughey et al. 2009)
- Lateral epicondylitis (SW) (Babaei-Ghazani et al. 2020)
- Postoperative movement restrictions (pulsed SW) (Draper 2011)
- CTS (SW and MW) (Fu et al. 2019)
- Subacromiodeltoid bursitis with calcification (SW) (Ginsberg 1961)
- Subacromial impingement (SW) (Akyol et al. 2012; Yilmaz Kaysin et al. 2018)
- Post-traumatic conditions (pulsed SW) (Wilson 1972, 1974; Pennington et al. 1993)

Such incomplete information makes it impossible to compare the results of the studies and to establish a dose-response relationship.

7.7 Pulsed High Frequency

The use of pulsed HF is very popular, although it is still unclear whether and how the method works. On the one hand, it is possible that this is a weak thermal stimulus, with all the known consequences (Lehmann 1990; Bricknell and Watson 1995; Low 1995; Malanga et al. 2015). The temperature only needs to be raised locally by 1 °C to stimulate metabolism. The patient does not feel anything. Does that make the treatment athermal? On the other hand, there are theories suggesting that electromagnetic EM energy directly influences processes at and within the cell membrane, whereby the membrane properties disturbed in an inflammatory process are "normalized" by the HF energy (Luben 1997; Cleary 1997). Investigators have been able to demonstrate that the energy is absorbed at the membrane and subsequently leads to an improvement in intracellular processes. This would occur either by influencing ion transport or by activating various pump mechanisms (Panagopoulos et al. 2002; Pall 2013). Here, a comparison with the use of electromagnetic waves in another field is compelling (see Chap. 6 on laser therapy/photobiomodulation).

7.8 Methodology

The treatment outcome is influenced by many factors. In addition to treatment duration, treatment frequency, treatment intensity, and number of treatments, the following variables are available to us:

- Frequency: 27.12 MHz (SWD), 433.92 MHz (MWD), or 2450 MHz (MW)
- Method:
  - capacitive or inductive
  - continuous or pulsed
- Type of application:
  - Electrodes
    - Disc electrodes, also known as Schliephake electrodes
    - Soft rubber electrodes (pads)
    - Solenoid cable
  - Coils, applicators
    - Minode, Monode, Diplode/Flexiplode, Circuplode®
    - Round field, long field, and concave applicators (Pyrodor)
    - Special electrodes: axillary, rectal, vaginal electrode

The Applicators

For the capacitive application of SWD, there are disc electrodes. These consist of a metal electrode plate housed in a plastic casing. The plates can be moved so that the electrode-skin distance (ESD) can be adjusted. A greater distance leads to a better distribution of the field lines, resulting in more homogeneous heating. A small ESD leads to a strong surface effect, which means only low intensities are possible. This limits the depth

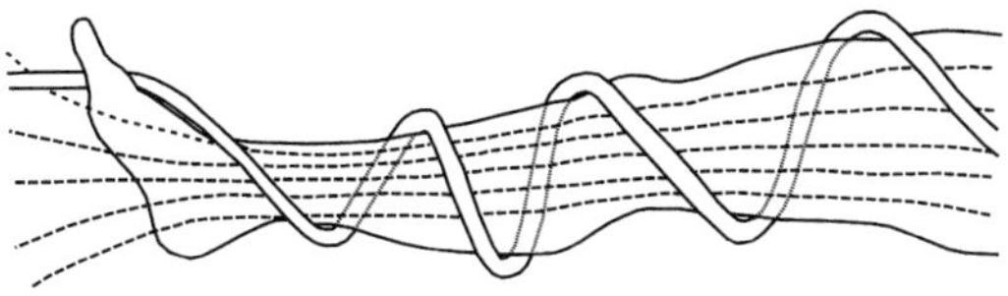

Fig. 7.5 Solenoid cable. © Enraf-Nonius, Delft, Netherlands, with kind permission

effect. One can attempt to concentrate the HF energy on one side of a joint by using an asymmetric setting. Of course, in such a case, it is easier to use a coil. There are also flexible plate electrodes (pads) made of rubber, which can be adapted somewhat to the body shape using fixation bands. The ESD here is set with felt pads about 1 cm thick (only when they are new!), see Fig. 7.6. For inductive application, there are coils in various designs. There is the relatively small Minode and the larger Monode. Some manufacturers equip a Monode with a metal grid so that part of the electric field is dissipated, thereby reducing the surface load; an example is the Circuplode®. The Diplode or Flexiplode is a coil made of movable parts and is therefore suitable for positioning, for example, around a shoulder or knee. The induction cable can be coiled into a "pancake" to treat a relatively large area, or it can be wrapped around a limb (Fig. 7.5).

One should not expect the entire limb to be heated evenly; the effect is very superficial. For MWD and MW, there are applicators that may also be called antennas or radiators. There are round field and long field applicators, as well as concave or hollow field applicators, which are suitable, for example, for large-area applications on the trunk. Some MW applicators are contact applicators (for example, the focus applicator), while others require a certain distance from the body, such as the long and round field applicators. Refer to the respective user manual for details.

The size of the area to be treated determines the size of the applicator. The inductive coil field method with a special electrode, in which the electric field is reduced, is best suited for the treatment of deeper structures and has been preferred for many years. In general: the higher the frequency, the more superficial the energy delivery. Therefore, MW with small, focused contact applicators are best suited for the treatment of local, rather superficial muscular pathologies (Fig. 7.6).

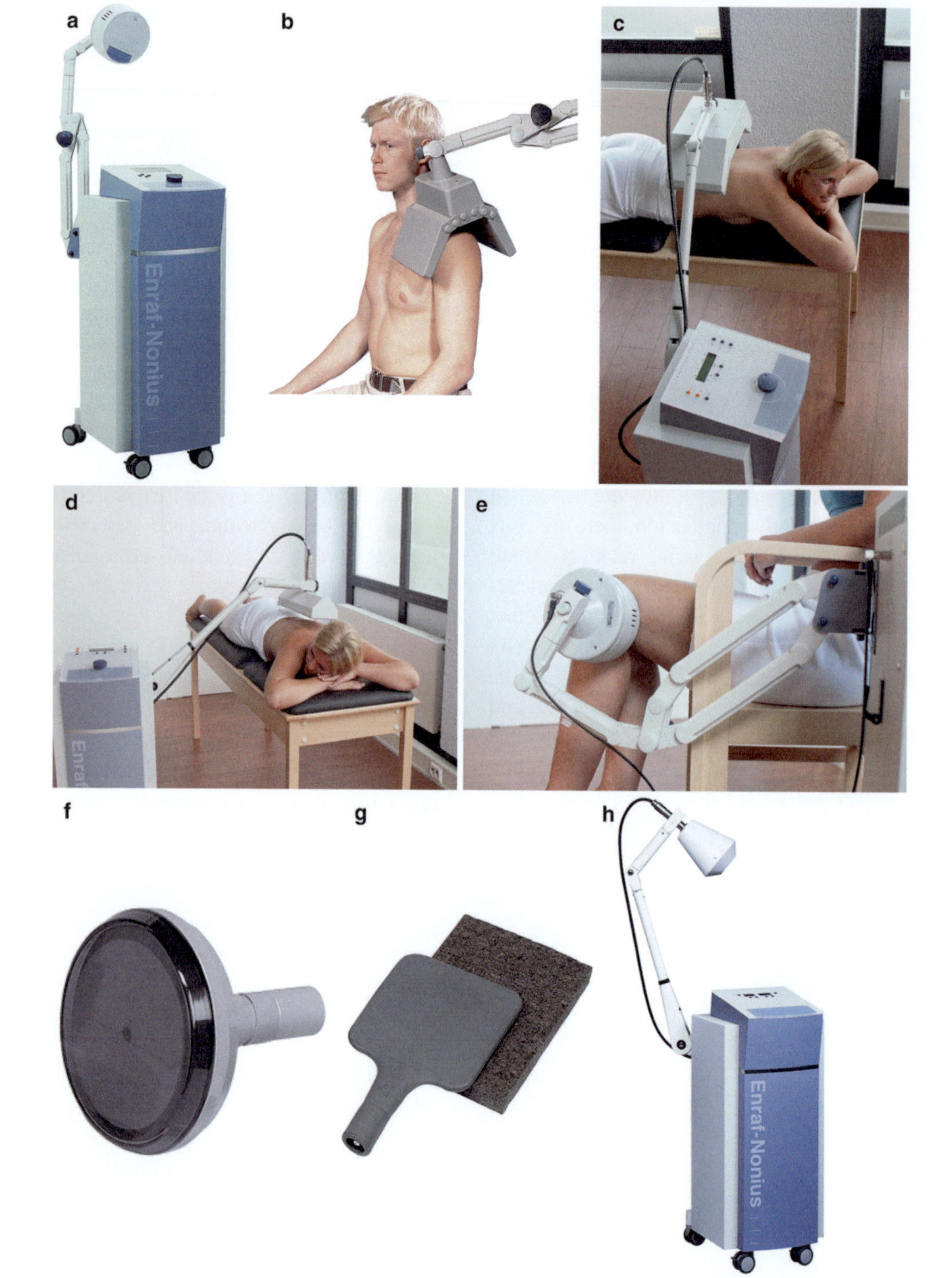

Fig. 7.6 (**a**) Modern SWD device; (**b**) Flexiplode or Diplode for SWD; (**c**) Cavity or concave applicator, microwave; (**d**) Long field applicator, microwave; (**e**) Coil, shortwave; (**f**) Disc or Schliephake electrode for SWD; (**g**) Flexible rubber electrode (pad) for SWD with felt pad; (**h**) Microwave device. © Enraf-Nonius, Delft, Netherlands, with kind permission

7.9 Dosage

There are various methods for setting the intensity, all of which are subjective and therefore unreliable. The biggest problem is that there are no heat receptors where the heat is supposed to be generated—in the deeper tissues. The sensation of warmth only occurs when convection and conduction stimulate the skin receptors. This requires intact sensation and is problematic in patients with cognitive deficits.

According to the classic Schliephake method (1960), there are 4 dosage levels (Table 7.4). After setting the intensity, the therapist must check every few minutes how the sensation of warmth is developing. This may seem cumbersome, but the risk of overdose is very real due to the unpredictable energy delivery.

Edel states that despite his efforts to create a nearly objective dosage matrix with healthy subjects—expressing the Schliephake levels in watts depending on the treatment area—there will still be dosing problems (Edel 1977). We still do not know how warm it gets at a certain depth with a certain setting and method.

Lehmann takes a rather aggressive approach in his dosage recommendations. He argues that normal blood flow is quite capable of compensating for a strong temperature increase (up to 44 °C) in the deeper tissues. In healthy individuals, this mechanism works (Lehmann 1990). He also argues that patients usually perceive pain caused by overheating quite well. If one wants to stimulate tissue with therapeutically effective temperatures, the desired temperature is 40–44 °C. (Exception: stimulation of metabolic processes, where 1–2 °C is sufficient). The relevant nociceptors of the TRPV family respond in healthy individuals at about 43 °C. If the patient reports mild pain during treatment, this means that a higher temperature has certainly been generated in the deeper tissues. It is high time to reduce the intensity!

The problem with this method is that many pathologies are associated with impaired blood flow, so the protective compensatory mechanism of circulation can only be trusted to a limited extent. Moreover, due to the inhomogeneity of the structures we treat, it is still completely unclear exactly where and how much heat is generated. If there is a local inflammatory process, the relevant nociceptors are sensitized and fire at much lower temperatures, sometimes even at body temperature. This also makes it more difficult to set the intensity.

With HF, we therefore have a modality that can efficiently heat larger areas up to 3–5 cm deep. However, we have a dosing problem.

In practice, we can only dose HF subjectively. But as already described, we cannot even rely on the statements of healthy subjects regarding the sensation of warmth. Nor do we know how skin temperature correlates with the temperature deeper in the tissue. There are carefully conducted clinical studies that attest to the effectiveness of HF therapy; the author has

Table 7.4 Dosage levels according to Schliephake (1960)

Dosage Level I	This is the weakest dosage, at which the patient feels no warmth. The intensity is increased until the patient perceives just a slight warmth after 1–2 min, after which the intensity is reduced slightly	This definitely does not mean that no heat is generated in deeper layers. It is simply not perceived
Dosage Level II	Schliephake calls this a "weak dosage." The patient feels a slight, just noticeable warmth	Al-Mandeel and Watson 2010 have shown that a fairly high temperature can already develop in deeper layers at this level. Details are discussed in the text
Dosage Level III	This is a "medium dosage." The patient feels a distinct, pleasant warmth	Here, more than a "distinct warmth" develops in the deeper tissues
Dosage Level IV	According to Schliephake, this is a "strong dosage," in which the patient feels a distinct but not unpleasant warmth	Here, one must expect that a very strong heating occurs in deeper layers

reviewed several hundred of them. However, if important information on method, intensity, and duration is missing, these studies are essentially worthless.

Large-scale reviews are useless if only the methodology is assessed and the parameters are insufficiently checked, even though the CONSORT statement explicitly requires this. In the list of Cochrane criteria, the parameters are not even mentioned. The outcome should also be correlated with the dosage. Researchers in the field of photobiomodulation can tell a sad tale about this (Stausholm et al. 2017). Bjordal already demonstrated in 2003 that studies with poor laser therapy outcomes were significantly underdosed (Bjordal et al. 2003, 2006) and that reviewers are by no means always neutral (Bjordal and Demmink 2004; Bjordal et al. 2008; Haslerud et al. 2015). The only solution is to study the original texts carefully yourself.

We know that certain therapeutic effects require a local temperature of 40–44 °C. The measurements by Lehmann (1990) show that this temperature in muscle tissue at about 2.5–3 cm depth can be reached with a coil and SWD at a power of 400 W after about 10 min. Draper has shown that at a depth of 3 cm in a muscle, with pulsed SWD after 20 min at an average power of 48 W, the temperature increases by about 3.5 °C; Draper also mentions the area of the applicator: 200 cm^2. That is at least something. Unfortunately, nothing is known about the heating of collagen, in contrast to ultrasound application. Nevertheless, if one wishes to use HF as thermotherapy, it can be cautiously stated that the temperature in the target tissue is in the therapeutic range when the patient feels a slight, pleasant warmth. This, of course, provided that all necessary precautions are taken and the patient is well monitored. Meanwhile, we await better studies.

Dosage (pulsed) SWD

But what about the pulsed, supposedly athermal application? Unfortunately, there are also very few publications with complete information on the parameters used. Of interest to us are the studies by Wilson from 1972 and 1974 and by Pennington et al. from 1991. Wilson treated patients with acute inversion injuries 36 h after injury with pulsed SWD or placebo, and his treatment parameters can be reconstructed with some calculation. His results: faster pain reduction, less swelling, and better function in the treatment group. One thing is especially important: his dosage. His patients received, converted, 140 kJ of HF energy per session, and the patients felt no warmth. His parameters: 975 W maximum power, 65 µs pulse duration, 600 Hz, 60 min, which corresponds to an average of 38 W, i.e., just under 140 kJ after 60 min. He used an inductive applicator with an area of about 300 cm^2, which corresponds to an energy density of about 120 mW/cm^2 or 460 J/cm^2 after 60 min.

Calculation: Pulse duration (s) × frequency (Hz) × maximum power (W) = average power (Ø W). Total energy: power (W) × time (s) = W/s = Joules. If the electrode area is known, the energy per cm^2 can be calculated, as is customary in ultrasound and low-level laser therapy.

Wilson had many successors who repeated his study in patients with comparable post-traumatic pathologies. One of them was Pennington, who in 1991 repeated Wilson's study exactly, with the same good result. The investigators were physicians in the US Army and were pleased to be able to return their soldiers with ankle injuries to the field more quickly. Other investigators used completely different parameters, unfortunately without success. Their conclusion: Pulsed SWD is ineffective for the mentioned pathologies. Now, however, dosage comes into play. Pasila et al. followed Wilson's protocol and found no significant changes (Pasila et al. 1978). Their parameters: average power 38 W and 40 W for 20 min, or 45 and 48 kJ, no further details, applicator unknown. About 30% of Wilson's dose. It was also 20 min of treatment time instead of 60. Laufer et al. (2005) compared the effect of "high-" and "low-" dosed pulsed SWD in patients with gonarthrosis and found no effect at all. Their parameters: a "high-dose thermal" group, Circuplode® (150 cm^2), 300 µs pulse duration, 300 Hz, 200 W max., average 18 W for 20 min. This corresponds to 21.6 kJ (144 J/cm^2), 30% of Wilson's dose. The patients felt a pleasant warmth. The "athermal" group: the same Circuplode®, 82 µs pulse duration, 110 Hz, 200 W max., average 1.8 W, 20 min. This corresponds to 2.1 kJ (10.5 J/cm^2), about 2% of Wilson's dose. These patients felt no warmth.

Babaei-Ghazani et al. (2020) treated patients with lateral epicondylitis; one group received, in addition to the "usual" treatment (stretching, strengthening, deep frictions, joint protection instruction), SWD, specifically "capacitive," 40–70 W for 15 min, which is 36 kJ to 63 kJ. The patients felt a "mild warmth." The SWD group clearly performed better. The difference from the gonarthrosis study lies in the method and the size of the applicators used. The researchers used disc electrodes, which normally have an area of either 130 cm^2, 50 cm^2, or 12 cm^2. This means that energy densities of about 480 J/cm^2 to 5200 J/cm^2 could be achieved. The 480 J/cm^2 correspond to Wilson's 460 J/cm^2; the 5200 J/cm^2 are rather unlikely, as the heating would have been too strong. The authors were not available for comment. The difference from Laufer's ineffective 144 J/cm^2 is clear. Is this the key to success?

One thing seems clear when using SWD and MW: Whether in pulsed or continuous mode—studies that judge HF application negatively were clearly underdosed.

Of course, a fresh inversion injury cannot be compared with tennis elbow or an arthritic knee joint. Until we have better studies, we can only adhere to promising dosages and should not be discouraged by researchers who, for unclear reasons, treat their participants with ineffective settings.

How much energy is actually absorbed in the tissue is unclear, but we have no other way to correlate the treatment outcome with the dose than with the calculations described above. The mentioned dosage data may serve as a basis for a more systematic approach to the use of HF therapy. Based on this information, one can then, over several therapy sessions and with careful monitoring of progress, gradually approach the optimal parameters for each individual patient.

What we urgently need are studies with precise information on the treatment parameters, with the specification of energy in joules per cm^2 being highly desirable (Table 7.5).

Table 7.5 Wish list for treatment parameters in high-frequency therapy

Parameter	Desired specification(s)
Frequency	SWD, MWD, or MW
Method	capacitive, inductive
Applicator, type and size	cm^2
Applicator position, placement	Describe, possibly with image
Electrode/applicator skin distance	cm
Treatment intensity	maximum and average, watts
Pulse duration	µs
Pulse frequency	Hz
Treatment duration	minutes
Treatment series	Total number of sessions
Treatment frequency	Number of sessions per day and per week
Energy per session or per 24 h	kJ
Energy per cm^2	J/cm^2
Patient sensation	Sensation of warmth, VAS?
Outcome measurement	Questionnaire, medication requirement, tests such as timed up and go, walking distance, etc.

7.10 Contraindications

In the following, no distinction is made between HF in pulsed or continuous mode when discussing contraindications. This is because, to date, it has not been definitively established whether pulsed HF applications are purely athermal. Due to the unclear patterns of heat development in tissue and the fact that devices do not always perform as they should (Shields et al. 2003a, b), it seems prudent to exercise caution. Many contraindications for therapeutic applications are not based on studies, but rather on assumptions and the use of common sense, see the parachute study by Smith and Pell (2006). In addition to contraindications, there are a number of precautions to consider with HF applications. These are discussed separately in Sect. 7.11:

- Metal in the treatment area. First of all: not all metals are the same. Stainless steel has different electrical and magnetic properties than titanium alloys. The latter are less responsive to magnetic fields (as in MRI) and should heat up less. However, this is by no means a carte blanche for HF application.
- Metal is an excellent conductor and does not heat up itself in the electric field. However, since the field lines concentrate on the metal, the surrounding tissue can become significantly heated, which can lead to local burns. Metal in a magnetic field can indeed heat up considerably, with the same result. Due to scattering, metal in the body near an applicator is also considered a contraindication. A safety distance of 1 m is recommended, as the wavelength of SW in the body is reduced to less than 1 m. Particularly problematic are cerclages made of metal wire, which function as coils in the body and can have a strong local effect.
- Intrauterine contraceptive devices (IUCs) containing metal are, according to some investigators, not a contraindication (Nielsen et al. 1979; Heick et al. 1991). Nielsen et al. calculated for a model of an SW application (capacitive, continuous, 150 W, 20 min, electrode placement unclear) an intrauterine temperature increase of 1.6 °C. Heick et al. found in a group of 6 subjects an intrauterine temperature of 38.1 °C after an application of 20 min on "Minode level 3" with a Diplode and a Siemens Ultratherm® 608. For measurement, the copper wire of an IUD was wrapped around a thermometer. The authors judged the application to be perfectly safe. However, the manufacturers of HF devices are decidedly of a different opinion. For the reasons mentioned above (unclear heat development, unclear output) and due to the lack of large-scale studies with various HF applications, the author considers the presence of an IUC to be an absolute contraindication for local HF application.
- How plastics in osteosynthesis material react to HF is unclear. Computational models suggest that heating is unlikely. However, whether the material is structurally altered is unknown. How resorbable osteosynthesis material reacts to HF is also unknown. Therefore, it is recommended to refrain from local HF applications in these cases as well.
- Draper has published case reports describing patients who, despite having osteosynthesis material in place, were treated with pulsed SW as preparation for mobilization. During an earlier study, treatment parameters had been determined in healthy subjects (Draper et al. 1999).
  - (Draper et al. 2004a) Female patient after comminuted elbow fracture, treated with plates and screws. Treatment parameters: 27.12 MHz, 800 Hz, pulse 400 µs, average power 48 W, 20 min, monode (200 cm^2) faradically shielded, 57.6 kJ, 288 J/cm^2. Since this was the first time Draper used HF with metal in the treatment area, the patient was closely monitored. The goal was to sufficiently heat the shortened tissue to make it more stretchable. For this, the temperature must be raised to at least 40 °C. No temperature measurements

were taken. The patient reported a gentle warmth. After about 6 sessions (not exactly clear from the publication), part of the osteosynthesis material was removed because it bothered the patient, and the surgeon could not detect any changes in the material or tissue.

- Seiger and Draper (2006) describe 4 patients after ankle fractures and postoperative movement restrictions with osteosynthesis material in place. The patients were treated with pulsed SW before mobilization, using the "Standard Draper" parameters as above. The patients reported no adverse events, and the mobilizations were successful.
- Draper (2011) describes successful mobilization treatment after pretreatment with pulsed SW in 7 patients with various fractures and dislocations, two of whom had metal in the treatment area. He always used the same parameters: 27.12 MHz, 800 Hz, pulse 400 µs, average power 48 W, 20 min, monode (200 cm^2), 57.6 kJ, 288 J/cm^2.
- (Draper 2013) Patient after humeral shaft fracture, treated with an intramedullary nail (verbatim "metal rod"). Two thermoelements were placed, one at a depth of 2.6 cm, supposedly in direct contact with the metal, which would have been difficult with an intramedullary nail, the second sensor was at the same depth in muscle tissue. Application: 27.12 MHz, 800 µs pulse, 400 Hz, average power 100 W, monode (200 cm^2), 120 kJ, 600 J/cm^2. After 20 min, both sensors indicated a temperature increase of 4.5 °C. The parameters here seem odd, and the author of this book believes there may be a typographical error. Draper has always used the same parameters; here, the values for pulse duration and frequency seem to be switched. Draper was not available for comment. A pity, as the temperature measurements are not irrelevant.

Draper's studies somewhat relativize the supposed risks of pulsed SW. Measurements in rabbits with titanium alloy implants (Ye et al. 2013) show no significant local heating after MW with 25 W/15 min, while Wang et al. (2015) claim the opposite and describe heat damage, albeit with a higher dose (40 W/20 min). However, apart from the one flawed measurement by Draper (2013), there are no serious in vivo studies in humans on this topic, so the author, for the time being, considers metal in the treatment area to be an absolute contraindication for HF application.

- The presence of a pacemaker or an implanted defibrillator (ICD) is an absolute contraindication. Although such devices are now particularly well shielded, warnings about interference with these devices in electric and magnetic fields continue to appear in the literature (Donnelly et al. 2007; Mattei et al. 2016; Samuels et al. 2020). Patients with implanted hearing aids or neurostimulators, such as in Parkinson's disease, must also not be treated. The electrodes can heat up significantly; this has led to death in a Parkinson's patient (Nutt et al. 2001; Ruggera et al. 2003) and in another case to temporary unilateral muscle cramps and visual disturbances (Roark et al. 2008).
- Circulatory disorders in the treatment area such as ischemia, pronounced edema, thrombosis, or increased bleeding tendency as in patients on anticoagulants, after recent injuries, or in hemophilia patients. If circulation cannot dissipate the generated heat, undesirably high local temperature increases may occur (Lehmann 1990). Zhang et al. (2011). Fang et al. (2015) describe several cases of penile necrosis after MW treatment following circumcision in this context.
- Pregnancy. We know from animal studies that high HF doses can lead to developmental disorders in the fetus (Brown-Woodman et al. 1988; Lary et al. 1982). Understandably, there are no studies in humans (Shields et al. 2003a, b). Whether this is a thermal or athermal effect

is unclear. There is only one publication in the literature in which the author describes three women who were unexpectedly treated with SW in the first trimester of pregnancy (Imrie 1971). Two had normal deliveries, and the children were reportedly healthy. One woman allegedly had a miscarriage, but no fetus was found. Imrie believes that the danger of such HF treatment is exaggerated, but nevertheless does not approve the use of SW therapy in pregnant women.

- Sensory disturbances in the treatment area. Since it is already very difficult for healthy subjects to perceive a temperature increase of up to 2 °C, it is obvious that patients with locally impaired warm-cold sensitivity should not be treated at all.
- Acute infections, fever. Bacterial infections could spread. Fever is a general contraindication for many therapeutic applications, as one does not want to put additional stress on the sick organism.
- Menstruation is not an absolute contraindication for treatment of the back or abdomen, but a relative one. A heat application (as with fango) could increase bleeding. There is some evidence that repeated SW treatment in the pelvic area can alter the menstrual cycle, but there is no solid proof of this (Shields et al. 2002).
- Rapidly dividing tissue such as epiphyseal plates and tumors. Regions with still active epiphyseal plates should not be treated until growth is complete, as growth disturbances could occur. The activity of the plates does not end simultaneously throughout the body. For example, the epiphyseal plates in the proximal shoulder area (humeral head, acromion, etc.) close only at about 20–21 years, around the elbow at 15–18, at the wrist at 17–19, and around the knee at about 19–20 years, similar to the upper ankle joint. In girls, the plates close 2–3 years earlier throughout. Tumors in the treatment area, whether malignant or benign, are an absolute contraindication, as one does not want to stimulate metastasis. Caution should be exercised with the testes, as a temperature increase could lead to infertility and it is not exactly known how rapidly dividing tissue reacts to HF application.
- Tissue that has been treated with X-rays. This does not refer to diagnostic procedures. It has been shown that such tissue reacts more strongly to X-rays after HF treatment in the sense of sensitization (van Rhoon and Visser 1988).
- Patients with cognitive impairments. If a patient is unable to understand what the treatment involves and how to react in the event of overheating, the application is absolutely contraindicated.
- No HF application in patients with pain of unclear origin. Tuberculosis is fortunately rare in Western Europe, but by no means eradicated. Patients with diffuse "bone pain" due to unrecognized chronic osteomyelitis can certainly be encountered. In case of doubt, do not treat and refer the patient back to the physician.

7.11 Precautions, General Safety Instructions

- When the skin is heated, sweating begins. The beads of sweat can become very hot in the HF field. This of course also applies to moist dressings in the treatment area. Garments made of synthetic fibers generally do not absorb sweat well and should be removed, as should any other clothing from the area to be treated. The advice to remove clothing that restricts circulation in the treatment area is probably superfluous. You want to see what you are doing. A scar may indicate surgery or, not to be ruled out these days, shrapnel or similar. There are patients who deny having had surgery and then enthusiastically talk about their new hip.

- For hygienic reasons and because of sweating, a terry cloth towel should be placed between the applicator and the skin. Especially in obese patients, sweat can accumulate in skin folds. Electrodes and applicators must, of course, be disinfected before each use.
- People with a hearing aid or an implanted hearing prosthesis should turn off their device as soon as they enter a room where an HF device is operating. Otherwise, the devices can start to whistle very loudly. During treatment, a hearing aid must be removed. Patients with implanted hearing prostheses must not be treated.
- Credit cards, ID cards with chips and the like, mobile phones, e-readers, personal pagers, etc. must be kept away from operating HF devices. Likewise, no other electrotherapy devices should be operated in the same room as an HF device, as they may be disrupted and unpleasant intensity surges could occur.
- Jewelry, wherever it is on the body, must be removed, including hair clips and watches, whether smart or classic, in fact anything made of metal. Please remove wallets with coins and credit cards from trouser pockets and be sure to place the removed items in the patient's line of sight. Have the patient put their own jewelry back on (in case something goes missing later).
- SW and probably MW can cause local overheating in wearers of contact lenses (Scott 1956). The publication is quite old, but unfortunately there is nothing more recent on this topic. Contact lens wearers should remove their lenses for SW and MW applications in the head area.
- Therapists who are pregnant or wish to become pregnant should not stay near an operating HF device; the safety distance is 1–2 m. The literature is clear on this. The devices emit large amounts of stray energy (Shields et al. 2004; Gryz and Karpowicz 2014; Shah and Farrow 2014; Andrikopoulos et al. 2017; Koutsojannis et al. 2018) and therapists unfortunately do not always take safety precautions seriously enough (Shields et al. 2002, 2003a, b) or are insufficiently informed about correct handling (Guirro et al. 2014). Poor maintenance is an important factor in stray values, especially with older devices (Guirro et al. 2014). There is no association between occupational exposure to electromagnetic waves and miscarriages, premature births, stillbirths, or fertility problems (Ouellet-Hellstrom and Stewart 1993). However, an association has been demonstrated with congenital malformations and low birth weight in male newborns (Ouellet-Hellstrom and Stewart 1993; Shields et al. 2003a, b). Larsen (1991) surveyed 4,021 female therapists in Denmark regarding their pregnancies and working conditions and also found that exposed therapists had male offspring with lower birth weights and that the sex ratio was slightly but significantly shifted toward girls. Since this figure depends on many different factors and has changed annually since 1985, the author points out that the result must be interpreted with caution. Feychting revisited the topic of SW and MW therapy and pregnancy in her review and stated that the available information is insufficient to draw any conclusions (Feychting 2005). The study groups were too small and the retrospective designs allowed too many opportunities for error.
- Therapists who frequently work with or near MW devices (> 5 hrs/day) seem to complain of fatigue more often (Anguera and Gianini 2014). The authors could not rule out that additional factors played a role. Only one in five therapists in their sample ($n = 193$) had observed any safety measures.
- Obesity is not a contraindication for HF treatment. However, due to the high energy losses in adipose tissue, significant deep effects cannot be expected in very overweight patients. There is also a risk of significant superficial overheating.

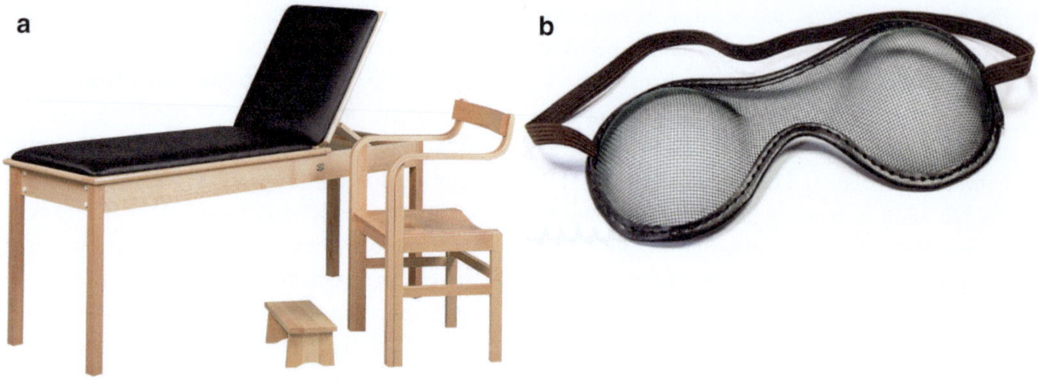

Fig. 7.7 (**a**) Special furniture for high-frequency applications; (**b**) Protective goggles for MW application. © Enraf-Nonius, Delft, Netherlands, with kind permission

- Due to the scattering of electromagnetic waves, special furniture must be used for HF therapy. There are chairs and couches constructed without metal parts for this purpose (Fig. 7.7a). The use of conventional couches or hospital beds is strongly discouraged.
- To protect the eyes during MW treatments in the head area, for example in sinusitis, there are special "glasses" made of wire that shield the eyes like a Faraday cage (Fig. 7.7b). The eyes are at risk, on the one hand, because they do not have a cooling circulation, and on the other hand, MW themselves, even without the thermal effect, seem to be able to damage the eye (Carpenter and van Ummersen 1968). Therapists should also be aware that high-dose MW could damage the eyes over time (Cutz 1989).

Electrode Placement

Instead of a more even energy distribution with two identical electrodes, one can attempt to localize the heating specifically. This is done either with different EHA, where the side with the lower EHA has greater surface heating, or by using two electrodes of different sizes. In this case, the energy is concentrated on the side of the smaller electrode. Figs. 7.8 and 7.9 show some examples of electrode placements. Please note that energy distribution in vivo is unpredictable due to the inhomogeneity of the human body.

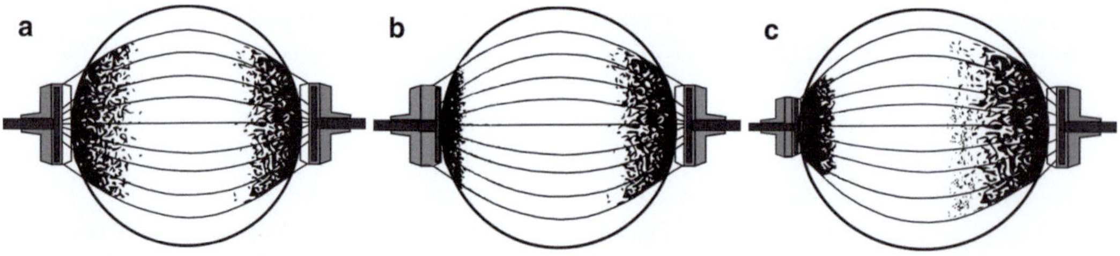

Fig. 7.8 (**a**) Theoretical energy distribution with two electrodes of equal size and equal EHA; (**b**) theoretical energy distribution with two electrodes of equal size and small (left) and large EHA; (**c**) theoretical energy distribution with two electrodes of different sizes and different EHA. © Enraf-Nonius, Delft, Netherlands, with kind permission

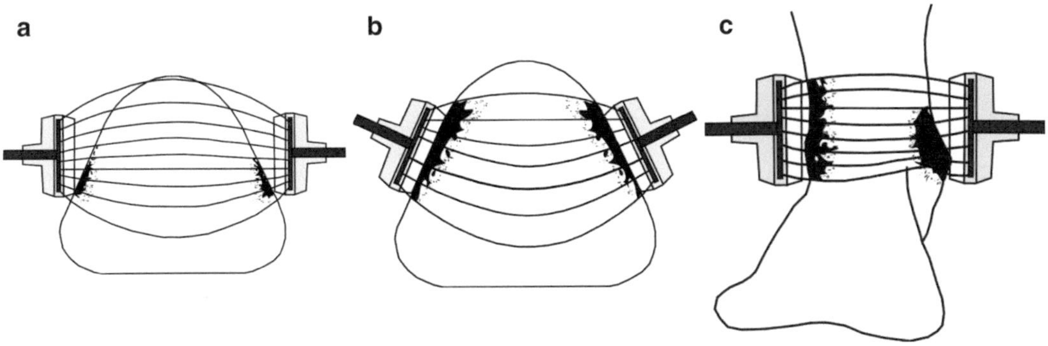

Fig. 7.9 (**a**) If the electrodes do not have uniform contact, the energy is localized to a small area. This can also be used intentionally; (**b**) even energy distribution with full contact; (**c**) point effect at the medial malleolus, beware of overheating! © Enraf-Nonius, Delft, Netherlands, with kind permission

References

Abramson DI, Belly Y, Tuck S Jr, Mitchell R, Chandrasekharappa G (1961) Changes in blood flow, oxygen uptake and tissue temperatures produced by therapeutic physical agents. III. Effect of indirect or reflex vasodilatation. Am J Phys Med 40:5–13

Akyol Y, Ulus Y, Durmus D, Canturk F, Bilgici A, Kuru O, Bek Y (2012) Effectiveness of microwave diathermy on pain, functional capacity, muscle strength, quality of life, and depression in patients with subacromial impingement syndrome: a randomized placebo-controlled clinical study. Rheumatol Int 32(10):3007–3016

Al-Mandeel MM, Watson T (2010) The thermal and nonthermal effects of high and low doses of pulsed short wave therapy (PSWT). Physiother Res Int 15(4):199–211

Andrikopoulos A, Adamopoulos A, Seimenis I, Koutsojannis C (2017) Microwave diathermy in physiotherapy units: a survey on spatial and time heterogeneity of the electromagnetic field. J Radiol Prot 37(2):N27–N41

Anguera M, Gianini RJ (2014) Prevalence of fatigue reported by physiotherapists operating diathermy equipment for microwave. Rev Bras Epidemiol 17(3):577–581

Atamaz FC, Durmaz B, Baydar M, Demircioglu OY, Iyiyapici A, Kuran B, Oncel S, Sendur OF (2012) Comparison of the efficacy of transcutaneous electrical nerve stimulation, interferential currents, and shortwave diathermy in knee osteoarthritis: a double-blind, randomized, controlled, multicenter study. Arch Phys Med Rehabil 93(5):748–756

Atkins PW, De Paula J (2014) Physical chemistry. Thermodynamics, structure, and change, 10. Aufl. W. H. Freeman, New York, ISBN-13: 978-1429290197

Babaei-Ghazani A, Shahrami B, Fallah E, Ahadi T, Forough B, Ebadi S (2020) Continuous shortwave diathermy with exercise reduces pain and improves function in lateral epicondylitis more than sham diathermy: a randomized controlled trial. J Bodyw Mov Ther 24(1):69–76

Bäcklund L, Tiselius P (1967) Objective measurement of joint stiffness in rheumatoid arthritis. Acta Rheumatol Scand 13(4):275–288

Bjordal J, Couppé C, Chow R, Tuner J, Ljunggren EA (2003) A systematic review of low laser therapy with location-specific doses for pain and chronic joint disorders. Australian J Physioth 49:107–116

Bjordal JM, Demmink JH (2004) Review of tennis elbow was biased. BMJ 328(7444):897–898

Bjordal JM, Johnson MI, Iversen V, Aimbre F, Lopes-Martins RAB (2006) Low-level laser therapy in acute pain: a systematic review of possible mechanisms of action and clinical effects in randomized placebo-controlled trials. Photomed Laser Surg 24(2):158–168

Bjordal JM, Lopes-Martins RA, Joensen J, Couppe C, Ljunggren AE, Stergioulas A, Johnson MI (2008) A systematic review with procedural assessments and meta-analysis of low level laser therapy in lateral elbow tendinopathy (tennis elbow). BMC Musculoskelet Disord 9:75

Bleakley CM, Costello JT (2013) Do thermal agents affect range of movement and mechanical properties in soft tissues? A systematic review. Arch Phys Med Rehabil 94(1):149–163

Bricknell R, Watson T (1995) The thermal effects of pulsed shortwave therapy. Br J Ther Rehab 2(8):430–434

Brown-Woodman PD, Hadley JA, Waterhouse J, Webster WS (1988) Teratogenic effects of exposure to radiofrequency radiation (27.12 MHz) from a shortwave diathermy unit. Ind Health 26(1):1–10

Carpenter RL, Van Ummersen CA (1968) The action of microwave radiation on the eye. J Microw Power 3(1):3–19

Charkoudian N (2010) Mechanisms and modifiers of reflex induced cutaneous vasodilation and vasoconstriction in humans. J Appl Physiol 109(4):1221–1228

Cleary SF (1997) In vitro studies of the effects of non-thermal radiofrequency and microwave radiation. Non-Thermal Effects of RF Electromagnetic Fields. Proceedings of the International Seminar on Biological Effects of Non-Thermal Pulsed and Amplitude Modulated RF Electromagnetic Fields and Related Health Risks, Munich, Germany, November 20–21, 1996. Munich: International Commission on Non-Ionizing Radiation Protection; 1997

Cutz A (1989) Effects of microwave radiation on the eye: the occupational health perspective. Lens Eye Toxic Res 6(1–2):379–386

Delpizzo V, Joyner KH (1987) On the safe use of microwave and shortwave diathermy units. Aust J Physiother 33(3):152–162

Donnelly P, Pal N, Herity NA (2007) Perioperative management of patients with implantable cardioverter defibrillators. Ulster Med J 76(2):66–67

Draper DO (2011) Injuries restored to ROM using PSWD and mobilizations. Int J Sports Med 32(4):281–286

Draper DO (2013) Comparison of shortwave diathermy and microwave diathermy. Int J Athl Ther & Train 18(6):13–17

Draper DO, Knight K, Fujiwara T, Castel JC (1999) Temperature change in human muscle during and after pulsed short-wave diathermy. J Ortho Sports Phys Ther 29(1):13–22

Draper DO, Castel CJ, Castel D (2004a) Low-watt pulsed shortwave diathermy and metal-plate fixation of the elbow. Athl Ther Today 9(5):28–32

Draper DO, Castro JL, Feland B, Schulthies S, Eggett D (2004b) Shortwave diathermy and prolonged stretching increase hamstring flexibility more than prolonged stretching alone. J Orthop Sports Phys Ther 34(1):13–20

Edel H (1977) Fibel der Elektrodiagnostik und Elektrotherapie, 4. Aufl. Verlag Theodor Steinkopff, Dresden

Fang DB, Shen YH, Zhu XW, Fang JJ, Mao QQ, Wang C-j, Tan FQ, He QW, Shen BH, Xie LP (2015) Penile necrosis resulting from post-circumcision microwave diathermy: a report of 9 cases. Zhonghua Nan Ke Xue 21(5):428–431

Feychting M (2005) Non-cancer EMF effects related to children. Bioelectromagnetics 7:69–74

Fu T, Lineaweaver WC, Zhang F, Zhang J (2019) Role of shortwave and microwave diathermy in peripheral neuropathy. J Int Med Res 47(8):3569–3579

Garrett CL, Draper DO, Knight KL (2000) Heat distribution in the lower leg from pulsed short-wave diathermy and ultrasound treatments. J Athl Train 35(1):50–55

Ginsberg AJ (1961) Pulsed short wave in the treatment of bursitis with calcification. Int Rec Med 174:71–75

Goldin JH, Broadbent NR, Nancarrow JD, Marshall T (1981) The effects of Diapulse on the healing of wounds: a double-blind randomised controlled trial in man. Br J Plast Surg 34(3):267–270

Gryz K, Karpowicz J (2014) Environmental impact of the use of radiofrequency electromagnetic fields in physiotherapeutic treatment. Rocz Panstw Zakl Hig 65(1):55–61

Guirro RR, Guirro EC, Alves de Sousa NT (2014) Lack of maintenance of shortwave diathermy equipment has a negative impact on power output. J Phys Ther Sci 26(4):557–562

Harris ED Jr, McCroskery PA (1974) The influence of temperature and fibril stability on degradation of cartilage collagen by rheumatoid synovial collagenase. N Engl J Med 290(1):1–6

Haslerud S, Magnussen LH, Joensen J, Lopes-Martins RA, Bjordal JM (2015) The efficacy of low-level laser therapy for shoulder tendinopathy: a systematic review and meta-analysis of randomized controlled trials. Physiother Res Int 20(2):108–125

Hébette C (2012) Diathermie contre hypothermie. Presentation 30 November 2012, La Léchère, Frankreich

Heggannavar A, Harugop A, Madhale D, Walavalkar L (2017) A randomised controlled study to evaluate the effectiveness of shortwave diathermy in acute sinusitis. Int J Physio Res 5(3):2066–2072

Heick A, Espersen T, Pedersen HL, Raahauge J (1991) Is diathermy safe in women with copper-bearing IUDs? Acta Obstet Gynecol Scand 70(2):153–155

Imrie AH (1971) Pelvic short wave diathermy given inadvertently in early pregnancy. J Obstet Gynaecol Br Commonw 78(1):91–92

Jan MH, Chai HM, Wang CL, Lin YF, Tsai LY (2006) Effects of repetitive shortwave diathermy for reducing synovitis in patients with knee osteoarthritis: an ultrasonographic study. Phys Ther 86(2):236–244

Jeziorski K (2018) Hyperthermia in rheumatic diseases. A promising approach? Reumatologia 56(5):316–320

Jo J, Lee SH (2018) Heat therapy for primary dysmenorrhea: a systematic review and meta-analysis of its effects on pain relief and quality of life. Sci Rep 8(1):16252

Kitchen S, Partridge C (1992) Review of shortwave diathermy continuous and pulsed patterns. Physiotherapy 78(4):243–252

Koutsojannis C, Andrikopoulos A, Adamopoulos A, Seimenis I (2018) Microwave diathermy in physiotherapy: introduction and evaluation of a quality control procedure. Radiat Prot Dosimetry 181(3):229–239

Kowarschik J (1926) Die Diathermie. Springer-Verlag, Berlin/Heidelberg, ISBN 978-3-662-02204-7

Lamina S, Hanif S, Gagarawa YS (2011) Short wave diathermy in the symptomatic management of chronic pelvic inflammatory disease pain: a randomized controlled trial. Physiother Res Int 16(1):50–56

Larsen AI (1991) Congenital malformations and exposure to high-frequency electromagnetic radiation among Danish physiotherapists. Scand J Work Environ Health 17(5):318–323

Lary JM, Conover DL, Foley ED, Hanser PL (1982) Teratogenic effects of 27.12 MHz radiofrequency radiation in rats. Teratology 26(3):299–309

Laufer Y, Dar G (2012) Effectiveness of thermal and athermal short-wave diathermy for the management of knee osteoarthritis: a systematic review and meta-analysis. Osteoarthritis Cartilage 20(9):957–966

Laufer Y, Zilberman R, Porat R, Nahir AM (2005) Effect of pulsed short-wave diathermy on pain and function of subjects with osteoarthritis of the knee: a placebo-controlled double-blind clinical trial. Clin Rehabil 19(3):255–263

Lehmann JF (1990) Therapeutic heat and cold, 4. Aufl. Williams & Wilkins, Baltimore, ISBN 0-683-04908-9

Low J (1995) Dosage of some pulsed shortwave clinical trials. Physiotherapy 81(10):611–616

Luben RA (1997) Effects of microwave radiation on signal transduction processes of cells in vitro. Non-Thermal Effects of RF Electromagnetic Fields. Proceedings of the International Seminar on Biological Effects of Non-Thermal Pulsed and Amplitude Modulated RF Electromagnetic Fields and Related Health Risks, Munich, Germany, November 20–21, 1996. Munich: International Commission on Non-Ionizing Radiation Protection; 1997

Machado AFP, Perracini MR, Rampazo ÉP, Driusso P, Liebano RE (2019) Effects of thermotherapy and transcutaneous electrical nerve stimulation on patients with primary dysmenorrhea: a randomized, placebo-controlled, double-blind clinical trial. Complement Ther Med 47:102188

Malanga GA, Yan N, Stark J (2015) Mechanisms and efficacy of heat and cold therapies for musculoskeletal injury. Postgrad Med 127(1):57–65

Martin GM, Herrick JF (1955) Further evaluation of heating by microwaves and by infrared as used clinically. J Am Med Assoc 159(13):1286–1287

Masayoshi I, Montemayor JS, Matsumoto E, Alice MPA, Lee MHM, Folk F (1991) Healing of pressure ulcers by pulsed high peak power electromagnetic energy (Diapulse). Decubitis 40:24–35

Mattei E, Censi F, Calcagnini G, Falsaperla R, Genovese E, Napolitano A, Cannatà V (2016) Pacemaker and ICD oversensing induced by movements near the MRI scanner bore. Med Phys 43(12):6621

McGaughey H, Dhamija S, Oliver L, Porter-Armstrong A, McDonough S (2009) Pulsed electromagnetic energy in management of chronic wounds: a systematic review. Phys Ther Rev 14(2):132–146

McMeeken J (1994) Tissue temperature and blood flow: a research-based overview of electrophysical modalities. Aust J Physiother 40S:49–57

Mense S (1978) Effects of temperature on the discharges of muscle spindles and tendon organs. Pflügers Arch 374:15–166

Nadler SF, Weingand K, Kruse RJ (2004) The physiologic basis and clinical applications of cryotherapy and thermotherapy for the pain practitioner. Pain Physician 7(3):395–399

Nielsen NC, Hansen R, Larsen T (1979) Heat induction in copper-bearing IUD'S during short-wave diathermy. Acta Obstet Gynecol Scand 58(5):495

Nutt JG, Anderson VC, Peacock JH, Hammerstad JP, Burchiel KJ (2001) DBS and diathermy interaction induces severe CNS damage. Neurology 56(10):1384–1386

Oosterveld FG, Rasker JJ, Jacobs JW, Overmars HJ (1992) The effect of local heat and cold therapy on the intraarticular and skin surface temperature of the knee. Arthritis Rheum 35(2):146–151

Ouellet-Hellstrom R, Stewart WF (1993) Miscarriages among female physical therapists who report using radio- and microwave-frequency electromagnetic radiation. Am J Epidemiol 138(10):775–786

Ozen S, Doganci EB, Ozyuvali A, Yalcin AP (2019) Effectiveness of continuous versus pulsed short-wave diathermy in the management of knee osteoarthritis: a randomized pilot study. Caspian J Intern Med 10(4):431–438

Palazzo E, Rossi F, Maione S (2008) Role of TRPV1 receptors in descending modulation of pain. Mol Cell Endocrinol 286(1–2 Suppl 1):S79–S83

Pall ML (2013) Electromagnetic fields act via activation of voltage-gated calcium channels to produce beneficial or adverse effects. J Cell Mol Med 17(8):958–965

Panagopoulos DJ, Karabarbounis A, Margaritis LH (2002) Mechanism for action of electromagnetic fields on cells. Biochem Biophys Res Commun 298(1):95–102

Pasila M, Visuri T, Sundholm A (1978) Pulsating shortwave diathermy: value in treatment of recent ankle and foot sprains. Arch Phys Med Rehabil 59(8):383–386

Pennington GM, Danley DL, Sumko MH, Bucknell A, Nelson JH (1993) Pulsed, non-thermal, high-frequency electromagnetic energy (DIAPULSE) in the treatment of grade I and grade II ankle sprains. Mil Med 158(2):101–104

Peres SE, Draper DO, Knight KL, Ricard MD (2002) Pulsed shortwave diathermy and prolonged long-duration stretching increase dorsiflexion range of motion more than identical stretching without diathermy. J Athl Train 37(1):43–50

Rabini A, Piazzini DB, Tancredi G, Foti C, Milano G, Ronconi G, Specchia A, Ferrara PE, Maggi L, Amabile E, Galli M, Bernabei R, Bertolini C, Marzetti E (2012) Deep heating therapy via microwave diathermy relieves pain and improves physical function in patients with knee osteoarthritis: a double-blind randomized clinical trial. Eur J Phys Rehabil Med 48(4):549–559

van Rhoon GC, Visser AG (1988) Hyperthermie bij de behandeling van kanker. Klinische Fysica 3:103–112

Roark C, Whicher S, Abosch A (2008) Reversible neurological symptoms caused by diathermy in a patient with deep brain stimulators: case report. Neurosurgery 62:E256

Robertson VJ, Ward AR, Jung P (2005) The effect of heat on tissue extensibility: a comparison of deep and superficial heating. Arch Phys Med Rehabil 86(4):819–825

Ruggera PS, Witters DM, von Maltzahn G, Bassen HI (2003) In vitro assessment of tissue heating near metallic medical implants by exposure to pulsed radio frequency diathermy. Phys Med Biol 48(17):2919–2928

Samuels JM, Overbey DM, Wikiel KJ, Jones TS, Robinson TN, Jones EL (2020) Electromagnetic interference on cardiac pacemakers and implantable cardioverter defibrillators during endoscopy as reported to the US Federal Drug Administration. Surg Endosc. https://doi.org/10.1007/s00464-020-07872-2. Epub ahead of print. PMID: 32804270

Schliephake E (1960) Kurzwellentherapie. Die medizinische Anwendung elektrischer Höchstfrequenzen. 6. überarbeitete Ausgabe. Gustav Fischer Verlag, Stuttgart

Schmicke P (1984) Die Wiedererwärmung von Menschen in tiefer Hypothermie mit einem Kurzwellentherapiegerät. Kasuistische Mitteilung über 3 Fälle Anasth Intensivther Notfallmed 19(1):27–29

Scott BO (1956) Effects of contact lenses on short-wave field distribution. Br J Ophthalmol 40(11):696–697

Seiger C, Draper DO (2006) Use of pulsed shortwave diathermy and joint mobilization to increase ankle range of motion in the presence of surgical implanted metal: a case series. J Orthop Sports Phys Ther 36(9):669–677

Shah SG, Farrow A (2014) Systematic literature review of adverse reproductive outcomes associated with physiotherapists' occupational exposures to non-ionising radiation. J Occup Health 56(5):323–331

Shields N, Gormley J, O'Hare N (2002) Short-wave diathermy: current clinical and safety practices. Physiother Res Int 7(4):191–202

Shields N, O'Hare N, Boyle G, Gormley J (2003a) Development and application of a quality control procedure for short-wave diathermy units. Med Biol Eng Comput 41(1):62–68

Shields N, O'Hare N, Gormley J (2003b) Short-wave diathermy and pregnancy: what is the evidence? Adv Physiother 5:2–4

Shields N, O'Hare N, Gormley J (2004) An evaluation of safety guidelines to restrict exposure to stray radiofrequency radiation from short-wave diathermy units. Phys Med Biol 49(13):2999–3015

Shinde N, Jayawant SK (2012) Efficacy of short wave diathermy in patients with sinusitis. Int J Health Sci Res 2(4):33–41

Smith GC, Pell JP (2006) Parachute use to prevent death and major trauma related to gravitational challenge: systematic review of randomised controlled trials. Int J Prosthodont 19(2):126–128

Stausholm MB, Bjordal JM, Lopes-Martins RAB, Joensen J (2017) Methodological flaws in meta-analysis of low-level laser therapy in knee osteoarthritis: a letter to the editor. Osteoarthritis Cartilage 4:e9–e10.

Takahashi K, Kurosaki H, Hashimoto S, Takenouchi K, Kamada T, Nakamura H (2011) The effects of radiofrequency hyperthermia on pain and function in patients with knee osteoarthritis: a preliminary report. J Orthop Sci 16(4):376–381

Tipler PA, Mosca G, Wagner J (Hrsg) (2019) Physik. 8., korr. u. erw. Aufl. Springer Spektrum, Heidelberg, ISBN 978-3-662-58280-0

Wang G, Xu Y, Zhang L, Ye D, Feng X, Fu T, Bai Y (2015) Enhancement of apoptosis by titanium alloy internal fixations during microwave treatments for fractures: an animal study. PLoS One 10(7):e0132046

Wang H, Zhang C, Gao C, Zhu S, Yang L, Wei Q, He C (2017) Effects of short-wave therapy in patients with knee osteoarthritis: a systematic review and meta-analysis. Clin Rehabil 31(5):660–671

Weinberger A, Fadilah R, Lev A, Levi A, Pinkhas J (1988) Deep heat in the treatment of inflammatory joint disease. Med Hypotheses 25(4):231–233

Wilson DH (1972) Treatment of soft-tissue injuries by pulsed electrical energy. Br Med J 2(5808):269–270

Wilson DH (1974) Comparison of short wave diathermy and pulsed electromagnetic energy in treatment of soft tissue injuries. Physiotherapy 60(10):309–310

Wright V, Johns RJ (1960) Observations on the measurement of joint stiffness. Arth Rheum 3(4):328–340

Ye D, Xu Y, Fu T, Zhang H, Feng X, Wang G, Jiang L, Bai Y (2013) Low dose of continuous-wave microwave irradiation did not cause temperature increase in muscles tissue adjacent to titanium alloy implants–an animal study. BMC Musculoskelet Disord 14:364

Yilmaz Kaysin M, Akpinar P, Aktas I, Unlü Ozkan F, Silte Karamanlioglu D, Cagliyan Hartevioglu H, Vural N (2018) Effectiveness of shortwave diathermy for subacromial impingement syndrome and value of night pain for patient selection: a double-blinded, randomized, placebo-controlled trial. Am J Phys Med Rehabil 97(3):178–186

Zhang H, Xiong EQ, Liu LM, Yan SX, Zhou ZS, Lu GS (2011) Penile necrosis after circumcision owing to inappropriate postoperative treatment. J Pediatr Surg 46(7):1469–1470

Risk Management 8

Systematic risk management has been an important topic in healthcare for several decades. Patient safety is of particular significance in this context. Treatment errors can, if at all, only be reversed with great effort and have consequences for all parties involved. Whether it concerns physical or psychological harm to the patient, financial or reputational damage to the hospital or practice, or legal consequences for the staff: risk management systems make it possible to develop reactive and proactive strategies to reduce risks and their consequences. Risk management essentially pursues the same goals as quality management, with measures, methods, and objectives often overlapping or complementing each other. Like quality management, risk management should be based on a continuous improvement process. Risk management can be considered an integral part of quality management. Good quality can lead to greater safety, and safety can lead to better quality (Paula 2007). The optimal care of the patient is always the primary focus.

8.1 Sources of Error

Physiotherapeutic practice includes the implementation of therapies that carry risks. This means, for example, that with active methods such as exercise therapy or with passive therapies such as heat and cold applications, adverse events may occur as side effects of the treatment. Technical equipment such as walking aids, exercise devices, or electrotherapy devices are potential sources of adverse events. The incorrect use of technically flawless aids can cause harm just as much as the correct use of defective equipment. Not only therapists (Crowcroft et al. 1996), but also electrotherapy devices (Lambert et al. 2000; Schabrun et al. 2006) can be vectors for nosocomial infections. The structure of the physiotherapy work environment is another reason why adverse events may occur. Physiotherapists in hospitals are deployed in very different areas and work in a highly interdisciplinary manner. Communication barriers can lead to serious errors even among recognized experts, a fact highlighted in 1999 by the failure of the Mars Climate Orbiter mission: one team performed calculations using SI units (Newton × second), another using imperial units (pound × second). The probe crashed on Mars (Mars Climate Orbiter Report 1999). Finally, the human factor plays a significant role in the occurrence of adverse events (Paula 2007; Reason 1997, 2008). For example, postoperative rehabilitation of elderly, multimorbid patients places ever-increasing demands on the professional, communicative, and organizational skills of therapists. In parallel with these increased demands, staff numbers are being reduced. There is a clear increase in workload for hospital staff with no prospect of improvement. This

P. van Kerkhof, *Evidence-Based Electrotherapy*, https://doi.org/10.1007/978-3-662-73019-5_8

leads, even among traditionally highly motivated healthcare professionals, to physical and psychological overload in the long term. The negative impact on patient safety has been described multiple times in the literature (Andersen et al. 2002; Clarke et al. 2002; Carlton and Blegen 2006; Halwani et al. 2006).

Risk management as part of quality management means identifying relevant risks and developing strategies to prevent and reduce harm. Identification is important because safety measures can only be developed if the risks are known. Electrotherapeutic applications carry risks. The practitioner must be aware of these risks in order to assess whether the expected therapeutic effect is reasonably proportionate to the risk. Unfortunately, we know very little about the true risks of many electrotherapeutic applications. Empirical studies are often not feasible. Many contraindications are based on experience or logical assumptions about possible biological or physical properties and effects. Many contraindications and supposed risks have been adopted from older books and relisted without empirical evidence or theoretical justification. For legal reasons, it is assumed that fewer harms are reported than actually occur. In Germany, Austria, and Switzerland, there is a legal obligation to report serious adverse events to the relevant authorities (see medical device regulations for Germany, Austria, and Switzerland in the bibliography). This applies to all medical device operators, including physiotherapists. Unfortunately, a SAE (Serious Adverse Event) is not uniformly defined. Generally, however, it refers to a serious deterioration in a patient's health, permanent bodily harm or lasting impairment of a bodily function, inpatient treatment or extension of inpatient treatment, or the patient's death. It is irrelevant whether the event was caused by a medical device. This definition also includes all reactions resulting from user error. The medical device in question also includes electrotherapy devices and their accessories. Since allergies and burns and the like are not particularly serious and therefore are generally not reported, there are no figures on the frequency and extent of such events, and there is no basis for scientific analysis of these risks. This means that general guidelines are inevitably incomplete and should be critically questioned when new findings become available. The risk for certain applications is probably lower than generally assumed. Nevertheless, sometimes the extent of potential harm argues against performing a treatment.

For the risk analysis, the author searched the literature in PubMed, Cochrane, and PEDro. All studies related to risks of electrotherapy applications published in English, German, or Dutch were included. Animal studies were included because the results can have clinical implications. The search was not limited by time, as this would have given an incomplete picture of the topic. Studies in which the treatment parameters clearly did not correspond to standard practice were excluded. The risks described are based on expert opinions regarding contraindications for the mentioned applications from current textbooks commonly used in German-speaking countries. The results of this research are discussed in detail in the relevant chapters.

8.2 Specific Risks

The aim of this discussion is to show which electrotherapies are actually associated with risks and how these risks can be substantiated. For most of the risks and contraindications mentioned in textbooks, there is no literature. The following risks can be substantiated by literature:

- Risk posed by high-frequency diathermy in patients with implanted brain stimulation electrodes (Nutt et al. 2001; Ruggera et al. 2003; Roark et al. 2008)
- Occurrence of contact allergies with TENS and NMES applications (Castelain and Chabeau 1986; Green and Pye 1991; Dwyer et al. 1994; Corazza et al. 1999)
- Interference with pacemakers and implanted cardioverter-defibrillators by TENS, NMES,

and high-frequency applications (Valtonen et al. 1975; Weitz et al. 1997; Vlay 1998; Pyatt et al. 2003; Crevenna et al. 2001, 2003; Occhetta et al. 2006; Holmgren et al. 2008; Carlsson et al. 2009; Mattei et al. 2016; Samuels et al. 2020)

- Occurrence of systemic allergic reactions after iontophoresis (Macchia et al. 2002; Foti et al. 2004).
- Occurrence of muscle damage with NMES applications (Mackey et al. 2008)
- Occurrence of thermal injuries with ultrasound applications (Frye et al. 2007).
- Risk posed by unmaintained ultrasound devices (Artho et al. 2002; Pye and Milford 1994; Pye 1996; Zeqiri 1997; Guirro and Britshcy Dos Santos 2002; Daniel and Rupert 2003; Holcomb and Joyce 2003)
- Occurrence of injuries with interferential current applications (Ford et al. 2005; Satter 2008).
- Occurrence of eye injuries with laser application (Barkana and Belkin 2000)
- Occurrence of eye injuries with MW applications (Carpenter and Van Ummersen 1968; Cutz 1989)
- The spread of nosocomial infections via electrotherapy devices and their accessories (Gaillot et al. 1998; Lambert et al. 2000; Schabrun et al. 2006; Quick-Alert No 5 2008)
- Effect of HF applications on an existing or planned pregnancy (Taskinen et al. 1990; Ouellet-Hellstrom and Stewart 1993; Lerman et al. 2001)
- Effect on bone growth by ultrasound and high-frequency therapy (Lyon et al. 2003; Doyle and Smart 1963)
- The risk of significant heating of metal-containing intrauterine contraceptives by HF cannot be ruled out with certainty (Nielsen et al. 1979; Heick et al. 1991).
- The risk of ultrasound in patients with vascular diseases is unclear, although the risk of embolism due to mechanical destabilization of a thrombus seems realistic. There is no literature on this. Nevertheless, Doppler sonography is used in vascular diseases. Atkins and Duck (2003) have shown that in this examination, tissue temperature increases significantly more than during a therapeutic ultrasound treatment. Treatment with ultrasound in such vascular diseases is considered contraindicated by almost all authors of German textbooks. Based on the facts, the risk posed by ultrasound treatment in such patients seems to be overestimated. However, since there are no data from large-scale studies, it is better to err on the side of caution here.
- The use of HF electrotherapy in the presence of osteosynthesis material is generally considered risky and therefore an absolute contraindication. The metal concentrates the electromagnetic field in a small area, which could lead to significant heating. Animal studies with implants made of a titanium alloy show contradictory results, albeit with different dosages; see Chap. 7. Seiger and Draper (2006) and Draper et al. (2004a, b), Draper (2011) used pulsed SWD (thermal) successfully as a pretreatment for mobilizations despite the presence of osteosynthesis material. As discussed in Chap. 7, however, the evidence remains unconvincing to this day. Until we have results from large-scale clinical studies with different HF applications, metal in the treatment area during HF therapy must be considered risky and therefore remains a contraindication.

Two contraindications must be critically questioned.

- TENS in pregnant women
  - Ketscher et al. published their results on lumbar TENS application in pregnant women in the third trimester in 1985 and 1987 (Ketscher et al. 1985, 1987). The parameters corresponded to standard therapeutic practice; see Chap. 3. No complications are mentioned. Pregnancy is considered an absolute contraindication for many applications in the lumbar and abdominal area. Based on the work

of Ketscher et al., this must be critically questioned for TENS in the last trimester. In pregnant women in the last trimester who suffer from lumbar pain, the pain can often not be satisfactorily managed with medication. Here, TENS would be a good alternative. See also Chap. 3.

- Interferential current with endoprosthesis
  - Some authors of German textbooks mention that interferential current could lead to loosening of an endoprosthesis. This is not supported by the literature and is also not physically plausible, except perhaps if, in a very early postoperative phase, extremely strong contractions of the relevant musculature were inadvertently triggered. In that case, however, it is not due to the current. This contraindication is unfounded.

There are probably several reasons for the lack of literature on injuries. The various laws for medical device operators in German-speaking countries require that incidents leading to death or serious deterioration in health must be reported. There is no reporting requirement for minor injuries, so no statements can be made about their occurrence. For certain possible risks, no studies have been conducted so far because such studies would be unnecessary or ethically unacceptable. Contraindications such as febrile conditions, infectious diseases, and unclear pathologies are generally accepted by experts even without proof, and the fact that high-frequency diathermy and ultrasound affect bone growth in rats and rabbits is sufficient to warrant caution in children. Physiotherapists are not accustomed to publishing on adverse events. With few exceptions (3 out of 42), the case reports found were published by physicians. It is possible that the observed injuries are so minor that publication does not seem necessary. This notion is incorrect. Even minor injuries or slight harm should be reported so that they can be scientifically evaluated. Otherwise, a false perception of the possible risks of electrotherapy would arise. For example, it is repeatedly claimed that interferential current is completely safe and can be used in the presence of osteosynthesis material. It is, of course, possible that injuries occur only rarely. According to many participants in electrotherapy courses, this seems unlikely. It is more likely that injuries that occur are not associated with an application due to lack of knowledge. Closing this gap is the responsibility of textbook authors. The following points show where there is room for improvement in the textbooks considered:

- Textbooks for physiotherapists and occupational therapists should emphasize measures for cleaning or disinfecting the materials used in connection with nosocomial infections.
- Patients with cognitive problems should be explicitly mentioned as a risk group.
- Physiotherapists traditionally use, in addition to exercise therapy in all its variations, soft tissue techniques and many different physical modalities. In order to prevent physiotherapy from developing into purely exercise therapy in the future, the foundations of these physical therapies must be thoroughly investigated. Only in this way can their use be justified according to the principles of evidence-based medicine and questionable applications be justifiably rejected. This also includes physiotherapists critically engaging with the risks of these applications and developing a culture that enables learning from their own mistakes and those of others.

8.3 Establishing a Risk Management System

Below are a few remarks on the structure and implementation of a risk management (RM) system. Not everywhere do therapists apply electrotherapy themselves; sometimes these applications are delegated. Why would one choose the electrotherapy department in particular to establish an RM system?

- It is a small, clearly defined subdepartment of physiotherapy. This reduces the personnel effort required.

- Applications in electrotherapy are largely standardized. This allows the results to be transferred to other hospitals and private physiotherapy practices, thus increasing the clinical relevance of the work.
- The electrotherapy department is networked with all departments relevant to physiotherapy in both inpatient and outpatient settings. In this way, many general processes can be observed and analyzed. This enables the transfer of risk management to the entire physiotherapy department.
- A risk analysis team should be established. The goal is for this team to continuously oversee risk management in (electro-)therapy. For this purpose, the team members are introduced by a project leader to the use of risk management tools such as creating a process landscape, failure mode and effects analysis (FMEA), and root cause analysis.
- The establishment and implementation of a risk management system in the electrotherapy department should serve as the foundation for risk management for the entire physiotherapy department in the clinic or practice.
- The publication of the results of this work should encourage physiotherapists to engage with the risks of their treatments.

8.4 Practical Implementation

What does the work of such a risk analysis team actually involve? A complete practical implementation of such work will not be discussed here, as it would go beyond the scope of this book. However, to give the reader a general impression, an incomplete summary follows.

After the project leader has clarified all organizational questions with the responsible management, the first task of the analysis team is to create the so-called process map or process landscape. This is not a diagram like an organizational chart that shows the structure of an organization or department. The process landscape essentially shows the workflows. An example: A patient registers. Who receives the registration? How and where is the registration recorded? Who creates the patient file? What forms are needed for this? Where can they be obtained? Where is the file stored? Who decides which therapist will take over the treatment? Are there specific criteria for this? How is the therapist informed? And so it continues, step by step, up to the moment when the case is closed and the file is stored somewhere (where? by whom? in what form? for how long?). "Along the way," the patient receives certain treatments, and various people are involved. Here, too, many questions need to be answered. With regard to electrotherapy, these could be questions such as: Where are the devices located? Who has access? When are they checked? Who is responsible for this? Where is the accessory equipment kept? Who orders consumables? How is cleaning done? How do we apply ultrasound? How is it documented? What do we do in the event of an allergic reaction? Is everyone up to date with life-saving emergency measures? Does everyone know how the defibrillator works? In a hospital, there are, among other things, contacts with nursing staff and the transport service; in a practice, there are contacts with physicians. How do these interactions take place? It makes sense to concretely imagine such a workflow step by step and to note each step, preferably together with several people. Surprises always come up, and it can be quite fun. Sometimes not.

After these workflows (the processes) have been recorded, the next phase is to search for sources of error. What could go wrong during registration? What happens if the secretary is absent? The therapist falls ill? The patient feels unwell? A burn occurs? An allergic reaction? Then all sources of error must be assessed in terms of a "reality check." What are the consequences if a particular step goes wrong, and how serious are they? How easy or difficult is it to correct the error? This is called an FMEA: a "Failure Mode and Effects Analysis," or in German, "Fehlermöglichkeits- und -einflussanalyse," or simply impact analysis, or also FMECA (Failure Mode and Effects and Criticality Analysis). It sounds complicated, but it is not. Experienced therapists can very quickly set priorities and use an FMEA to assess the sources of error.

After this assessment has been carried out and priorities have been set, the next step is to look for solutions for the two or three most important issues. It would be a mistake to try to tackle too much at once. In the famous PDCA cycle (Plan, Do, Check, Act), or Deming circle, this analysis is the "Plan" phase (Fig. 8.1). For the possible errors, solutions are proposed and then implemented in practice; this is the "Do" phase. Then, things are observed for a while, and after a certain predetermined period, the result is checked—the "Check" moment. And then action is taken. If necessary—and it is always necessary—the process is adjusted somewhat and new goals are formulated; this is the "Act" phase. And then the whole thing starts all over again.

Risk management is like quality management: it is never finished. Therefore, an analysis team should also be a permanent part of a therapist team.

8.5 Questions

What is the benefit of risk management in an electrotherapy department in a hospital?
The electrotherapy department is a small subunit of a physiotherapy department. The department is usually structured in such a way that all described processes can be applied to the entire department. In this way, the whole department can benefit from the work of just a few individuals. With very simple and cost-effective means, measures to reduce risk can be introduced in the short term, with the literature providing scientific justification for most of these measures. Treatment procedures can be largely standardized and can be clearly represented graphically using flowcharts. The introduction of a documentation form and a treatment algorithm can lead to the standardization of applications and their documentation. The introduction of risk management in electrotherapy will likely raise awareness of risk among the staff of the entire physiotherapy institute. Topics such as handling patient data, slip resistance of the floor in the therapy pool area, or the often poor footwear of patients with gait disorders should be addressed. The experiences gained from this work can be used to analyze such and other risks in physiotherapy and to develop strategies to eliminate these risks or reduce their consequences.

What aspects need to be considered when establishing risk management in an electrotherapy department in a hospital?
This book lists many publications on the subject of risks and harm. These are necessary when justifying the establishment of RM to the responsible authorities. However, to ensure that such an application is based on current facts, it is essential to conduct a thorough literature review in advance regarding the risks of electrotherapy.

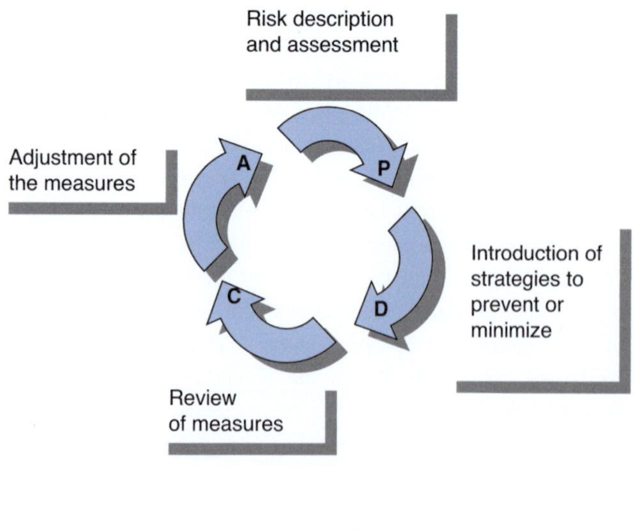

Fig. 8.1 The Deming circle or PDCA cycle

The process work should be carried out with experienced staff from different areas who are familiar with the structure of the entire physiotherapy department. This is because electrotherapy is interconnected with all departments, and not all processes run the same way in the various wards and departments. These different procedures should, where possible, be standardized to avoid undesirable events. This requires staff willingness to implement changes. Without the support of management, this is not possible. Before even the most rudimentary risk management can be introduced, it is essential to ensure management support. The commitment to support should be documented in writing, with specific goals formulated regarding personnel and financial resources. This includes defining responsibilities, the number of working hours allocated for the task (with a time buffer absolutely necessary!), and the amount of expenditure one is willing to invest in optimizations.

What is the financial and personnel effort required to establish risk management?
The author carried out such work in a larger hospital (500 beds) in Switzerland. The analysis was conducted over 4 months with 5 employees. There were 9 meetings of one hour each with these individuals, although not all 5 were always present. In addition, there were interviews with other professional groups such as physicians, secretaries, nursing staff, laboratory staff, and technical service personnel. The total time required was just under 58 working hours. The calculation of personnel effort was based on information from the HR director regarding average annual salaries including 21% social security contributions, a weekly working time of 42 h, and 252 working days per year. Added to this is the work involved in this project. Had this work been carried out as part of an employment relationship, the effort for literature research, clarifications regarding the legal situation, clarifications with the Institute of Metrology and with other hospitals, time for developing the process landscape, creating flowcharts for treatment procedures, creating checklists, developing the treatment algorithm, bacteriological investigations, and staff training would have to be included. This shows that the establishment and maintenance of risk management can only be carried out seriously if a person is released for this additional work. In a department with 30 employees, a weekly workload of 4 h, corresponding to a 10% position, seems appropriate. For the subsequent maintenance and expansion of RM, members of the "risk team" must plan at least 1–2 h per month. The size of the risk team depends on the size of the therapy department, but there should be no fewer than 3 people from different areas (orthopedics, surgery, internal medicine, outpatient).

The personnel and financial effort required to establish risk management can be justified by the increased safety. Pittet et al. estimated in their 2000 study the cost of a hospital-acquired infection conservatively at SFr 3500 (at that time about €3000). With their hand hygiene campaign in a Geneva university hospital, the authors were able to prevent 900 nosocomial infections annually and thus save about SFr 3,000,000. Kilgore and Brossette analyzed 58,381 nosocomial infections from 55 clinics in 2008. The authors calculated the additional costs incurred for various types of infections. Urinary tract infections, the most common, cause the lowest additional costs: $3936 per case. The most expensive infections are also the rarest. Infections of the cerebrospinal tract cause additional costs of $31,573 per case. Broex et al. (2009) concluded in their 2009 review that the treatment costs for patients with nosocomial infections after surgical procedures were on average twice as high as for patients without infections ($4163–56,607). The personnel effort mentioned above for establishing and implementing the risk management system was about 58 working hours. According to the hospital administration, this roughly corresponds to a one-time expenditure of SFr 3000. If the measures introduced can prevent even a single infection in a patient in the coming years, this work has already paid off.

What are the consequences of establishing and implementing risk management in an electrotherapy department in a hospital?

Right at the beginning of the aforementioned work, it became apparent that almost all optimization potentials for electrotherapy could be transferred to the entire physiotherapy institute. This applies in particular to measures for preventing nosocomial infections, standardized documentation, and data protection. It also became clear that it is sensible to carry out an annual performance check on therapeutic ultrasound heads. Although measurement with such an ultrasound scale is rough, it still allows a statement as to whether further, more precise testing is necessary. Discussions with therapists showed that the risk awareness of all physiotherapists had changed, not only regarding electrotherapy but also other applications. For example, in the case mentioned above, the lack of slip resistance of the floors in the therapy pool area and the poor accessibility of treatment cubicles in an emergency were addressed.

What are the optimization potentials in establishing and implementing risk management in an electrotherapy department in a hospital?

This question can only be answered in very general terms. Based on many discussions with professional colleagues, the author has compiled the following list. This enumeration is not intended as criticism, but as food for thought. The order is arbitrary:

- The lack of a suitably trained quality management officer for physiotherapy. It is absolutely necessary to have a person with a clearly defined area of responsibility and competence and a defined workload, who works across departments with other quality management officers in a clinic. In a hospital physiotherapy department, this is logically a physiotherapist. In a physiotherapy practice, an employee or the owner should take on this task and be given time for it.
- Lack of risk awareness due to insufficient information about risks in physiotherapy in general and, in this case, about electrotherapy. Textbooks must point out risks and measures to prevent their consequences. Training institutions must address quality and risk management in their curricula.
- Lack of awareness regarding the handling of patient data. Patient cards must not be left lying around accessible to everyone. It is unacceptable for a patient to see "HIV" or "NO CPR" written in bold on their roommate's card. Passwords do not belong on Post-it notes on the monitor. When handing over patients for the weekend, one should carefully consider which information is necessary for treatment and which is not.
- Insufficient measures to prevent the transmission of nosocomial infections via electrotherapy devices and positioning materials. Experience shows that a 15-min instruction is sufficient in this case. However, this must be repeated regularly.
- Lack of measures for performance control of therapeutic devices such as ultrasound and high frequency. The legislator is unequivocal in all German-speaking countries: we are obliged to do so.
- The lack of a standardized documentation method. Experience shows that in a hospital, therapists from different departments usually use different documentation methods (if any at all). This complicates patient handover in the absence of the treating therapist.
- Patients must be informed about their treatment, and risks and side effects must be mentioned, even if it is only a "normal" muscle ache. Patients should consent to the treatment. In our part of the world, fortunately, we do not have a culture of litigation, but the wiser person takes precautions.
- The lack of a healthy "error reporting culture." Near misses must also be considered.

It is important in physiotherapy to address occupational risks. The consequences of these risks are rarely very serious, but in the complex hospital system, as part of a chain of errors, they could lead to serious harm. As an example of such serious consequences, the spread of nosocomial infections was discussed in this work. Other known risks may individually have less serious consequences. How their effects would play out in an unfortunate chain of events is unpredictable. Therefore, it is still worthwhile to analyze these risks and develop prevention strategies. Less obvious risks and their consequences should also be considered. The lack of awareness regarding the protection of patient data is, in the author's opinion, an underestimated problem, as is the fact that patients are not systematically informed about the risks and side effects of a therapy application before treatment. To avoid unnecessary legal problems in this era, which is characterized by increasing patient self-confidence, these topics must be incorporated into the professional self-understanding of physiotherapists. With little effort, measures to reduce risk can be introduced in a physiotherapy department in a short time. This increases staff risk awareness and, as a result, improves patient safety. The introduction of corresponding laws and binding regulations, including sanctions, could help physiotherapists engage more intensively with the topic of patient safety. This can only benefit the profession.

References

Andersen BM, Lindemann R, Bergh K, Nesheim BI, Syversen G, Solheim N, Laugerud F (2002) Spread of methicillin-resistant Staphylococcus aureus in a neonatal intensive unit associated with understaffing, overcrowding and mixing of patients. J Hosp Infect 50(1):18–24

Artho PA, Thyne JG, Warring BP, Willis CD, Brismée LNS (2002) A calibration study of therapeutic ultrasound units. Phys Ther 82:257–263

Atkins T, Duck F (2003) Heating caused by selected Doppler and physiotherapy ultrasound beams measured using thermal test objects. Eur J Ultrasound 16:243–252

Barkana Y, Belkin M (2000) Laser eye injuries. Surv Ophtalmol 44:459–478

Broex EC, van Asselt AD, Bruggeman CA, van Tiel FH (2009) Surgical site infections: how high are the costs? J Hosp Infect 72(3):193–201

Carlsson T, Andrell P, Ekre O, Edvardsson N, Holmgren C, Jacobsson F, Mannheimer C (2009) Interference of transcutaneous nerve stimulation with permanent ventricular stimulation: a new clinical problem? Europace 11:364–369

Carlton G, Blegen MA (2006) Medication-related errors: a literature review of incidence and antecedents. Annu Rev Nurs Res 24:19–38

Carpenter RL, Van Ummersen CA (1968) The action of microwave radiation on the eye. J Microw Power 3(1):3–19

Castelain PY, Chabeau G (1986) Contact dermatitis after transcutaneous electric analgesia. Contact Dermatitis 15:32–35

Clarke SP, Sloane DM, Aiken LH (2002) Effects of hospital staffing and organizational climate on needlestick injuries to nurses. Am J Public Health 92(7):1115–1119

Corazza M, Maranini C, Bacilieri S, Virgili A (1999) Accelerated allergic contact dermatitis to a transcutaneous electrical nerve stimulation device. Dermatology 199:281

Crevenna R, Quittan M, Wiesinger GF, Nuhr MJ, Nicolakis P, Pacher R, Fialka-Moser V (2001) Elektrostimulationstherapie bei Patienten mit Herzschrittmachern. Phys Med Rehab Kuror 11:159–164

Crevenna R, Stix G, Pleiner J, Pezawas T, Schmidinger H, Quittan M, Wolzt M (2003) Electromagnetic interference by transcutaneous neuromuscular electrical stimulation in patients with bipolar-sensing implantable cardioverter defibrillators. Pace 26:626–629

Crowcroft N, Maguire H, Fleming M, Peacock J, Thomas J (1996) Methicillin-resistant Staphylococcus aureus: investigation of a hospital outbreak using a case-control study. J Hosp Infect 34:301–309

Cutz A (1989) Effects of microwave radiation on the eye: the occupational health perspective. Lens Eye Toxic Res 6(1–2):379–386

Daniel DM, Rupert RL (2003) Calibration and electrical safety status of therapeutic ultrasound used by chiropractic physicians. J Manipulative Physiol Ther 26(3):171–175

Doyle JR, Smart BW (1963) Stimulation of bone growth by short-wave diathermy. J Bone Joint Surg Am 45:15–24

Draper DO (2011) Injuries restored to ROM using PSWD and mobilizations. Int J Sports Med 32(4):281–286

Draper DO, Castel CJ, Castel D (2004a) Low-watt pulsed shortwave diathermy and metal-plate fixation of the elbow. Athl Ther Today 9(5):28–32

Draper DO, Castro JL, Feland B, Schulthies S, Eggett D (2004b) Shortwave diathermy and prolonged stretching increase hamstring flexibility more than prolonged stretching alone. J Orthop Sports Phys Ther 34(1):13–20

Dwyer CM, Chapman RS, Forsyth A (1994) Allergic contact dermatitis from TENS gel. Contact Dermatitis 30:305

Ford KS, Shrader MW, Smith J, Mclean TJ, Dahm DL (2005) Full-thickness burn formation after the use of electrical stimulation for rehabilitation of unicompartmental knee arthroplasty. J Arthroplast 20:950–953

Foti C, Cassano N, Conserva A, Vena GA (2004) Allergic contact dermatitis due to diclofenac applied with iontophoresis. Clin Exp Dermatol 29:91

Frye JL, Johns LD, Tom JA, Ingersoll CD (2007) Blisters on the anterior shin in 3 research subjects after a 1-MHz, 1.5 W/cm^2, continuous ultrasound treatment: a case series. J Athl Train 42(3):425–430

Gaillot O, Maruéjouls C, Abachin E, Lecuru F, Arlet G, Simonet M, Berche P (1998) Nosocomial outbreak of Klebsiella pneumoniae producing SHV-5 extended-spectrum beta-lactamase, originating from a contaminated ultrasonography coupling gel. J Clin Microbiol 36(5):1357–1360

Green T, Pye RJ (1991) Skin reactions to TENS equipment used for pain relief. Br J Dermatol 125(suppl 38):35

Guirro R, Britshcy Dos Santos SC (2002) Evaluation of the acoustic intensity of new ultrasound therapy equipment. Ultrasonics 39(8):553–557

Halwani M, Solaymani-Dodaran M, Grundmann H, Coupland C, Slack R (2006) Cross-transmission of nosocomial pathogens in an adult intensive care unit: incidence and risk factors. J Hosp Infect 63(1):39–46.

Heick A, Espersen T, Pedersen HL, Raahauge J (1991) Is diathermy safe in women with copper bearing IUDs? Acta Obstet Gynecol Scand 70:153–155

Holcomb WR, Joyce CJ (2003) A comparison of temperature increases produced by 2 commonly used ultrasound units. J Athl Train 38:24–27

Holmgren C, Carlsson T, Mannheimer C, Edvardsson N (2008) Risk of interference from transcutaneous electrical nerve stimulation on the sensing function of implantable defibrillators. Pace 31:151–158

Ketscher KD, Retschke U, Kindt J (1985) Die transkutane elektrische Nervenstimuation zur Behandlung der Plazentainsuffizienz. Methodenprinzip und Gerätekombination. Zbl Gynaekol 107:500–502

Ketscher KD, Retschke U, Kindt J (1987) Die transkutane elektrische Nervenstimuation zur Behandlung der Plazentainsuffizienz. Ergebnisse der Behandlung im Vergleich zu einer speziellen Infusionsbehandlung. Zbl Gynaekol 109:850–853

Lambert I, Tebbs SE, Hill D, Moss HA, Davies AJ, Elliott TSJ (2000) Interferential therapy machines as possible vehicles for cross-infection. J Hosp Infect 44:59–64

Lerman Y, Jacubovich R, Green MS (2001) Pregnancy outcome following exposure to shortwaves among female physiotherapists in Israel. Am J Ind Med 39:499–504

Lyon R, Liu X, Meier J (2003) The effects of therapeutic vs. high-intensity ultrasound on the rabbit growth plate. J Orthop Res 21:865–871

Macchia L, Caiaffa MF, Vacca A (2002) General adverse reaction to aspirin administered by transdermal iontophoresis. Eur J Pharmacol 58:641–642

Mackey AL, Bojsen-Moller J, Qvortrup K, Langberg H, Suetta C, Kalliokoski KK, Kjaer M, Magnusson SP (2008) Evidence of skeletal muscle damage following electrically stimulated isometric muscle contractions in humans. J Appl Physiol 105:1620–1627

Mars Climate Orbiter Mishap Investigation Board Phase I Report. https://llis.nasa.gov/llis_lib/pdf/1009464main1_0641-mr.pdf. Zugriff April 2021 10.09.1999. ftp://ftp.hg.nasa,gov./pub/pao/reports/1999/MCO report

Mattei E, Censi F, Calcagnini G, Falsaperla R, Genovese E, Napolitano A, Cannatà V (2016) Pacemaker and ICD oversensing induced by movements near the MRI scanner bore. Med Phys 43(12):6621

Medizinprodukte-Betreiberverordnung in der Fassung der Bekanntmachung vom 21. August 2002 (BGBl. I S. 3396), zuletzt geändert durch Artikel 386 der Verordnung vom 31. Oktober 2006 (BGBl. I S. 2407) 27. http://bundesrecht.juris.de/mpbetreibv/BJNR176200998.html. Zugriff Juni 2020

Medizinprodukteverordnung (MepV) Schweiz vom 1. Juli 2020. https://www.fedlex.admin.ch/eli/oc/2020/552/de. Zugriff Juni 2020

Medizinprodukteverordnung Österreich, Fassung vom 19.02.2021, StF: BGBl. II Nr. 129/2003 https://www.ris.bka.gv.at/GeltendeFassung.wxe?Abfrage=Bundesnormen&Gesetzesnummer=20002557. Zugriff Juni 2020

Nielsen NC, Hansen R, Larsen T (1979) Heat induction in copper-bearing IUD'S during short-wave diathermy. Acta Obstet Gynecol Scand 58(5):495

Nutt JG, Anderson VC, Peacock JH, Hammerstad JP, Burchiel KJ (2001) DBS and diathermy interaction induces severe CNS damage. Neurology 56:1384–1386

Occhetta E, Bortnik M, Magnani A, Francalacci G, Marino P (2006) Inappropriate implantable cardioverter-defibrillator discharches unrelated to supraventricular tachyarrhythmias. Europace 8:863–869

Ouellet-Hellstrom T, Stewart WT (1993) Miscarriages among female physical therapists who report using radio- and microwave-frequency electromagnetic radiation. Am J Epidemiol 138:775–786

Paula H (2007) Patientensicherheit und Risikomanagement im Pflege- und Krankenhausalltag. Springer Medizin Verlag, Heidelberg, ISBN-10 3-540-33726-1

Pyatt JR, Trenbath D, Chester M, Connelly DT (2003) The simultaneous use of a biventricular implantable cardioverter defibrillator (ICD) and transcutaneous electrical nerve stimulation (TENS) unit: implications for device interaction. Europace 5:91–93

Pye S (1996) Ultrasound therapy equipment: does it perform? Physiotherapy 82:39–44

Pye S, Milford C (1994) The performance of ultrasound physiotherapy machines in Lothian Region, Scotland, 1992. Ultrasound Med Biol 4:347–359

Quick-Alert No 5 (2008) Kontaminiertes Ultraschallgel. Stiftung für Patientensicherheit, Schweiz. https://www.patientensicherheit.ch/publikationen/quick-alert/?tx_news_pi1%5B%40widget_0%5D%5BcurrentPage%5D=3&cHash=a5976491d6b3fb10d930e813b265feb1. Zugegriffen im Dezember 2009.

Reason JT (1997) Managing the risks of organizational accidents. Ashgate Publishing Limited, Aldershot England, ISBN: 978-1-84014-105-4

Reason JT (2008) The human contribution: unsafe acts, accidents, and heroic recoveries. Ash- gate Publishing Limited, Surrey England, ISBN: 978-0-7546-7402-3

Roark C, Whicher S, Abosch A (2008) Reversible neurological symptoms caused by diathermy in a patient with deep brain stimulators: case report. Neurosurgery 62:E256

Ruggera PS, Witters DM, von Maltzahn G, Bassen HI (2003) In vitro assessment of tissue heating near metallic medical implants by exposure to pulsed radio frequency diathermy. Phys Med Biol 48:2919–2928

Samuels JM, Overbey DM, Wikiel KJ, Jones TS, Robinson TN, Jones EL (2020) Electromagnetic interference on cardiac pacemakers and implantable cardioverter defibrillators during endoscopy as reported to the US Federal Drug Administration. Surg Endosc. PMID: 32804270

Satter E (2008) Third-degree burns incurred as a result of interferential current therapy. Am J Dermatopathol 30:281–283

Schabrun S, Chipchase L, Rickard H (2006) Are therapeutic ultrasound units a potential vector for nosocomial infection? Physiother Res Int 11(2):61–71

Seiger C, Draper DO (2006) Use of pulsed shortwave diathermy and joint mobilization to increase ankle range of motion in the presence of surgical implanted metal: a case series. J Orthop Sports Phys Ther 36(9):669–677

Taskinen H, Kyyrönen P, Hemminki K (1990) Effects of ultrasound, shortwaves, and physical exertion on pregnancy outcome in physiotherapists. J Epidmiol Community Health 44:196–201

Valtonen EJ, Lilius HG, Tiula E (1975) Disturbances in the function of cardiac pacemaker caused by short wave and microwave diathermies and pulsed high frequency current. An Chir Gynaecol Fen 64:284–287

Vlay SC (1998) Electromagnetic interference and ICD discharge related to chiropractic treatment. Pace 21:2009

Weitz SH, Tunick PA, McElhinney L, Mitchell T, Kronzon I (1997) Pseudoatrial flutter: artifact simulating atrial flutter caused by a transcutaneous electrical nerve stimulator (TENS). Pace 20:3010–3011

Zeqiri B (1997) Calibration and safety of physiotherapy ultrasound equipment. Physiotherapy 83:559–560

MIX
Papier aus verantwortungsvollen Quellen
Paper from responsible sources
FSC® C105338

If you have any concerns about our products, you can contact us on
ProductSafety@springernature.com

In case Publisher is established outside the EU, the EU authorized representative is:
Springer Nature Customer Service Center GmbH
Europaplatz 3, 69115 Heidelberg, Germany

Printed by Libri Plureos GmbH
in Hamburg, Germany